DATE DUE

MAR 2 1 2013		
NOV 3 0 2016		

Demco, Inc. 38-293

HEART DISEASE IN WOMEN

HEART DISEASE IN WOMEN

BENJAMIN V. LARDNER
AND
HARRISON R. PENNELTON
EDITORS

Nova Science Publishers, Inc.
New York

NOTICE TO THE READER

The Publisher has taken reasonable care in the preparation of this book, but makes no expressed or implied warranty of any kind and assumes no responsibility for any errors or omissions. No liability is assumed for incidental or consequential damages in connection with or arising out of information contained in this book. The Publisher shall not be liable for any special, consequential, or exemplary damages resulting, in whole or in part, from the readers' use of, or reliance upon, this material. Any parts of this book based on government reports are so indicated and copyright is claimed for those parts to the extent applicable to compilations of such works.

Independent verification should be sought for any data, advice or recommendations contained in this book. In addition, no responsibility is assumed by the publisher for any injury and/or damage to persons or property arising from any methods, products, instructions, ideas or otherwise contained in this publication.

This publication is designed to provide accurate and authoritative information with regard to the subject matter covered herein. It is sold with the clear understanding that the Publisher is not engaged in rendering legal or any other professional services. If legal or any other expert assistance is required, the services of a competent person should be sought. FROM A DECLARATION OF PARTICIPANTS JOINTLY ADOPTED BY A COMMITTEE OF THE AMERICAN BAR ASSOCIATION AND A COMMITTEE OF PUBLISHERS.

Library of Congress Cataloging-in-Publication Data

Heart disease in women / [edited by] Benjamin V. Lardner and Harrison R. Pennelton.
        p. ; cm.
  Includes bibliographical references and index.
  ISBN 978-1-60692-066-4 (hardcover)
  1. Heart diseases in women. I. Lardner, Benjamin V. II. Pennelton, Harrison R.
  [DNLM: 1. Heart Diseases. 2. Women's Health. WG 210 H43475 2009]
  RC682.H3836 2009
  616.1'20082--dc22
                    2008041207

Published by Nova Science Publishers, Inc. ✛ *New York*

Contents

Preface

Heart disease is an umbrella term for a number of different diseases affecting the heart. As of 2007, it is the leading cause of death in the United States,England, Canada and Wales, killing one person every 34 seconds in the United States alone.Heart disease is synonymous with cardiac disease but not with cardiovascular disease which is any disease of the heart or blood vessels. Among the many types of heart disease are, for example: Angina; Arrhythmia; Congenital heart disease; Coronary artery disease (CAD); Dilated cardiomyopathy; Heart attack (myocardial infarction); Heart failure; Hypertrophic cardiomyopathy; Mitral regurgitation; Mitral valve prolapse; and Pulmonary stenosis. This new book brings together important recent research on heart disease with a focus on women and heart disease.

Chapter I - Over the past decade progress has been made toward education and increasing awareness, in both patients and physicians, of the risks of cardiovascular disease in women. There has also been an increase in federally funded initiatives in the area of gender-specific cardiovascular research. However, cardiovascular disease continues to be the primary cause of death among women in the United States. Each year more women than men die of cardiovascular disease. Gender-based differences in the prevalence, risk factors, presentation, treatment, and outcomes of cardiovascular disease remain important areas of active research. A frequently overlooked, yet vitally important, component of treatment for the secondary prevention of cardiovascular disease in women is participation in cardiac rehabilitation. Cardiac rehabilitation programs are comprehensive secondary prevention programs which contain specific core components that aim to optimize cardiac risk reduction, teach and develop healthy behaviors, decrease disability, and promote an active lifestyle for patients with cardiovascular disease. Research has documented the efficacy and effectiveness of cardiac rehabilitation with reductions in mortality and improvements in clinical and behavioral outcomes. Despite this, cardiac rehabilitation is under prescribed and underutilized, especially in women. In this review, the current evidence-based findings, research, and recommendations for cardiac rehabilitation in the treatment of cardiovascular disease in women is addressed with a focus on those areas specific to the needs of women. Persistent gaps in our knowledge regarding the role of cardiac rehabilitation in women with cardiovascular disease are presented as research initiatives for the future.

Chapter II - The higher cardiovascular risk in men and post-menopausal women implies a protective action of estrogen. A large number of experimental studies have provided strong evidence indicating that estrogen has protective effect in the process of myocardial infarction (MI). Estrogen may prevent deterioration of cardiac function post-MI through improving heart failure of cadiocyte biology and also through mediating arrhythmia. The alternations by estrogen in immune function, apoptosis and endothelial progenitor cells after MI may be the most important mechanisms for cadiocyte survival. For the control of cardiac hypertrophy, estrogen acts as both a potent vasodilator and a direct mediator for cadiocyte. The major mechanisms underlying arrhythmia effect may involve affecting neural remodeling, electrical remodeling and structural remodeling. In this article, we mainly focus on the current mechanisms underlying the estrogen effects after MI through genomic pathway and non-genomic pathway. A further understanding of estrogen and estrogen receptors function and regulation may lead to the development of highly specific prevention and treatment of cardiovascular diseases.

Chapter III - *Preeclampsia* (PE) is a pregnancy-specific syndrome characterised by the appearance of hypertension (systolic blood pressure $\geq$ 140 mmHg or diastolic blood pressure $\geq$ 90 mmHg) and proteinuria ($\geq$ 300mg per 24 hours) during the second half of pregnancy (after 20 weeks of gestational age). It may be variously associated with a myriad of other signs and symptoms, such as oedema, visual disturbances, headache, seizures (eclampsia), epigastric pain, HELLP syndrome (haemolysis, liver dysfunction and low platelet count), and it typically resolves after delivery.

PE is to be differentiated from other hypertensive disorders in pregnancy, both from a prognostic and a pathophysiological point of view. Under this respect, the NHLBI Working Group on Research on Hypertension During Pregnancy distinguishes PE from:

-    *gestational hypertension*: de novo hypertension arising after midpregnancy, in the absence of proteinuria. This category includes women who later satisfy diagnostic criteria for preeclampsia. However, in most cases, proteinuria never occurs, the course is relatively benign, and blood pressure normalizes postpartum;

-    *chronic hypertension*: maternal hypertension recognised before pregnancy; it can also be assumed when hypertension is detected before mid-pregnancy and when it fails to normalize 12 weeks after delivery. Women with chronic hypertension are at increased risk to develop *superimposed preeclampsia* (25% risk) and the outcomes for the mother and infant with preeclampsia superimposed on existing hypertension are worse than with de novo preeclampsia.;

-    *eclampsia* is a life-threatening complication of PE characterised by new-onset of seizures in a woman with PE. Such convulsions usually occur after mid-pregnancy, or during delivery, but about one third of eclamptic convulsions occur during the first 48 hours of the postpartum period.

The exact incidence of PE is uncertain, but it has been reported to be approximately 5-8% and to be substantially higher in nulliparous women, and in women with multifetal pregnancies, history of PE in previous pregnancies, family history of PE, chronic hypertension, pregestational diabetes, antiphospholipid antibodies, obesity, age > 40 years. Paradoxically, cigarette smoking reduces the risk.

PE is one of the leading causes of maternal mortality in the developing countries and a cause of neonatal morbidity and mortality worldwide. Mortality from PE is largely preventable by delivery that stops the progression of the disease, so that the high rate of maternal mortality in developing countries is a marker of low quality of care, rather than disease frequency. Anyway, even in developed countries, PE puts the mother at risk for abruptio placentae, renal failure, pulmonary oedema, stroke and seizures (eclampsia).The reason for neonatal risks depends on the fact that, given the absence of an effective treatment, the only possibility to prevent further deterioration of maternal conditions is delivery, and preterm birth is associated with increased mortality and neurological disabilities. It is estimated that 15% of all preterm births are iatrogenic deliveries for preeclampsia. Moreover, preeclampsia also increases the risk of fetal growth restriction (FGR) that, in turn, is an important cause of neonatal mortality and morbidity and a recognised risk factor for long-term pathologies in adulthood, such as cardiovascular disease and insulin-resistance syndrome.

Chapter IV - The number of diabetic patients in the world has been estimated to at least double during the next 30 years. Coronary heart disease is the leading cause of death among patients with type 2 diabetes. The associations of type 2 diabetes and hyperglycemia with the risk of coronary heart disease have been assessed by a number of prospective studies and the results are consistent. Patients with type 2 diabetes have a 2-4 times higher risk of coronary mortality than those without diabetes. Among the middle-aged general population, men have a 2 to 5 times higher risk of coronary heart disease than women. However, women with diabetes will lose their relative protection against coronary heart disease compared with men. In recent years, several studies compared the gender specific impact of diabetes and myocardial infarction at baseline on coronary mortality. These studies found that both diabetes and myocardial infarction at baseline increased coronary mortality. In women, prior myocardial infarction at baseline confers a lower risk on coronary mortality than prior diabetes does. The results of these studies have important implications for clinical practice. For future coronary heart disease risk we need to consider carefully the treatment strategies on individual disease status, particularly type 2 diabetes, in women.

Chapter V - An elevated heart rate can indicate a patient's risk for cardiovascular disease. A large number of population-based studies have demonstrated an association between elevated heart rate and cardiovascular disease as well as all-cause mortality with and without diagnosed cardiovascular disease. Despite accumulating evidence of its significance, elevated heart rate remains neglected as a cardiovascular risk factor. From the preventive point of view, heart rate may be a useful biomeasurement for identifying subjects at risk for hypertension, metabolic syndrome, and cardiovascular events. By identifying subjects with these conditions, targeted and cost-effective cardiovascular disease prevention programs can be planned. Previous findings also suggest that heart rate modulation should be considered in the treatment of cardiovascular disease. There is a linear relationship between heart rate reduction and a reduction in mortality rate. Tachycardia is a strong marker of widespread abnormality of the autonomic control of the circulation. This autonomic nervous system imbalance could explain the association between elevated heart rate and hypertension, metabolic syndrome, and cardiovascular events. Unfortunately, lowering the heart rate is not currently a clinically recognized therapeutic goal. Prospective trials are needed to investigate the heart rate levels that should be considered hazardous and whether treatment of high heart rate can prevent cardiovascular events.

Chapter VI - The central purpose of the study was to examine differences between women and men, ages 30-50 years, in their responses to heart disease, and to identify the factors influencing them in the fields of health and illness. The study was conducted using a qualitative method. The participants in the study included 30 men and 30 women who suffered from coronary heart disease. The study findings suggest that women delayed seeking treatment and that when they did seek treatment they were not initially diagnosed as suffering from heart disease due to physicians' perceptions that heart disease is a men's disease. The recovery period for women was characterized by their quick return to daily home making before their physical condition permitted it. Conversely, the men extended their recovery period and received support from their families. As part of the return to normal life, the men were strict in following the instructions of the health regimen, whereas most of the women ignored it. The women, compared to the men, received less support from their spouses and families, and they noted that social expectations concerning their role were high. Our study concludes that heart disease varies between men and women in the characteristics of its symptoms and in the attitude of medical staff and the public, as well as of patients themselves, towards the disease. The role of the cardiac patient is based on male characteristics and, as a result, men are legitimized and receive social support in all that relates to the disease; consequently, men adhere to the health regimen, whereas women are less inclined to. This study can advance insights on the influence of the gender variable on responses to heart disease, as well as supply information on therapeutic intervention for male and female cardiac patients and the nature of the different measures used for each.

Chapter VII - Young women are at a 3-fold higher risk of experiencing venous thromboembolism compared to young men. This risk is further increased by oral contraceptives, smoking, hereditary thrombophilia and/or low socioeconomic status. There are also hints for gender specific differences in the arterial system. Coronary heart disease which is particularly important develops in women 10-15 years later than in men. However, the clinical course in women is often more complicated. In women, thrombophilic predispositions play a more important role before menopause and metabolic risk factors after menopause, compared to men.

Thrombus formation needs to be initiated by disturbances of at least one element of the Virchow trias. There is principally no difference between men and women. However, all three elements are influenced by estrogen, resulting in gender specific differences. There is a favourable influence on blood flow by the inhibition of atherogenesis and on the endothelial function by increased NO release, and an unfavourable influence on hemostasis resulting in hypercoagibility. Thus, particularly non-selective hormone replacement therapy for the inhibition of atherogenesis may be questionable due to increased thrombogenicity. The solution may be more selective estrogen receptor modulators. Clinical trials are still needed for both, hormone replacement therapy and the therapy of venous and arterial thromboembolism which has been thus far studied in predominantly male patient cohorts.

Chapter VIII - Aging, a natural process in human life, begins at conception, continues with growth and development and finishes with dysfunction of various organs towards the end of life. Coronary heart disease (CHD) is one of the most common cardiovascular diseases, leading to death in women and is responsible for more deaths each year than all other diseases together. The incidence of myocardial infarction (MI) in women, although lower than in men, increases dramatically after the menopause. This increase is at least partly due to aging, although men also have a progressive increase in MI with age. The role of the menopause itself is not very clear. The evaluation of chest pain, the main symptom of CHD, is less straightforward in women than in men, because the language used to describe symptoms differs between the sexes. In fact, symptoms in women are slightly different from those in men. Until now, medical data published in literature was based on research done on male patients. However, there are numerous differences in the epidemiology and primary manifestation of CHD in women and men. In addition, the diagnosis of angina pectoris in women is more difficult than in men for several reasons, which are mentioned later in this chapter. The clinical usefulness of some non-invasive tests is lower in women than in men. A number of studies have shown gender-based differences in frequency rates of coronary angiography and revascularization, even among those with acute MI. It should be stressed that women with angina are much more likely than men to have normal coronary arteries on angiography. On the other hand, the risk of complications after coronary angiography in women is higher than in men. This may explain why physicians fail to refer women for subsequent invasive tests. Several case reports included in this paper show the difficulties in diagnosis and treatment of women with CHD.

In conclusion, it could be said that difficulties in diagnosis and limited data on the treatment of CHD in women, have led to a situation in which women with CHD often remain under-investigated and under-treated.

Chapter IX - Background. Participation of women in studies of acute coronary syndromes, including acute ST-elevation myocardial infarction (MI) as well as unstable angina and/or non-ST-elevation MI is about 30-40% and is remaing constant during last 20 years. It is well known that in ST-elevation MI women, who are older than men and are mostly less agressively treated, experience worse outcome than men. The results of studies of unstable angina and/or non-ST-elevation MI also demonstrated that women are significantly older and with significantly more comorbidities. However, the results of the studies are controvesial, regarding the short- and long term prognosis. Some studies demonstarted significantly increased risk of 30-day and six-month adverse outcomes in women, when compared to men in spite of their similar treatments, but others similar outcomes with similar treatments in spite of older age.

Conclusions. In this review article the results of studies, regarding the outcomes of women compared to men in acute coronary syndromes are discussed, especially the use of treatments, including coronary interventions, misuse or errors in medical treatments, as well as future perspectives in women with coronary artery disease in the new millenium.

Chapter X - Introduction: The presence of electrophysiological abnormalities of the atrial myocardium with increasing age could explain the differences in the genesis of atrial fibrillation in women with paroxysmal atrial fibrillation (PAF). Aging could influence not only the atrial response to premature atrial depolarizations but also the morphology of atrial electrograms.

Material and Methods: Programmed atrial stimulation with single extrastimulus was performed in 102 female patients, 48 of them had normal sinus node function and did not have PAF (Group I), and 54 of them had PAF, idiopathic or associated to other arrhythmias (Group II). Programmed atrial stimulation was performed from the right atrial appendage at double diastolic threshold with stimulus duration of 2 ms with a computarized cardiac stimulator.

Results: The incidence of induction of repetitive atrial firing (68% vs 36%; p<0.02), fragmented atrial activity (85% vs 47%; p<0.005), and sustained PAF (43% vs 5%; p<0.001) was significantly higher in Group II than in Group I. The zone of induction of repetitive atrial firing (34±33 vs 10±19 ms; p<0.005), fragmented atrial activity (49±40 vs 12±15 ms; p<0.001), and interatrial conduction delay (51±32 vs 26±28 ms; p<0.02) was significantly wider in Group II than in Group I. The induction rate and the respective zones of these electrophysiologic parameters had a significantly positive correlation with age in Group II.

Conclusions: The authors' results shed light on the mechanisms responsible for developing atrial fibrillation in aging women. The electrophysiological indicators of augmented atrial vulnerability are significantly altered with increasing age in women with paroxysmal atrial fibrillation. There is a significantly greater predisposition to atrial fibrillation in aging women because they develop a significantly greater augmented atrial vulnerability with increasing age.

Chapter XI - Background: Angina pectoris is the result of myocardial ischemia caused by an imbalance between myocardial blood supply and oxygen demand. In women, often than men, coronary heart disease may manifest with atypical presentations. Beside conventional, psychosocial factors are especially expressed in our country as risk factors which come to disease of coronary arteries, separately in women. Diagnosis this conditions in emergency department (ED) at such circumstances where electrocardiogram (ECG) is only one exact method that may show myocardial ischemia is very difficult. Methods and Results: In undeveloped community of municipal Zivinice living about 70.000 people. About 20% of them are refuges from East Bosnia, mainly women and younger people. We analyzed data in 2007th from Emergency Department (ED) of Health center Zivinice. ED in this year accepted 32.570 or about 46,5% population of this community, respectively 89 patients per day. We investigate number of patients who had diagnosis of angina pectoris, symptoms, risk factors and co morbidity, and entirely part of female. During time of investigation, number of patients with conditions and risk factors to originate of CHD, and symptoms who may be seen in angina pectoris, were 6.937 or 21,3%. Almost two-thirds of these patients was female with average age 61,5 (±11,2) years. During period of research in ED were registered 910 women with diagnosis of stable angina pectoris. Even in 275 of these women electrocardiogram was performed first time in their life on the occasion of an examination. In eleven of all them, without significant ECG changes, biomarkers of cardiac damage (troponin and creatin kynaze) were elevated and they were hospitalized under diagnoses of acute coronary syndrome. At an average, refuge women become angina pectoris for 5,4 years before domicile women. The most frequent three risk factors were menopause, hypertension and psychosocial factors; smoking was relatively rare risk factor. Leadings symptoms in these women were weakness and breathless, frequently than palpitation, and in only one woman angina pectoris was presented with chest pain. At more of two-third of female patients with established diagnosis of angina pectoris leadings symptoms were atypical, in difference than men where atypical symptoms had been less at one-third of them. Conclusions: Beside of presence of conventional risk factors, big role for origin to angina pectoris have psychosocial factors whose especially are expressed in women that refuge from Eastern Bosnian.

Possibility of establishing of missed diagnoses of angina pectoris and inappropriate medical decision impartially is high, and their percentage in such circumstances is approximately about 15%. We need adequately approach to reorganization of emergency medical services in sense to quality and quantify, together with strongly support of local community and state.

In: Heart Disease in Women
Editor: B. V. Larner and H. R. Pennelton

ISBN 978-1-60692-066-4
© 2009 Nova Science Publishers, Inc.

Chapter I

Cardiac Rehabilitation: Secondary Prevention of Cardiovascular Disease in Women

Richard Snow[1,2], Michelle LaLonde[1,2], Cheryl Graffagnino[1,2], Kathy Spencer[1,2], and Teresa Caulin-Glaser[1,2,]*

[1]Riverside Methodist Hospitals, Columbus, Ohio, USA
[2]McConnell Heart Health Center, Columbus, Ohio, USA

Abstract

Over the past decade progress has been made toward education and increasing awareness, in both patients and physicians, of the risks of cardiovascular disease in women. There has also been an increase in federally funded initiatives in the area of gender-specific cardiovascular research. However, cardiovascular disease continues to be the primary cause of death among women in the United States. Each year more women than men die of cardiovascular disease. Gender-based differences in the prevalence, risk factors, presentation, treatment, and outcomes of cardiovascular disease remain important areas of active research. A frequently overlooked, yet vitally important, component of treatment for the secondary prevention of cardiovascular disease in women is participation in cardiac rehabilitation. Cardiac rehabilitation programs are comprehensive secondary prevention programs which contain specific core components that aim to optimize cardiac risk reduction, teach and develop healthy behaviors, decrease disability, and promote an active lifestyle for patients with cardiovascular disease. Research has documented the efficacy and effectiveness of cardiac rehabilitation with reductions in mortality and improvements in clinical and behavioral outcomes. Despite this, cardiac rehabilitation is under prescribed and underutilized, especially in women. In this review, the current evidence-based findings, research, and recommendations for cardiac rehabilitation in the treatment of cardiovascular disease in women is addressed with a focus on those areas specific to the needs of women. Persistent gaps in our knowledge

[*] Corresponding Author: Teresa Caulin-Glaser, M.D. McConnell Heart Health Center 3773 Olentangy River Road, Columbus, Ohio 43214-3646, Phone:(614) 566-5777; Fax:(614) 566-6907; e-mail: tcauling@ohiohealth.com.

regarding the role of cardiac rehabilitation in women with cardiovascular disease are presented as research initiatives for the future.

Introduction

Coronary heart disease (CHD) is the most common form of cardiovascular disease. Atherosclerotic plaque is composed of cells with a range of regulatory functions that in turn influence the progressive growth of the plaque. It is the continued presence of the deposited lipids causing an inflammatory response that can become injurious. The chronic inflammatory response eventually results in a "walling off" of the damaged arterial segment, which then negatively impacts the function of that segment and becomes a part of the progressive atherosclerotic process itself. As CHD continues to progress to a more advanced stage, ongoing immunological processes can precipitate acute coronary syndromes and myocardial infarction. [1]

With the exception of 1918, cardiovascular disease (CVD) has been the leading cause of death in the United States since 1900. National Health and Nutrition Examination Survey (NHANES) data from 1999-2004 suggests that as of 2004, CVD accounts for one of every 2.8 deaths in the United States annually. Cardiovascular disease is estimated to cost approximately $431.8 billion a year in direct and indirect healthcare costs. [2] The American Heart Association (AHA) reports that 1 in 3 female adults suffer from CVD and the number of CVD deaths in females has exceeded the number of CVD deaths in males since 1984. African American females have the highest prevalence of deaths from CVD with a greater percentage of those deaths occurring at a younger age than in white females. [3]

Heart Disease is often mislabeled as a "man's disease" because the risk factors and symptoms for women are less likely to be recognized or treated as compared to those of men. Heart disease is the most common cause of disability and death in the United States. Of the 14 million Americans living with heart disease today, 49% are women. Reports indicate that women under the age of 50 who suffer an acute myocardial infarction (AMI) are twice as likely to die as men in the same age group. [4] Within one year after a heart attack, 38 percent of women, compared to 25 percent of men will die.[5] Early diagnosis and primary prevention of CHD is critical given the fact that 64% of women and 50% of men who died suddenly of CHD had no previous symptoms of this disease.[6,7]

Gender Differences in Cardiac Risk Factors

Risk factors for the development of CHD have been identified through observational studies such as the Framingham study and include non-modifiable risk factors: genetic predisposition, age and male gender, and modifiable risk factors: high blood pressure, high cholesterol, cigarette smoking and diabetes mellitus (DM). Recent studies have also demonstrated that obesity, physical inactivity, inflammation, and depression are likely independent risk factors for the development and progression of heart disease. With the exception of cigarette smoking, obesity has been identified as a risk factor for the all of the modifiable risk factors listed above.

Coronary disease presents approximately ten years later in women than in men and may be misdiagnosed in younger women if clinicians have a lower index of suspicion. Other factors that increase risk in women are a family history of a father or brother who developed heart disease before age 55 and a mother or sister who developed heart disease before age 65. Race is another factor with black women being at increased risk of dying from CVD. The 2004 overall death rate from CVD for black women was 333.6 deaths per 100,000 versus a death rate in white females of 238.0 per 100,000. [6]

Smoking

The majority of factors contributing to CHD can be controlled or modified through lifestyle change and if necessary utilization of pharmacologic therapy. Tobacco use is the leading preventable cause of death among women. Smoking has been associated with one-half of all coronary events in women.[7] Furthermore, coronary risk is elevated even in women with minimal use (relative risk 2.4 for 1.4 cigarettes/day).[7] Heavy smokers (defined as those who smoke 20 or more cigarettes per day), have a risk of heart disease two to four times higher than women who do not smoke.[8] Women who smoke suffer their first myocardial infarction 19 years earlier than a non-smoker and smoking cessation reduces the risk to baseline within 3 years.[8,10] An overall higher prevalence of smoking is found in both men and women who live in low-income households, have low-status jobs or are unemployed, have low levels of education, or are divorced or single parents.[11,12]

Dyslipidemia

The lipoprotein risk factors for CHD are somewhat different in women compared to men. The primary lipoprotein in the development of atherosclerosis is low-density lipoprotein (LDL). Elevated LDL cholesterol levels are more predictive of CHD risk in men but only when compared to premenopausal women. However, after age 50 years LDL levels have been found to stabilize in men and increase in women possibly due to declining estrogen levels.

Low levels of high-density lipoprotein (HDL), rather than high LDL cholesterol, is more predictive of coronary risk in women. High-density lipoprotein has been shown to be an independent predictor of CHD in both men and women with a greater predictive potential in women than men. [13,14] The Framingham Heart Study found that a 0.025-mmol/L increase in HDL cholesterol was associated with a 3% decrease in the incidence of CHD in women and a 2% decrease in men.[12]

Elevated triglycerides are commonly accompanied by other metabolic disturbances that may predispose to CHD, including lower HDL cholesterol, increased very low-density lipoprotein cholesterol (VLDL) and insulin resistance all of which makes it difficult to assess the independent risk that hypertriglyceridemia has on CVD. Angiographic studies have shown that overall lipid modification therapies have slowed the progression of coronary atherosclerosis and prevented the development of new coronary lesions. [15]

Diabetes Mellitus

Diabetes mellitus (DM) is an established risk factor for the development of CHD and is a stronger risk factor for CHD in women than men. The importance of this difference was demonstrated in a meta-analysis of 37 studies of approximately 450,000 patients with type 2 DM: the summary relative risk for fatal CHD in patients with DM was 3.5 in women and 2.1 in men.[16] Individuals with DM have a 2- to 4-fold greater risk of developing CHD compared with those individuals without DM.[17] Among those living with CHD, DM is the leading cause of morbidity and mortality and is considered the equivalent of already having an MI when assessing risk. DM counteracts the ten-year advantage in the development of CHD between men and women, increases the effects of current coronary risk factors, and may impair estrogen binding. The excess cardiovascular risk in women is at least in part due to DM being more commonly accompanied by other cardiovascular risk factors in women. [18]

Hypertension

The prevalence of hypertension is approximately 75 percent in women above age 70 years. [19] Hypertension is a strong predictor of cardiovascular risk in women. Among the elderly, hypertension in women compared to men is a stronger predictor of cardiovascular risk and is more commonly seen in women with CHD.[20] Hypertension in premenopausal women is associated with up to a 10 fold increase in cardiovascular mortality.[21] Hypertension also increases the risk of cardiovascular events in women who have known CHD.

Obesity

As rates of overweight (BMI = 25.0-29.9) and obesity (BMI $\geq$ 30.0) in the United States have reached epidemic proportions, the need to address this risk factor for CVD has become paramount. As such, the AHA has issued a call to action to treat obesity as a major risk factor for CHD. [22] Obesity has been identified as an independent risk factor for CHD in both men and women. [23] In addition, the AHA and American Association of Cardiovascular and Pulmonary Rehabilitation (AACVPR) have included guidelines and recommendation for treating overweight and obesity in secondary prevention and cardiac rehabilitation programs. [24]

Obesity, especially Class II (BMI $\geq$ 35) and III (BMI $\geq$ 40) obesity, has been associated with an increase in mortality as compared to normal weight individuals.[25] The mechanism by which this increase in mortality occurs is thought to be related to a higher risk of comorbid conditions such as type 2 DM, hypertension, hyperlipidemia and some cancers. In addition to these physical co-morbid conditions, psychological morbidity has been associated with obesity as well. A study by Meunnig et al. evaluated sociodemographic variables as they related to chronic health conditions, health related quality of life , annual deaths, years of life lost and quality adjusted years of life for men and women. The study found that obese women lost 1.8 million quality adjusted life years versus 270,000 years lost by men when compared to normal weight subjects. This discrepancy appears to result from a lower health-related quality of life and late life mortality suggesting that women experience a greater share of the disease burden associated with overweight and obesity as compared to men. [26]

In addition to the personal costs of overweight and obesity in American society, the economic costs are extensive as well. Healthcare costs related to obesity increased from $3.6 to $36.5 billion between 1987 and 2002.[27] In 2000, it was estimated that healthcare costs of morbidly obese individuals (BMI $\geq$ 40 kg/m^2) were more than $11 billion dollars, almost 81% higher than the healthcare costs of normal weight individuals.[28]

Cardiovascular disease is one of the many disease states and co-morbid conditions associated with the increased morbidity, mortality and economic burden of overweight and obesity. The mechanism by which body weight affects cardiovascular health is multifactorial in nature. Overweight and obesity affects both the structure and function of the heart and is an independent predictor of coronary atherosclerosis.[29] Obesity is also a factor in the development of other cardiovascular risk factors such as hypertension, type 2 DM, heart failure and sleep apnea. Overweight women are 44% more likely to develop at least one of the following risk factors: hypertension, hyperlipidemia or type 2 DM. Obese women are 46% more likely to develop at least 1 of these risk factors. Body fat distribution as measured by waist circumference is also of importance. Compared to overweight women with a normal waist circumference, overweight women with a high waist circumference (> 35 inches), are 2 times more likely to develop hypertension and 4 times more likely to develop type 2 DM. While each of these risks is of independent importance for CVD, the tendency for risk factor clustering in overweight and obese individuals is of even greater concern as multiple risk factors in the same individual can produce an additive effect greatly increasing the risk of CVD. In the presence of at least 3 of the following risk factors an individual is considered to have metabolic syndrome and an increased risk for CHD. These risk factors include increased waist circumference, hypertension, impaired fasting blood glucose, elevated triglycerides and low HDL cholesterol. [30]

It has been estimated that 40% of coronary heart disease in all women can be attributed to overweight and weight gain.

Depression

In the general population, depression affects 6% of men and 18% of women. [Kemp] The lifetime risk of depression is 20% to 25% for women and 7% to 12% for men. [32] There is increasing evidence that emotional stress is associated with adverse outcomes from medical illnesses. In particular, clinical depression and adverse cardiovascular outcomes have been studied and well defined by several authors (Borowicz et al., 2002; Glassman and Shapiro,

1998; Lauzon et al., 2003; Pignay-Demaria, Lesperance, Demaria, Frasure-Smith, and Perrault, 2003).[33-36] Depression has also been defined as a risk factor for both ischemic heart disease and AMI.[37]

Over the last decade, several studies have investigated the connection between heart disease and depression. In a study by Frasure-Smith and colleagues (2000), 887 patients were followed for one year after an AMI. Approximately one week after discharge from intensive care units, subjects were evaluated using the Beck Depression Inventory (BDI), a standardized measure for symptoms of depression. [38] They were also queried about the emotional support they received from family and friends based on another standardized test, the Perceived Social Support Scale. The BDI showed about 32 percent of these patients were experiencing mild to moderate symptoms of depression. During the first year after their heart attacks, about 8 percent of the patients with symptoms of depression died of heart-related problems compared to less than 3 percent of those who did not exhibit symptoms of depression. However, the relationship between depression and cardiac mortality decreased with high scores on the social support inventory. Those patients with symptoms of depression who also reported high levels of social support from friends and family members were more likely to overcome their symptoms of depression. Approximately half of the patients who exhibited symptoms of depression immediately after an AMI remained symptomatic a full year after their illness. Short-term symptoms of depression are common after an AMI, according to Frasure-Smith, but these findings suggest that if the depressive symptoms linger and there is no strong social support system present for the patient, a second AMI is more probable.

Another study by Murberg (1999) confirms the concern that patients with both depression and CHD are at greater risk for heart disease related complications. [39] In this study of 119 clinically stable Norwegian patients with congestive heart failure (CHF), patients with severe depressive symptoms were about four times more likely to die within two years compared with patients without symptoms of depression. During the study 20 patients died, all from heart disease related complications. Twenty-five percent of patients with depressive symptoms died as compared with 11.3 percent of patients without symptoms. However, depression may not only place heart disease patients at risk for further heart disease-related illness. Depression may also be an independent risk factor for having a first heart attack.

Women with CHD are twice as likely to die if they exhibit symptoms of depression, when compared to women who do not show such signs, according to an analysis by Blumenthal et al. (1999).[40] This study was one of the first to look specifically at depression as a predictor of mortality in women with CHD. Most previous studies have only included small numbers of women. Specific studies that look only at women are crucial because CHD may manifest itself differently in women. For their analysis, the researchers enrolled 265 women admitted for a cardiac catheterization. Patients were given the BDI. The patients were followed for up to 3.5 years, with a median follow-up of 1.8 years. The researchers compared the BDI scores of the women who died to those who were alive, and found that women whose BDI score was 12 (the top 25th percentile in terms of symptoms of depression) were twice as likely to have died when compared to women with a score of 4 (the bottom 25th percentile).

Wassertheil-Smoller et al. (2004) investigated the association between depressive symptoms and cardiovascular events in 93,676 healthy, older women who participated in the Women's Health Initiative observational study. [41] The women were evaluated for depressive symptoms and cardiovascular disease risk factors upon enrollment, between 1993-1998, and were then followed for an average of 4 years. The study found that depressive symptoms were reported by 15.8% of these women and depressive symptoms were significantly related to CHD risk. Women were 12% more likely to have hypertension and 60% more likely to have a history of stroke or angina if they had depressive symptoms. Among women with no history of CHD, symptoms of depression were an independent predictor of death from CVD (50% more likely) or death from any other cause (32% more likely). Depressive symptoms were an independent risk factor for subsequent cardiovascular death at a lower level than DM or hypertension but at a higher level than body mass index, income, education, race, or ethnicity.

In a study by Agatisa et al. (2005), the investigators, using electron-beam tomography, evaluated 210 women with a history of depressive symptoms for evidence of arterial and aortic calcification.[42] One quarter of the women studied had a history of recurrent major depression. The authors report that coronary calcium was present in approximately 50% of the 210 women, and aortic calcification in 54%, with both coronary calcium and a high degree of calcification being associated with a history of recurrent major depression. After adjustment for other cardiovascular risk factors, a history of major recurrent depression was associated with an odds ratio of 2.46 for any coronary calcium, 2.71 for high coronary calcification, and 3.39 for high aortic calcification. A number of pathways may contribute to the link between depression and calcification including poor nutrition, sedentary behavior, obesity and perhaps central adiposity. Depressive symptoms are also predictive of the development of metabolic syndrome which has been associated with heart disease in women.

Although the precise causal mechanism between depression and heart disease has not been definitively identified, evidence has clearly demonstrated that depression in patients with CHD is harmful and needs to be recognized and treated. Physicians and other caregivers need to be particularly vigilant to recognize the presence of depression in their cardiac patients. A mechanism should be in place to screen cardiac patients for depression and to provide scheduled follow-up one month after a patient's heart attack to determine if the depression has abated. If it persists, caregivers should refer cardiac patients for treatment.

Gender Differences in Diagnosis of Cardiovascular Disease

There are differences between the genders in terms of the development, presentation, diagnosis and treatment of CHD. Women are approximately 10 years older than men at the time of presentation with cardiovascular disease. [43-47] In addition, women are more likely to initially present with angina as opposed to AMI. [48] Unfortunately, women who present to the emergency department with complaints of new onset chest pain/discomfort are often evaluated and diagnosed less aggressively than men. Studies have shown that compared to men, women are less likely to be evaluated with an electrocardiogram and cardiac enzyme measurements. [49, 50] The presentation and symptoms of CHD can be different in women compared to men. It has been reported that dyspnea (58%), weakness (55%) and fatigue (43%) are more common presentations of AMI than chest pain in women.[51] In another study comparing symptoms of men and women presenting with AMI, women more often presented with neck, jaw, or back pain/discomfort and nausea in addition to chest pain as compared to men.[52] A recent analysis performed from the Clopidogrel in Unstable Angina to Prevent Recurrent Events (CURE) trial found high risk women with acute coronary syndrome (ACS) underwent fewer invasive procedures including angiography, angioplasty, and coronary artery bypass graft surgery (CABG) (47.6% vs. 60.5%; p = 0.0001) compared to men. The women studied were more likely than men to develop refractory ischemia and to be re-hospitalized for chest pain during follow-up (16.6% vs. 13.9%; p = 0.0001).[53] This may be partially due to decreased awareness by treating physicians of the different presentation and clinical course of acute coronary syndrome in women as compared to men.

A recent national survey conducted by the AHA found that even though minority women have one of the highest rates of CVD, they are least aware (Caucasian women 62% vs. African American women 38% and Hispanic women 34%). [54] In this study that included a random and nationally representative sample of 1,008 women ≥25 years old, only 55% of women recognized cardiovascular disease as their leading killer. Fifty-four percent of women who were evaluated by a healthcare professional on a regular basis reported having a discussion of their risk factors for CVD. Thirty eight percent of women said they did not discuss their risk for the development of heart disease because their healthcare provider did not bring it up. [54] Only 24% of Caucasian women, 12% of African American women and 14% of Hispanic women were aware of the appropriate level for LDL cholesterol. Women were somewhat better informed about appropriate blood pressure goals however the higher at-risk minority women were less aware (Caucasian women 52%, African American women 40% and Hispanic women 37%, p<0.05).[54] These are important observations because awareness of risk is the first step toward prevention. These data highlight the need for health care providers to help raise awareness of the real versus perceived threat of CVD in women. However, in an AHA random online survey of 500 primary care physicians, obstetricians/gynecologists and cardiologists, less than 1 in 5 physicians knew more women than men die each year from CVD. The physicians who participated also tended to rate women at lower risk for CVD than men even when their Framingham risk level was the same as men. [55]

Gender Differences in Prevention of Cardiovascular Disease

Excess weight and physical inactivity have an adverse impact on other risk factors for cardiovascular disease including blood glucose levels, blood pressure and lipid profiles. Participants in the Framingham study who lost at least 2.25 kg over a span of 16 years had a 40%-50% reduction in their total cardiovascular risk factor score. [56]

Low levels of physical activity are directly related to an increased risk for CHD. In a study examining the impact of physical activity on mortality, women in the lowest tertile of physical activity had a greater than 5-fold increased risk of mortality than compared with women in the highest tertile of physical activity. When comparing men of the same groupings, the increased risk of mortality was only 3-fold when comparing the lowest tertile of physical activity with the highest tertile of physical activity. [57] The Nurses' Health Study of over 70,000 women between the ages of 40 and 65 years demonstrated that moderate intensity walking or vigorous exercise was inversely related to the risk of a cardiovascular event. Multivariate analysis demonstrated that women in increasing quintile groups for energy expenditure had age-adjusted relative risks for coronary events of 0.88, 0.81, 0.74, and 0.66, showing a graded cardiovascular benefit from exercise.[58] Women who initiated exercise in mid life or later had a lower incidence of cardiovascular events compared to those who did not exercise.

To reduce or prevent the development of obesity-related risk factors for coronary heart disease, intentional weight loss for overweight and obese patients is recommended. However, effective treatment options for dramatic, sustained weight loss in overweight and obese individuals remains elusive. However, even modest weight losses can effectively improve risk factors for coronary heart disease. For example, meta-analysis indicates that a 1 kg weight loss can reduce total cholesterol, LDL cholesterol and serum triglycerides by 2.28 mg/dl, 0.91mg/dl and 1.54 mg/dl respectively. Anderson et al suggests that a 5 kg weight loss may improve average fasting blood glucose levels in patient with DM by as much as 18 mg/dl, similar to the reductions produced by some oral hypoglycemic agents. [59] It is also important to recognize prevention of weight gain as an effective prevention strategy. A recent study found that individuals who gained approximately 1 pound per year over 15 years of follow-up experienced significant increases in blood pressure, triglycerides, insulin, fasting blood glucose and a decrease in HDL-cholesterol. Individuals who were overweight at baseline but whose weight remained stable had stable risk factors during the same time period. [30]

Cardiac Rehabilitation Programs

Cardiac rehabilitation (CR) programs are an important venue for the delivery of effective secondary preventive care. CR programs deliver coordinated, multifaceted interventions including baseline patient assessments, risk factor management, nutritional counseling, psychosocial counseling, physical activity and exercise training in addition to the use of cardioprotective medications. Participation by women in CR programs have shown rates of improvement in functional capacity and relief of angina symptoms similar to those of men.[60] Women may benefit by participation in a CR program to a greater extent than men due to overall greater improvements in women's exercise capacity as well as quality of life pre-rehabilitation to post-rehabilitation.[61,62]

Although the benefits of CR programs have been demonstrated, studies have shown low rates of enrollment of women into outpatient CR programs after a coronary event. Although nearly 40% of all coronary events occur in women and women tend to have a greater burden of death and disability following a cardiac event, participation rates among eligible women range from 15-20% compared with 25-31% among men. [60,63-67] Some of this can be attributed to the fact that women are less likely than men to be instructed on secondary prevention strategies or to receive a physician referral to CR after revascularization.[68]

Cardiac rehabilitation has been recognized as one of the primary methods of secondary prevention and is recommended as an integral component of care for patients with CVD. The goal of CR is to provide an intervention that will optimize the cardiac patient's functional capacity in all areas of life, including physical, psychological and social aspects and to slow, stop or reverse the progression of CVD. [69]

Historically, CR programs were developed in response to lengthy hospitalizations and extreme deconditioning associated with AMI and surgical interventions for CHD in the 1960's and 1970's. Initially, the focus of CR was on exercise to improve functional capacity and to achieve a decrease in mortality. [70] Exercise training has long been the cornerstone of CR programs and to date, exercise training has been the most effectively studied component of these programs. Its benefits in improving functional capacity, quality of life and reducing morbidity and mortality have been well-documented. Over the past 40-50 years, exercise in a CR setting has also been shown to be exceedingly safe with only 2 fatalities per 1.5 million hours of patient exercise. [69] The health benefits of CR for AMI, CABG and stable angina are well-established and have been the primary diagnoses for which third party payers have approved reimbursement. While the evidence continues to mount for the benefits of CR for these diagnoses, a growing body of evidence for health benefits associated with other CVD states continues to develop. There is a clear evidence of benefit associated with CR after percutaneous coronary intervention, CHF, heart transplant and heart valve replacement.[71] Given the safety and benefits associated with supervised exercise, criteria for participation in CR programs has expanded to include not only post myocardial infarction and surgical revascularization, but also percutaneous coronary interventions, recent valvular heart surgery, chronic heart failure, heart transplantation and peripheral artery disease.[70] A meta-analysis based on a review of 48 randomized trials found that when compared to usual medical care, patients participating in exercise-based rehabilitation had a significant reduction in all-cause mortality and in cardiac mortality.[69]

Multiple factors have been identified that may account for the cardioprotective effects of exercise training. Supervised exercise training after a cardiovascular event along with regular daily activity has been shown to increase peak oxygen uptake by 11% to 36%. This improvement in fitness leads to improvements in quality of life and physical function. It has also been shown to improve submaximal heart rate and hypertension. This improvement, demonstrated by improvements in endurance on exercise testing, has also been associated with a significant decrease in both fatal and non-fatal cardiac events regardless of the presence of other risk factors for CVD.[69] Exercise has been associated with a significant improvement in endothelial function as a result of increased flow-mediated shear stress on artery walls during exercise. This is also associated with an improvement in the synthesis, release and action of nitric oxide which inhibits the progression of atherogenesis and thrombosis. Exercise may also reduce myocardial ischemia and improve coronary flow. It may also reduce the risk of sudden cardiac death secondary to ventricular tachyarrhythmia by increasing heart rate variability and baroreceptor sensitivity through reduced sympathetic and enhanced parasympathetic activity. Exercise training may also reduce the risk of thrombosis and subsequent occlusion of coronary arteries through increased plasma volume, decreased platelet aggregation and blood viscosity and enhanced thrombolytic ability. Exercise training may also reduce plasma levels of fibrinogen. Exercise training also decreases C-reactive protein levels suggesting that exercise has an anti-inflammatory effect. Other cardioprotective mechanisms through which exercise training and CR may decrease the morbidity and mortality of cardiovascular disease include weight loss and loss of fat mass, decreases in blood pressure and in triglycerides. Increases in HDL cholesterol, insulin sensitivity and glucose control also offer protective benefits. Exercise training also improves the elasticity and vasodilatation of coronary arteries thereby improving blood flow. It may also increase blood flow through arteriogenesis and angiogenesis. Exercise training also reduces the risk of sudden cardiac death and lethal ventricular tachycardia by reducing sympathetic and parasympathetic activity and making the myocardium more tolerant to ischemic stress. Exercise training also may reduce the risk of thrombosis and occlusion after plaque is disrupted through increased plasma volume and thrombolytic activity and decreased blood viscosity and platelet aggregation. [69]

Although CR programs have been founded on the principles of supervised exercise and the clear benefits associated with exercise, several randomized-controlled clinical trials have demonstrated that a combination of exercise, low-fat diets and lipid management therapies can slow the progression of atherosclerotic disease and decrease the incidence of cardiac events and hospitalizations. Multiple clinical trials have shown that intensive risk factor management through lifestyle and nutrition counseling and prescribed drug therapies are also effective in reducing mortality. However, research suggests that few patients with CVD are achieving desired risk factor status in traditional patient care settings. For example, as few as 9-25% of patients treated in physician practices met the National Cholesterol Education Program (NCEP III) goals for treatment. [70] In light of this and evidence that focused risk factor management interventions can slow the progression of the cardiovascular disease process, CR programs have been called upon to expand their focus beyond exercise and to focus on targeted interventions for risk factor modification.[70]

A joint scientific statement offered by the AHA and AACVPR in 2007, in agreement with the 2006 update of the AHA/American College of Cardiology (ACC) secondary prevention guidelines, identified core components that should be included in any CR program. These include baseline patient assessment, nutritional counseling, physical activity training, exercise counseling and psychosocial interventions (including depression). Additional recommendations for intensive risk factor management include counseling and treatment of obesity, hypertension, lipids, DM and tobacco cessation. Recommendations for the use of antiplatelet agents, rennin-angiotensin-aldosterone system blockers, beta blockers and influenza vaccine included in guidelines for secondary prevention may also impact the direction of CR programs.[24] These statements and guidelines emphasize the importance of programs focusing on lifelong behavior change, incorporating strategies to maximize patient adherence and working in conjunction with the patient's primary care provider and/or cardiologist for sustained benefits.[24]

A variety of models for delivery of cardiac rehabilitation programs designed to address the issue of intensive risk factor modification have been proposed. A case management system of care can help focus CR programs to manage multiple risk factors for cardiovascular disease in patients. Case management includes: screening, risk stratification, assignment to a case manager (usually a nurse or exercise physiologist), intensive risk-reduction interventions based on clinical practice guidelines, medical monitoring for safety, efficacy and patient adherence, measurement of outcomes and satisfaction, follow-up and modification of treatment plans as appropriate.[70] This type of directed intervention has been shown to produce clinical benefits, an increase in utilization and adherence to medical therapies, and a decrease in recurrent coronary events and hospitalizations.[70] Traditionally, most CR programs have been delivered in hospitals or community centers. However, geographic limitations, poor patient referrals and inadequate reimbursement have led to efforts to create alternative delivery sites and systems for CR programs.[69] Alternative models include home and community-based programs coordinated by a nurse or other healthcare providers.[69] As technological advances impact the delivery of healthcare, opportunities for telemedicine and telehealth may enhance the delivery of programs as an adjunct or provide an alternative when direct contact is not an option. The AACVPR defines telemedicine as using electronic communication such as e-mail to provide and support clinical care. Telehealth is identified as using electronic communication for educating healthcare professionals and the community and for public health and research activities. The AACVPR has published standards of practice for the appropriate use of telemedicine and telehealth. These standards focus on access, safety, and that communication methods should adhere to the same standards of ethics, professional conduct, documentation, regulation and communication as face-to face-interactions.[72] However, little research is available to document the effectiveness of these alternative methods for providing a CR program.[69]

Gender Differences in Utilization of Cardiac Rehabilitation

While evidence of the health benefits of CR and intensive risk factor management is extensive and continues to grow, CR remains a greatly underutilized resource in secondary prevention of patients with CVD. A study of Medicare beneficiaries found that only 18.7% of eligible patients participated in CR after an AMI or CABG surgery. While overall utilization of CR is poor, it is even more underutilized in females with only 14.3% of women in the cohort receiving CR services as compared to 22.1% of eligible men in the same cohort. Being older, nonwhite and having a lower income, less education and a higher level of disability also decreased the likelihood that Medicare eligible patients participated in CR.[73] These findings are consistent with those of other researchers who have found that women and ethnic minorities are less likely to be referred to and to participate in CR.[74] The cause of this underutilization of CR, particularly among women and ethnic minorities, in spite of the conclusive evidence as to the benefits is multifactorial in nature. Lack of physician and other healthcare provider referral and endorsement has consistently been shown to negatively impact participation in CR. Women, particularly those with lower incomes and lacking medical insurance, are less likely to be referred to CR by a physician.[75] Completion of a CR program is inherent to its effectiveness in providing benefits. When women are referred to CR, they are more likely to drop out of the program before completion if they are older, obese, more deconditioned as evidenced by a 6-minute walk test and if they show greater evidence of depressive symptoms as measured by the Beck Depression Inventory (BDI-II) or if they have poorer mental health scores on the SF-36.[76] In addition to a lower referral rate and increased risks for drop-out in women, increasing distance from a CR program also reduced participation in both men and women. This suggests accessibility is a deterrent to participation regardless of gender. A significant difference in CR participation rates by region in eligible Medicare participants was also identified. North Central states had the highest rates of utilization with Nebraska having 53.5% of eligible Medicare patients participating in CR. The authors suggest that if this rate was achieved in all other states it would result in a 26-31% decrease in cardiac mortality among those patients. [73

Gender Differences on Entry to a Cardiac Rehabilitation Program

We have performed a detailed analysis on patient characteristics of those participating in our CR program at the McConnell Heart Health Center. Data used for the analyses were drawn from a free standing community hospital based CR program between 2003 to 2007. This program provides comprehensive secondary prevention services to patients referred from the inpatient setting as well as outpatient private physician practices. Retrospective data was analyzed only on those patients completing a minimum of 7 weeks of a 12 week CR program. The program components include structured and supervised exercise, individual counseling, and group education classes. The supervised exercise program consisted of work intensity and goals consistent with the AHA and AACVPR recommendations. [24] The topics of education included nutrition, exercise, managing heart health and risk factors, stress management, and lifestyle modification. Patients attended three exercise sessions per week which included forty minutes of cardiovascular exercise and ten minutes of stretching and strength training. An individualized plan of care was developed for each patient based on the initial medical and lifestyle assessment. Each patient in the program had a health coordinator (a registered nurse or exercise physiologist) who set mutual goals with the patient and coordinated the care throughout the program. The health coordinator triaged patients to a registered dietitian for individual nutrition counseling based on criteria of BMI over 30, DM and/or uncontrolled dyslipidemia. Diabetics were defined as such if they gave a history of DM or if they were taking diabetic medication. Registered nurses, exercise physiologists, registered dietitians, cardiologists, and the social worker circulated among patients during the exercise sessions to provide ongoing guidance and feedback.

During this time frame, a total of 2546 individuals were enrolled in CR at the McConnell Heart Health Center. A total of 125 individuals who enrolled but never started the program were excluded from analysis. Of the remaining 2421 participants, 386 (15.9%) quit prior to program completion and 229 (9.5%) completed CR but had incomplete outcomes data.

The remaining 1806 individuals had complete data and were included in the analysis. Data collection was considered complete if the individual had complete demographics, co-morbidities, as well as pre and post lipid profiles, and stress tests.

Women entering the CR program were older than the men. The mean age of women was 65.8 ± 12.0 yrs compared to a mean age of 63.4 ± 10.8 yrs in men (table 1). Although the difference between the mean ages for men and women is small, 39.5% of women were 70 years old or older upon program entry compared to only 30.0% of men (p=0.0001).

Table 1. Entry Characteristics by Gender

Entry Characteristics	Males (n=1335)	Females (n=471)	p value
Age (yrs ± SD)	63.4 ± 10.8	65.8 ± 12.0	0.0001
Age ≥ 70 yrs (%)	30.0	39.5	0.0001
Caucasian (%)	87.7	88.1	0.82
Married/Partner (%)	83.5	54.6	<.0001
Education > 12 yrs (%)	67.8	47.8	<.0001
Currently Employed (%)	47.1	30.8	<.0001
Diabetes (%)	28.4	27.4	0.68
Current Smoker (%)	6.1	4.3	0.13
Hypertension (%)	71.5	80.5	0.0001
Obesity (%)	39.5	40.8	0.62

Table 2. Cardiac Rehabilitation Diagnoses by Gender

Entry Characteristics	Males (n=1335)	Females (n=471)	p value
PTCA (%)	37.6	44.0	0.02
CABG (%)	39.5	23.3	< 0.0001
Myocardial Infarction (%)	12.1	12.1	0.98
Valve Replacement/Repair (%)	4.8	10.0	< 0.0001
Angina (%)	1.9	3.2	0.10
Other (%)	4.1	7.4	0.008

While there were gender differences in age, there were no significant gender differences in race (table 1). Although it has bee reported in the literature that females participating in CR are more likely than males to come from a racial/ethnic minority group. [77]

Gender differences extend into martial status, level of education, employment status, referring diagnosis and co-morbidities. Approximately 50% to 60% of women report being married/cohabitating vs. 60% to 90% of men. [77] Similar percentages were found in our analysis (table 1). Women in our program were significantly less likely to have more than a high school education compared to men (47.8% vs. 67.8%, respectively) and significantly less likely to report current employment than men (30.8% vs. 47.1%, respectively). Gender differences were also apparent in the diagnoses for referral of men and women to CR (table 2) (p < 0.0001). Women were significantly more likely than men to be referred after angioplasty and/or stenting or valve surgery but were less likely to have undergone CABG.

In our CR program, men and women entering CR have a similar prevalence of DM with slightly more than a quarter of participants entering with a diagnosis of DM. However, a large national survey of gender differences in CR performed in 1996 did report significant gender differences in the prevalence of DM (23.4% women vs. 15.9% men). [77] The differences between the prevalence of DM in our program and the prevalence reported in 1996 by Thomas, et al may be attributable to the rise in obesity and DM rates in the U.S. over this time period. Results from the 1999-2002 NHANES showed a 16% increase in obesity and a 35.1% increase in hyperinsulinemia compared to the 1988-1994 NHANES. [78, 79]

There was no significant difference in the prevalence of tobacco use between men and women in our program with approximately 5% of participants reporting current tobacco use. Reported prevalence of tobacco use by gender from Thomas et al in 1996 was higher than reported in our program (9.2% women vs. 11.6% men). Differences could be due to societal changes in acceptance of smoking and the general continued decrease in tobacco use since 1996. [80]

Significant gender differences were noted in the prevalence of a history of hypertension upon entry to our CR program. Among women, 80.5% had a history of hypertension compared to 71.5% of men entering CR (p = 0.0001). Evaluation of mean blood pressures upon entry to CR in our program showed no distribution of gender by blood pressure classification. Based on JNC VII guidelines, approximately 35% of all participants had blood pressures in the normal range (systolic blood pressure < 120 and diastolic blood pressure < 80), 55% had blood pressures in the prehypertension range (systolic blood pressure between 120 and 139 or diastolic blood pressure between 80 to 89), and 10% were classified as Stage 1 hypertension or higher (systolic blood pressure ≥ 140 or diastolic blood pressure ≥ 90.

Although there were no apparent gender differences in the prevalence of obesity by gender upon entry to CR, differences become apparent when BMI was stratified by BMI classifications (table 3). There were significantly more women entering CR with a BMI ≥ 40 kg/m^2 (Class III obesity) compared to men (10% vs. 4.9%, respectively).

Data is sparse and study sample sizes are small with regard to gender differences in lipid profile among CR participants. In our analysis, significant gender differences were noted with women having higher entry total cholesterol, HDL, LDL and non HDL cholesterol. A significantly lower percentage of women met ATP III guideline goals compared to men. There was no significant difference in entry triglyceride levels between men and women or in the percentage meeting ATP III recommended levels for triglycerides (table 3). A 2004 study by Savage et al evaluated gender specific differences in entry lipid profiles on a sample of 77 women and 263 men. They reported significantly higher entry HDL and triglyceride levels in women, but no statistically significant differences in entry total cholesterol, or entry LDL as we found in our CR program. Differences between our CR program entry lipids and the entry lipids reported by Savage et al are most likely due to differences in sample size. [81]

Gender differences were also observed in maximal functional capacity upon program entry. Maximal functional capacity is often estimated upon entry to a CR program using graded exercise testing and is commonly expressed in METs. MET is an abbreviation for metabolic equivalent and expresses oxygen consumption relative to resting requirements. For example, an activity requiring a 3 MET capacity requires three times the oxygen consumption required sitting quietly at rest. Upon CR program entry, maximal functional capacity was significantly higher for men compared to women. Relative to the mean entry MET level for women, the mean entry MET level for men was 38.5% higher than the mean entry MET level for women. This is similar to the 33.1% difference reported by Ades et al. [82].

Table 3. Entry Clinical Variables by Gender

Mean Entry Clinical Variables	Males (n=1335)	Females (n=471)	p value
Weight (lbs ± SD)	203.0 ± 41.1	172.2 ± 41.2	<.0001
BMI (ml/kg^2 ± SD)	29.7 ± 5.5	30.2 ± 6.8	0.18
% Not obese	58.4	56.3	0.41
% Class I Obesity	26.1	23.1	0.21
% Class II Obesity	10.6	10.6	1.0
% Class III Obesity	4.9	10.0	<.0001
Cholesterol (mg/dl ± SD)	156.7 ± 35.6	175.4 ± 39.7	<.0001
LDL (mg/dl ± SD)	83.5 ± 29.1	89.5 ± 31.7	0.0003
HDL (mg/dl ± SD)	44.3 ± 11.5	55.8 ± 15.9	<.0001
Triglycerides (mg/dl ± SD)	149.1 ± 95.4	152.8 ± 85.2	0.42
Non HDL cholesterol (mg/dl ± SD)	112.5 ± 34.5	119.6 ± 38.4	0.0004
% Chol at goal	88.9	77.7	<.0001
% LDL at goal	74.0	70.3	0.12
% HDL at goal	62.7	61.2	0.55
% Trigs at goal	64.1	62.2	0.46
% Non HDL at goal	72.6	66.9	0.02
Systolic Blood Pressure (mm Hg)	126.1± 21.1	125.0 ± 15.4	0.31
Diastolic Blood Pressure (mm Hg)	74.0 ± 8.2	71.6 ± 7.6	< 0.0001
Fasting Blood Glucose (non diabetics)	101.0 ± 14.5	97.9 ± 12.7	0.0006
Fasting Blood Glucose (diabetics)	137.5 ± 42.3	139.9 ± 48.8	0.64
A1C (diabetics)	6.9 ± 1.1	7.2 ± 1.2	0.07
MET Level (mean ± SD)	6.6 ± 2.9	4.8 ± 2.1	<.0001
BDI (mean ± SD)	6.7 ± 6.2	8.5 ± 7.6	<.0001

Table 4. Entry Characteristics for Women by Age Group

Entry Characteristics Variables	< 70 yrs (n=285)	≥ 70 yrs (n=186)	p value
Age (yrs)	58.2 ± 8.8	77.3 ± 4.6	<0.0001
Caucasian (%)	86.0	91.4	0.08
Married/Partner (%)	59.3	47.3	0.01
Catchment Area (%)	35.1	51.1	0.0006
Education > 12 yrs (%)	48.8	46.2	0.59
Currently Employed (%)	47.7	4.8	<.0001
Diabetes (%)	28.1	26.3	0.68
Current Smoker (%)	6.3	1.1	0.006
Hypertension (%)	79.0	82.8	0.30
Obesity (%)	49.8	26.9	<.0001

To examine age differences for women, age was dichotomized into older women (≥ 70 yrs) and younger women (< 70 yrs) based on age upon program entry. In our CR program, older women accounted for 60.5% of all women with a mean age of 77.3 ± 4.6 yrs; 39.5% of all women were in the younger age group with a mean age of 58.2 ± 8.8 yrs (table 4). Analysis of demographic data demonstrated no difference in race or education level between older and younger women. However, there were significant differences in marital and employment status (table 4). Older women were significantly less likely to be married or have a live in partner and were more likely to be separated, divorced or have a deceased spouse. Younger women were significantly more likely to report current employment upon program entry compared to older women (47.8% vs. 4.8%) (table 4). Interestingly, when zip code of residence of the participants was used as a proxy for distance from our center, a significantly higher percentage of older women lived within our facility's catchment area compared to younger women (51.1% vs. 35.1%, respectively). This is suggestive that distance from our facility potentially poses a greater barrier to participation for older women compared to younger women.

There were also age differences among women in referring diagnosis. Older women were significantly more likely than younger women to be enrolled in CR with a diagnosis of CABG or angina, while younger women were significantly more likely to be enrolled with a referral of valve replacement/repair or other diagnoses such as heart failure or cardiomyopathy (table 5).

There was no significant difference between younger and older women in the prevalence of hypertension or DM. Differences were noted in the prevalence of smoking. Relative to older women, younger women participating in CR were nearly 5 times more likely to be a current smoker (6.3% vs. 1.1%, respectively). Younger women were also significantly more likely to be obese compared to older women. Stratification of entry BMI measurements by obesity classification levels indicate that this finding persists through each level of obesity classification (table 6).

Age differences for women were also apparent in their clinical entry variables. Although mean total cholesterol, LDL cholesterol, triglycerides and non-HDL cholesterol levels were similar for both younger and older women, mean HDL levels in older women were 8% higher relative to mean entry HDL levels of younger women. Similar findings were reported by Beckie, et al. in their age stratified comparison of women in CR. [83] There were no differences in the number of younger women vs. older women at NCEP III goal for lipid levels with the exception of entry HDL level. Differences were also noted in mean entry fasting blood glucose by age group of individuals with DM. Relative to the younger women, the older women with DM had a 17.9% lower blood glucose level. The younger women with DM had a higher A1C level than the older women reflecting poorer glucose control.

Similar to the results reported by Beckie, et al, younger women in our program had a significantly higher entry MET level than older women (table 6).[83] Relative to the entry MET level of older women, the mean MET level for older women was 55% lower than the mean MET level for younger women. Although not gender specific, Lavie et al reported a difference in entry MET levels between younger and older participants upon CR entry of 27% between CR participants under 55 yrs of age and over 70 years of age. [84]

Table 5. Cardiac Rehabilitation Diagnoses for Women by Age Group

Entry Characteristics	< 70 yrs (n=285)	≥ 70 yrs (n=186)	p value
PTCA (%)	45.3	41.9	0.48
CABG (%)	18.6	30.7	0.003
Myocardial Infarction (%)	11.6	12.9	0.67
Valve Replacement/Repair (%)	12.6	5.9	0.02
Angina (%)	1.8	5.4	0.03
Other (%)	9.8	3.2	0.007

Table 6. Clinical Variables on Entry to Cardiac Rehabilitation for Women by Age Group

Mean Entry Clinical Variables	< 70 yrs (n=285)	≥ 70 yrs (n=186)	p value
Weight (lbs)	181.8 ± 43.7	157.4 ± 32.0	<.0001
BMI (kg/m^2)	31.4 ± 7.3	28.2 ± 5.4	<.0001
% Not obese	46.7	71.0	<.0001
% Class I Obesity	26.3	18.3	0.04
% Class II Obesity	14.0	5.4	0.003
% Class III Obesity	13.0	5.4	0.007
Cholesterol (mg/dl ± SD)	175.4 ± 41.7	175.5 ± 36.5	1.0
LDL (mg/dl ± SD)	90.5 ± 32.6	87.9 ± 30.3	0.39
HDL (mg/dl ± SD)	54.1 ± 15.6	58.5 ± 16.0	0.003
Triglycerides (mg/dl ± SD)	154.9 ± 92.4	149.7 ± 73.1	0.50
Non HDL cholesterol (mg/dl ± SD)	121.3 ± 40.2	117.0 ± 35.3	0.23
% Chol at goal	77.2	78.5	0.74
% LDL at goal	69.5	71.5	0.64
% HDL at goal	54.7	71.0	0.0004
% Trigs at goal	61.8	62.9	0.80
% Non HDL at goal	65.3	69.4	0.36
Systolic Blood Pressure	121.7 ± 14.3	129.9 ± 15.6	< 0.0001
Diastolic Blood Pressure	72.2 ± 7.5	70.7 ± 7.5	0.05
Fasting Blood Glucose (non diabetics)	96.7 ± 12.4	99.9 ± 13.1	0.03
Fasting Blood Glucose (diabetics)	150.2 ± 54.6	123.3 ± 31.9	0.002
A1C (diabetics)	7.4 ± 1.4	6.7 ± 0.7	0.0006
MET Level	5.6 ± 2.0	3.6 ± 1.5	<.0001
BDI	9.4 ± 8.5	7.1 ± 5.8	0.0007

Younger women in our program had significantly higher scores on the BDI-II indicating symptoms of depression. Although, Beckie, et al. utilized different measurement tools, they also reported significantly higher levels of depressive symptoms and anxiety in younger women compared to older women. [83]

Gender Differences in Clinical Outcome in Cardiac Rehabilitation

Morbidity and Mortality:

Exercise training has beneficial hemodynamic effects in patients following AMI, with an improvement in aerobic capacity averaging 20 percent. More important are reductions in both mortality and recurrent AMI. Participation in comprehensive CR programs has been associated with cardiovascular benefits that include weight loss, improved functional capacity, improved lipid profile, a reduction in blood pressure, and improved control of type 2 DM. A 2005 meta-analysis included 11 randomized trials of 2285 patients with CHD assigned to an exercise-based CR program or control therapy.[85] Participation in an exercise-based CR program was associated with a significant reduction in all-cause mortality (6.2% vs. 9.0%, summary risk ratio 0.72, 95% CI 0.54-0.95). There was also a 24% reduction in recurrent AMI in the CR group (summary risk ratio 0.76, 95% CI 0.57-1.01). The meta-analysis also included 15 trials of 4655 patients who were randomly assigned to a CR program that combined exercise and risk factor education program or to control therapy. Cardiac rehabilitation was associated with an almost significant reduction in all-cause mortality (9.3% vs. 10.8 %, summary risk ratio 0.88, 95% CI 0.74-1.04) and a significant reduction in recurrent AMI (summary risk ratio 0.62, 95% CI 0.44-0.87).

Similar findings were noted in a 2004 meta-analysis of 24 trials that included patients following myocardial revascularization procedures; 20 percent of patients were women as well as patients older than 65 years. [86] Exercise-based rehabilitation was associated with lower total and cardiac mortality rates, with favorable trends for nonfatal AMI and the need for myocardial revascularization. Compared with usual care, CR was associated with reduced all-cause mortality (odds ratio = 0.80; 95% confidence interval 0.68 to 0.93) and cardiac mortality (odds ratio = 0.74; 95% CI: 0.61 to 0.96); greater reductions in total cholesterol level (mean difference, -14.3 mg/dL; 95% CI:-24.3 to -4.2 mg/dL), triglyceride level (mean difference,-20.4 mg/dL; 95% CI:-34.5 to -6.2 mg/dL), and systolic blood pressure (mean difference, -3.2 mm Hg; 95% CI: -5.4 to -0.9 mm Hg); and lower rates of self-reported smoking (odds ratio = 0.64; 95% CI: 0.50 to 0.83).The benefits of exercise were independent of the dose of exercise intervention or the CHD subset.

Diabetes Mellitus:

Type 2 DM and metabolic syndrome are important disease processes associated with the development of CHD. One of the critical steps in the treatment and prevention for both of these conditions is therapeutic lifestyle interventions in addition to traditional pharmacologic therapy. The goals of comprehensive CR programs are to prevent disability resulting from CVD, improve cardiac risk profile, prevent subsequent cardiovascular events, hospitalizations and death from CHD. The benefit seen with CR in patients with type 2 DM and metabolic syndrome is likely related to the impact these programs have on the common pathophysiologic background of atherosclerosis shared in type 2 DM and metabolic syndrome. Lipoprotein abnormalities are a major contributor to accelerated atherosclerosis in type 2 DM and metabolic syndrome. After a first AMI, 1-year mortality rates in men with DM are nearly twice as high as men without DM and women with DM have a 3.5 fold higher mortality rate than women without DM. [87] In addition, women with DM are four times more likely to develop CHD than women who do not have DM. Patients with both clinical heart disease and DM are at especially high risk, with an incidence of AMI of nearly 50% at 7 years.[88]

The Nurses' Health Study included 5125 women with reported type 2 DM. [89] The women with DM who performed moderate (including walking) or vigorous exercise had a 40 percent lower risk of developing CVD (including CHD and stroke) than those who did not. The age-adjusted relative risks according to average hours of moderate or vigorous activity per week (<1, 1 to 1.9, 2 to 3.9, 4 to 6.9, >/=7) were 1.0, 0.93 (95% CI, 0.69 to 1.26), 0.82 (CI, 0.61 to 1.10), 0.54 (CI, 0.39 to 0.76), and 0.52 (CI, 0.25 to 1.09) (P < 0.001 for trend). This improvement in risk remained after adjustment for smoking, BMI, and other cardiovascular risk factors.

There have been few studies on the impact of CR in CHD patients with type 2 DM and the results reported vary. Landmark research published by Lavie and Milani demonstrated improvements in exercise capacity (+38%; p<0.0001), quality of life (p<0.001), anxiety (p<0.0001) and somatization (p<0.0001) in a cohort of 70 patients with DM who participate in CR but with non-significant improvements in lipid profile.[90, 91] In addition, Banzer et al reported on a cohort of 250 DM patients who achieved a +26% improvement in exercise capacity after completing a CR program.[92] However in contrast, in a study by Verges et al in a group of 59 patients with DM compared to 36 patients without DM, the investigators reported that while baseline exercise capacity parameters were similar between the two groups, after CR, improvement in exercise capacity was significantly less in patients with DM compared to those without DM (peak work load 19% vs. 29%; p=0.02; peak VO2 13% vs. 30%; p=0.002).[93] We have reported the detailed analysis on the patient characteristics and treatment modalities of those participating in our CR program previously.[94] Retrospective data was analyzed only on those patients completing a minimum of 7 weeks of a 12 week CR program. Analysis was reported on 1,831 patients with type 2 DM (n=395) and without DM (n= 1436). There were significant improvements in total cholesterol

(-3.3%; p=0.003), LDL-cholesterol (-4%; p=0.01), HDL- cholesterol (+2.8%; p=0.0003), triglycerides (-6%; p=0.05), glucose (-4.3%; p=0.003), BMI (-0.6; p=0.02) and MET level (+24.6%; p<0.0001) in each group after CR as compared to pre-CR. As shown in Table 7 on completion of CR, men with DM, men without DM, and women without DM were at NCEP III goals in total cholesterol, LDL-cholesterol, HDL-cholesterol and triglycerides and were at a higher rate as compared to pre-CR. However, this only reached significance in the men without DM. The women without DM did not achieve NCEP III goals as effectively as men with DM, men without DM and women without DM when comparing pre versus post CR outcomes.

Table 7. Effects of Cardiac Rehabilitation by Gender to Achieve NCEP ATP III Goals in Diabetics and Non-Diabetics

	Men (n=285)			Women (n=110)		
Diabetics	Entry (%)	Exit (%)	p	Entry (%)	Exit (%)	p
TC < 200	84.6%	87.0%	0.40	72.7%	70.9%	0.76
LDL-C < 100	69.5%	75.4%	0.11	63.6%	62.7%	0.89
HDL-C 40 ♂, >50♀	49.1%	55.0%	0.15	67.3%	76.4%	0.13
Triglycerides < 150	51.2%	53.3%	0.61	38.2%	43.6%	0.41

	Men			Women		
Non-diabetics	Entry (%)	Exit (%)	P	Entry (%)	Exit (%)	P value
TC < 200	83.2%	87.6%	0.004	72.2%	75.8%	0.27
LDL-C < 100	62.2%	68.7%	0.002	60.0%	64.9%	0.17
HDL-C > 40 ♂, >50♀	53.0%	59.8%	0.001	85.0%	87.2%	0.39
Triglycerides < 150	58.5%	66.0%	0.0003	54.2%	60.5%	0.09

Abbreviations: TC, total cholesterol; HDL-C, high-density lipoprotein; LDL-C, low density lipoprotein; To convert cholesterol to millimoles per liter, multiply by 0.0259; for triglycerides multiply by 0.0113.

Pre-CR exercise capacity (METs) was greater in the group without DM at entry to CR however the exercise capacity (METs) did improve significantly in both the group with DM (24.6%, p< 0.0001) and the group without DM (27.1%, p< 0.0001) at completion of the CR program compared to pre-CR. Our findings of improved exercise capacity with completion of a CR program concur with previous studies demonstrating improved METs level in patients with DM participating in CR. [90,92]

The improvement in lipid profile we report may play a role in clinical outcomes. A prior study reported outcomes in patients with CHD randomized to exercise training and a low fat diet or to usual care. Repeat coronary angiography was performed at one-year. In patients participating in the exercise and diet group, body weight decreased by 5% (p< 0.001), total cholesterol by 10% (p< 0.001), and triglycerides by 24% (p< 0.001); HDL-cholesterol increased by 3% (p = NS). Stress-induced myocardial ischemia decreased, indicating improvement of myocardial perfusion. Based on minimal lesion diameter, progression of coronary lesions was noted in nine patients (23%), no change in 18 patients (45%), and regression in 13 patients (32%). In the control group, metabolic and hemodynamic variables remained essentially unchanged, whereas progression of coronary lesions was noted in 25 patients (48%), no change in 18 patients (35%), and regression in nine patients (17%). These changes were significantly different from the intervention group (p<0.05). [95]

In addition, HDL-cholesterol levels are also predictive of coronary events in patients with known CHD. An analysis of patients in the LIPID and CARE trials found that low HDL-cholesterol was a strong predictor of cardiac events in patients with an LDL-cholesterol <125. For a 10 mg/dL increase in HDL-cholesterol, the event rate decreased by 29%. [96]

Lipids

Comprehensive CR programs have been shown to produce favorable changes in the lipoprotein profile in patients with CHD.[97-100] The majority of reports have shown a significant increase in serum HDL-cholesterol and a decrease in serum triglycerides compared with baseline values.[101,102] Several investigators have also shown a reduction in serum total cholesterol and LDL-cholesterol in patients participating in these programs.[100] These improvements in lipid profile in part, correlated with weight loss.[103] While the majority of CR studies demonstrate improvement in lipid profile, they have not investigated the effects of CR on lipid profile independent of the improvements observed with the use of pharmacologic agents in this population. In a prior study we reported on participants (n=766; ♂=547 (71.4%), ♀219 (28.6%), age 61.6±10.6 years) who completed 20 or more sessions in our CR program. [104] This study demonstrated the independent effect of participation in a CR program on lipid profile in patients with comparable risk factors and indications for participating in the program who were being treated with lipid lowering agents. In our investigation, we demonstrated that while initiation of a lipid altering agent, changes in the lipid altering agent, or increase in dosing of the lipid altering agent during the CR program results in a larger improvement in lipid levels, participation in CR alone in both men and women on lipid altering agents also adds a significant benefit independent of pharmacologic changes. (table 8).

Effective control of LDL-cholesterol to levels less than 100 mg/dL in patients with pre-existing CHD has been demonstrated to reduce subsequent cardiac events through randomized clinical trials.[105, 106] Methods of achieving similar rates of control in community settings are of increasing interest. Direct recommendations to primary care physicians in the CHAMP study resulted in 58% of post AMI patients achieving an LDL level of less than 100 mg/dL; nursing driven management of post AMI patients demonstrated an increase to 97% in those patients having an LDL less than <3.2 mmol/L.[107, 108] In a previous report our group has demonstrated that a fairly simple, physician directed intervention in a CR population with CHD was associated with a 55.8% relative increase in the percentage of CR participants achieving LDL goal on CR exit.

Table 8. Absolute Change Pre and Post Lipid Levels in Patients Completing CR Program

	Mean Lipid Value Change Post-Pre with no medication change [mg/dl] (p-value)	Mean Lipid Value Change Post-Pre with medication change [mg/dl] (p-value)
LDL-C	-4.12 (<0.0001)	-10.05 (0.0003)
HDL-C	2.13 (<0.0001)	1.16 (0.14)
TC	-5.13 (<0.0001)	-9.39 (0.0027)
Triglycerides	-22.38 (<0.0001)	-6.75 (0.61)
Non-HDL-C	-7.25 (<0.0001)	-16.49 (0.0006)

Abbreviations: TC, total cholesterol; HDL-C, high-density lipoprotein; LDL-C, low density lipoprotein; non-HDL-C, non-high density lipoprotein.

This improvement is greater than the response to elevated cholesterol in patients with DM at 44 separate clinical practices in the USA from 2000-2002 where it was noted 55.9% of patients with LDL>100mg/dL were not on lipid altering therapy and of those not receiving treatment only 5.6% were started on a lipid altering agent during the clinic visit.[109] Use of systematic reminders directed at the primary care physician during CR can substantially increase the percentage of patients achieving nationally recognized goals.

Obesity

Given the growing prevalence of overweight and obesity in the United States and its role in the development of CHD and related risk factors, it is not surprising that the rate of overweight and obesity in individuals with diagnosed CHD are greater than the rates identified in the general population. It has been estimated in the United States and Canada over 80% of individuals with newly diagnosed CHD is overweight while 36-53% is obese. In addition, more than 50% of the participants enrolled in CR are classified as having metabolic syndrome as compared to 24% of the general public. [27] As a result, CR programs have been called upon to address the epidemic of overweight and obesity. Traditional rehabilitation programs have focused on exercise training and are relatively short in duration (3 months). This approach has been ineffective in producing significant weight loss. With reported weight losses of 0.5-1.0 kg over 3 months, CR has not produced substantial weight loss in obese individuals. This disappointing weight loss statistic is likely related to the fact that most programs result in a modest increase in caloric expenditure through physical activity but do not specifically target reduction in caloric intake through nutrition counseling. It has been suggested that CR programs should implement behavioral weight loss techniques. A study by Savage et al implemented a weight loss intervention during a CR program that included a daily caloric goal 500-1000 calories less than maintenance energy requirements, exercise including 45 minutes of aerobic conditioning, a weekly session to discuss behavior modification techniques focused on eating behaviors and a 1 hour treatment group that met weekly led by a registered nurse trained in behavior modification techniques. Upon completion of the program, the weight loss intervention group lost 4.3 ± 2.8 kg as compared to 1.7 ± 2.6 kg in the group participating in the traditional CR program. This study demonstrated that a behavioral weight loss intervention, implemented in a CR program, can result in significant weight loss in overweight and obese individuals. [110]

Depression

We previously reported on the impact on CR on symptoms of depression in our CR program. In our cohort, 48% of women entering CR had BDI-II scores ≥10 compared to 28% of men. Within the group of men and women scoring ≥10 on the BDI-II, women had significantly higher non-completion rates when compared to men (48% vs. 20.8% p=0.003, respectively). The women not completing the program were more likely to be African American, never married or divorced. Prior studies have shown that women are significantly less likely to participate in and complete CR programs compared to men; depressive symptoms may be one of the factors contributing to these observations. [111] Additionally, those participants with an enrollment BDI-II score ≥10 who were able to adhere and complete the program demonstrated significant improvements in BDI-II score as well as clinical outcomes such as lipid profile and exercise capacity after CR. This was true regardless of gender. The clinical improvement in women with a BDI-II score ≥10 was similar in proportion to women with a BDI-II score<10 on completion of the CR program. Women with high BDI-II scores had an overall lower exercise capacity pre and post CR. However, based on previous studies, an improvement of 1 MET level in both men and women yield activity changes that would enhance daily living. [112-116] The finding that patients with depressive symptoms and BDI-II scores ≥10 at enrollment to CR were significantly more likely to not complete the program compared to those with a BDI-II scores <10 is a clinically important observation. Numerous studies have shown depression to be an independent risk factor for increased post AMI morbidity and mortality, even after controlling for the extent of CHD, infarct size, and the severity of left ventricular dysfunction.[117, 118] Approximately half of patients recovering from an AMI have either major or minor depression and major depression alone occurs in approximately one in five of these patients.[119] Our study highlights that screening and interventions to prevent drop-out should be implemented to close the gap that continues to exist in cardiovascular management in patients with depressive symptoms. Combination screening for depressive symptoms, referral for behavioral therapy and/or medication when indicated, and CR programs addressing and educating patients on depression/depressive symptoms are some of the interventions that may be necessary to address these gaps. This is especially important since prior studies having demonstrated depression to be associated with poor compliance with overall medical recommendations after a cardiac event as well as being associated with a poor prognosis. It has been reported that those with depressive symptoms are significantly less likely to exercise, participate in weight management, take medications and stop smoking. [120] In our cohort, clinically significant improvements in lipid profile, exercise capacity and BDI-II scores were observed in those who completed the program. These results lend further support for the development of a process for screening and referral of patients with significant symptoms of depression that hinder their participation in CR for further evaluation, recommendations and treatment from mental health professionals.

Hypertension:

Data regarding gender specific changes in blood pressure specific to CR are limited. However, lifestyle recommendations such as weight reduction, dietary modification, moderation of alcohol intake and regular physical activity that are all key components to CR programs have demonstrated reductions in systolic blood pressure ranging from 2 to 20 mm Hg (JNC VI Guidelines). In our CR program, we define our goal for blood pressure as mean systolic readings < 140 mm Hg or diastolic readings < 90 mm Hg. There was no difference in the prevalence of hypertension by gender upon program entry and program exit in our CR program. Both men and women had a significant improvement in blood pressure when comparing program entry to program exit mean blood pressures (Figure 1).

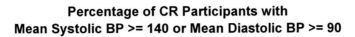

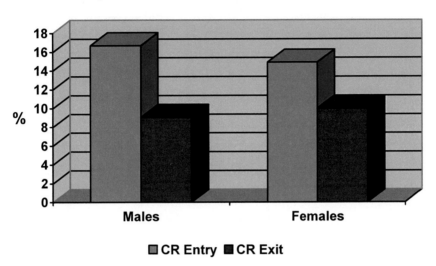

Figure 1.

Conclusion

Coronary heart disease, currently the leading cause of death in the United States, has been traditionally under-diagnosed and under treated in women. This is in spite of the equal distribution of heart disease between men and women and increased cardiovascular death rates for women over men. The disparity in recognition of the occurrence of CHD in women can mislead clinicians and healthcare workers when evaluating females for risk factors of heart disease, diagnosing latent or clinically apparent CVD and the development of treatment strategies.

Traditional risk factors for CHD occur in both men and women include smoking, dyslipidemia, DM, hypertension, and obesity although the association of these risk factors with clinical disease varies by gender. Smoking in females, as in males, is associated with an increased risk for cardiac event regardless of age. This risk starts at even low exposure to tobacco products and is consistent across all age categories. Smoking cessation has been associated with a substantial reduction in CHD risk and should be aggressively pursued regardless of gender. Dyslipidemia, as measured by LDL, is more predictive of CHD risk in men versus pre-menopausal women. Low HDL levels tend to be more predictive of CHD risk in women than in men. DM is an established CHD risk factor and is considered the equivalent of a cardiac event when evaluating patients for aggressiveness of risk reduction strategies. The association between type 2 DM and fatal CHD is stronger in women than in men with women with DM having a 66% increased rate of mortality compared to men with DM according to a recent meta-analysis. After a first myocardial infarction, women with DM experience a 3.5 fold higher mortality risk than men with DM. Hypertension in elderly women is a stronger predictor of cardiovascular risk than in men.

Obesity has been associated with increased risk of cardiovascular mortality. This is especially important with the continuously increasing number of individuals suffering from obesity in this country. The association of obesity with dyslipidemia, hypertension and glucose intolerance has been demonstrated and defined in the clinical syndrome know as Metabolic Syndrome. One risk factor of Metabolic Syndrome is central obesity, which reflects visceral fat that may be active in many of the cardiac risk factors discussed. A recent evaluation of obesity trends in the United States found that the rate of increase in central obesity in women over the past several decades has been much higher than in men. This study found that whereas the prevalence of central obesity, as demonstrated by increasing waist circumference, in men increased from 12.7% to 38.3% between 1960 and 2000, it increased much more significantly from 19.4% to 59.9% in adult women.[121] Recent studies suggest that CHD risk is associated more closely with Metabolic Syndrome than with obesity in women suggesting that meticulous attention to CHD risk factors in addition to the lifestyle changes necessary for weight reduction would be a prudent approach in obese women.[122] Recent studies have shown that reversal of type 2 DM, the strongest CHD risk factor, can occur with substantial and sustained weight loss.

Observational studies have demonstrated a growing association between depressive symptoms and CHD mortality. This is of special interest in the treatment of women since the point and lifetime prevalence of depression is 2 to 3 times higher in women than in men. Definitive studies assessing the effect of treatment of depression on the outcomes of CHD have yet to be completed. The need for recognition and treatment of depressed women with CHD should be in the forefront of all healthcare providers caring for women.

Differences in diagnosis of CHD between men and women have been addressed through numerous studies. Women are known to present with CHD symptoms later in life than men and more commonly with 'atypical' symptoms sometimes confusing diagnosis in chronic and acute CHD events. In addition, there is evidence that even with appropriate diagnosis of CHD women undergo therapeutic interventions less frequently than men.

The above discussion is important in understanding where the gaps are in the care of women with CHD. Identification of opportunity gaps can lead to the development of systematic methods of improving care for women at risk of CHD. This approach works well when healthcare providers have a target population such as within a medical practice. As a method of providing secondary prevention, CR programs provide an ideal focus for the reduction of risk factors in women after coronary event or revascularization. Cardiac rehabilitation programs were originally developed to transition patients from acute cardiac events back to normal activities of daily living. Over the past several decades CR programs have evolved and expanded their focus to include secondary prevention and lifestyle modification. The effectiveness of the current structure of CR was demonstrated in a recent meta-analysis showing a significant reduction in all-cause and cardiac mortality associated with participants with the effect ranging from a 12 to 27 percent risk reduction in all cause mortality associated with CR. Improvements in exercise tolerance, reduction in weight, improved lipid profile, reduction in blood pressure and improved control of type 2 DM have all been associated with CR. These studies usually enrolled more men than women although the effects of CR should be similar in both genders.

In addition to the improvement in metabolic parameters of patients enrolled in CR, there is also an improvement in patient's exercise tolerance. Increased levels of exercise have been associated with a reduction in cardiac events and a reduction of inflammation as demonstrated by decreases in C-reactive protein. The association of weight loss with exercise promotes less insulin resistance, lower blood pressure and improved levels of HDL.

Cardiac rehabilitation can be delivered across a variety of settings as long as the basic tenets of care are intact. These include a case management system of care directed to the identification of cardiac risk factors and the application, in a controlled setting, of intensive risk reduction interventions based on evidence based practice. Traditionally these have been delivered in healthcare facilities although distributed models of care, such as telemedicine, are surfacing.

Continuing the trend towards under treatment of cardiac disease in women, enrollment of women in outpatient CR programs after cardiac events lags the frequency of enrollment of men with one study showing participation rates among eligible women between 20 and 52 percent less than men. Causes of this may be lower rates of referral or reduced reinforcement of the importance of prevention strategies to women from healthcare providers. Referral rates can be affected by individual bias or by systematic issues such as transportation or insurance covering CR.

When referred to CR, women are more likely to drop out of the program reducing any benefit they may receive from CR. Risk factors for women to not complete a prescribed course of CR include age, obesity, de-conditioning and depressive symptoms.

In our own experience with CR we have found that women entering CR were older than men, consistent with their expression of cardiac disease later in life, less likely to have a high school education or current employment and having different diagnoses for referral. Women were more likely to be referred after angioplasty and/or stenting or valve surgery and men were more likely to be referred after CABG. Women entering our program had a significantly different metabolic profile with higher levels of total cholesterol, HDL, LDL and non-HDL cholesterol than men. Among diabetics, men were more likely to have higher fasting blood glucose than men. These differences may reflect different levels of aggressiveness in lipid control between men and women prior to enrollment.

We evaluated the effect age has on women in CR and found differences in marital and employment status with younger women having higher levels of both. Older women were more likely to be referred after CABG or angina and younger women were more likely to be referred for valve replacement. In terms of risk factors older and younger women had the similar frequency of hypertension and DM, but younger women were more likely to smoke, be obese, have lower levels of HDL and, if DM, had worse blood glucose control. Consistent with reports in the literature, younger women had higher levels of depressive symptoms in our program.

With the increased risk DM confers to women with CHD we evaluated the outcomes of patients with DM in our program. This study demonstrated significant improvements in total cholesterol, triglycerides, glucose, BMI, and MET level in CR participants regardless of presence of DM. We did note that women with DM were less likely to be at NCEP-III goal at the end of the CR program. This may have been due to sample size although it reinforces the need to pay special attention to this high-risk group.

With the increased frequency of central obesity in women over men demonstrated over the past several decades we need to determine if this is visceral, metabolically active, fat and, if so, pay special attention to the role of weight reduction in the management of women for both primary and secondary prevention. Incorporating a behavioral weight loss program as part of CR can result in sustained weight loss in obese individuals and may assume a special place in the treatment of women.

In our program we have found that as many as 48% of women have symptoms of depression as compared to 28% of men, and that the rate of non-completion in those patients with symptoms of depression was higher in women. Adequate attention to depression and its treatment may improve CR completion in women, although this needs to be evaluated.

Primary and secondary prevention of cardiac events in women requires special attention to the unique challenge presented by differences in risk factors, awareness of presentation and participation and response to CR between men and women. Solutions to the issues that may be unique to women need to be developed and implemented at the community level to improve the care delivered to women in this country. These solutions should be pursed with enough scientific integrity to provide evidence of the value of systematic changes in health care for women. This can be done using standard experimental (randomized clinic trials) or observational methods.

References

[1]   Ross, R. Atherosclerosis – an inflammatory disease. *New England Journal of Medicine*. 1999;340:115-126.

[2]   American Heart Association. Heart Disease and Stroke Statistics --- 2007 Update. Dallas, Texas: American Heart Association; 2007.

[3]   American Heart Association. Women and Cardiovascular Diseases - Statistics. Dallas, Texas: American Heart Association; 2007.

[4]   Vaccarino, V; Krumholz, HM; Yarzebski, J; et al. Sex Differences in 2 year Mortality after Hospital Discharge for Myocardial Infarction. Annals of Internal Medicine. 2001;134:173-181.

[5]   American Heart Association. Heart disease and stroke statistics – 2006 update: A report from the American Heart Association statistics committee and stroke statistics subcommittee. Circulation. 2007; 85-151.

[6]   American Heart Association. Heart Disease and Stroke Statistics 2008 Update: A Report from the American Heart Association Statistics Committee and Stroke Statistics Subcommittee. Circulation. 2008; 117; e25-e146.

[7]   Willett, WC; Green, A; Stampfer, MJ; et. al. Relative and absolute excess risks of coronary heart disease among women who smoke cigarettes. *New England Journal of Medicine*. 1987 Nov 19; 317(21):1303-1309.

[8] Hansen, EF; Andersen, LT; Von Eyben, FE. Cigarette smoking and age at first acute myocardial infarction, and influence of gender and extent of smoking. *American Journal of Cardiology*. 1993 Jun 15;71(16):1439-1442.

[9] US Department of Health and Human Services. Women and Smoking: A Report of the Surgeon General. Rockville, Md: US Department of Health and Human Services, Public Health Service, Office of the Surgeon General; 2001.

[10] Rosenberg, L; Palmer, JR; Shapiro, S. Decline in the risk of myocardial infarction among women who stop smoking. *New England Journal of Medicine*. 1990;322:213-217.

[11] Kirkland, S; Greaves, L; Devichand, P. Gender differences in smoking and self reported indicators of health. BMC Womens Health. 2004;4(Suppl 1):S7.

[12] Watson, JM, Scarinci, IC, Klesges, RC; et. al. Relationships among smoking status, ethnicity, socioeconomic indicators, and lifestyle variables in a biracial sample of women. Prev Med. 2003 Aug; 37(2):138-147.

[13] Castelli, WP; Anderson, K, Wilson, PW; et. al. Lipids and risk of coronary heart disease. The Framingham Study. Annals of Epidemiology. 1992 Jan-Mar; 2(1-2): 23-28.

[14] Castelli, WP. Epidemiology of triglycerides: a view from Framingham. *American Journal of Cardiology*. 1992;70:3H-9H .

[15] Waters, D; Higginson, L; Gladstone, P; et. al. Effects of cholesterol lowering on the progression of coronary atherosclerosis in women. A Canadian Coronary Atherosclerosis Intervention Trial (CCAIT) substudy. *Circulation*. 1995 Nov 1;92(9):2404-2410.

[16] Huxley, R; Barzi, F; Woodward, M. Excess risk of fatal coronary heart disease associated with diabetes in men and women: meta-analysis of 37 prospective cohort studies. *British Medical Journal*. 2006 Jan 14;332(7533):73-78.

[17] Haffner, S.M., Alexander, C.M., Cook; et. al. Reduced coronary events in simvastatin-treated patients with coronary heart disease and diabetes or impaired fasting glucose levels: subgroup analyses in the Scandinavian Simvastatin Survival Study. Archives of Internal Medicine. 1999; 159, 2661-2667.

[18] Zuanetti, G; Latini, R. Influence of diabetes on mortality in acute myocardial infarction: data from the GISSI-2 study. *Journal of the American College of Cardiology*. 1993; 22(7), 1788-1794.

[19] Burt, VL; Whelton, P; Roccella, EJ; et. al. Prevalence of hypertension in the US adult population. Results from the third national health and nutrition examination survey: 1988-1991. Hypertension, 1995; 25, 305-313.

[20] Rich-Edwards, JW; Manson, JE; Hennekens, CH; et. al. The primary prevention of coronary heart disease in women. *New England Journal of Medicine*. 1995 Jun 29;332(26):1758-1766.

[21] Cornoni-Huntley, J; LaCroix, AZ. Race and sex differentials in the impact of hypertension in the United States. The National Health and Nutrition Examination Survey I Epidemiologic Follow-up Study, Archives of Internal Medicine. 1989; 149(4), 780-788.

[22] Eckel, RH; Krauss, RM. American heart association call to action: obesity as a major risk factor for coronary heart disease. Circulation. 1998; 97: 2099-2100.

[23] Eckel, RH. Obesity and Heart Disease: A statement for the Healthcare Professional from the Nutrition Committee, American Heart Association. Circulation. 1997; 96:3248-3250.

[24] Balady, GJ; Williams, MA; et. al. Core Components of Cardiac Rehabilitation/Secondary Prevention Programs: 2007 Update. A Scientific Statement from the American Heart Association Exercise, Cardiac Rehabilitation, and Prevention Committee, the Council on Clinical Cardiology; the Councils on Cardiovascular Nursing, Epidemiology and Prevention, and Nutrition, Physical Activity, and Metabolism; and the American Association of Cardiovascular and Pulmonary Rehabilitation. Circulation. 2007; 115: 2675-2682.

[25] Flegal, KM; Graubard, BI. Excess deaths associated with underweight, overweight, and obesity. Journal of the American Medical Association. 2005; 293: 1861-1867.

[26] Meunnig, P; Lubetkin, E; Jia, H; et. al. Gender and the Burden of Disease Attributable to Obesity. *American Journal of Public Health.* 2006 Sep; 96(9): 1162-1668.

[27] Savage, PD; Ades, PA. The obesity epidemic in the United States: role of cardiac rehabilitation. Coronary Artery Disease. 2006; 17: 227-231.

[28] Arterburn, DE; Maciejewski, ML. Impact of morbid obesity on medical expenditures in adults. *International Journal of Obesity.* 2005; 29: 334-339.

[29] Poirier, P; Giles, TD. Obesity and cardiovascular disease: pathophysiology, evaluation, and effect of weight loss: an update of the 1997 American Heart Association scientific statement on obesity and heart disease from the Obesity Committee of the Council on Nnutrition, Physical Activity, and Metabolism. *Circulation.* 2006; 113: 898-918.

[30] Berry, JD; Lloyd-Jones, DM. The clinical implications of obesity for cardiovascular disease. Obesity Management. 2007; 64-68.

[31] Kemp, DE; Malhotra, S; Franco, KN; et. al. Heart Disease and Depression: Don't Ignore the Relationship. *Cleveland Clinic Journal of Medicine.* 2003 Sep 70; (9): 745-761.

[32] Kay, J. (2000). Psychiatry: Behavioral science and clinical essentials. Philadelphia: W.B. Saunders

[33] Borowicz, L Jr; Royall, R; Grega, M. et. al. Depression and cardiac morbidity 5 years after coronary artery bypass surgery. *Psychosomatics.* 2002 Nov-Dec; 43(6): 464-471.

[34] Glassman, AH; Shapiro, PA. Depression and the course of coronary artery disease. *Am. J. Psychiatry.* 1998 Jan; 155(1): 4-11.

[35] Lauzon, C; Beck, CA; Huynh, T; et. al.Depression and prognosis following hospital admission because of acute myocardial infarction. *Canadian Medical Association Journal.* 2003 Mar 4; 168(5): 570-571.

[36] Pignay-Demaria, V; Lespérance, F; Demaria, RG; et. al. Depression and anxiety and outcomes of coronary artery bypass surgery. *Annals of Thoracic Surgery.* 2003 Jan; 75(1):314-321.

[37] Jiang, W, Krishnan, RR, O'Connor, CM. Depression and heart disease: evidence of a link, and its therapeutic implications. CNS Drugs. 2002; 16(2):111-127.

[38]   Frasure-Smith, N; Lesperance, F. Social Support and Depression, and mortality during the first year after myocardial infarction. *Circulation.* 2000; 101: 1919-1924.

[39]   Murberg, TA; Bur, E. Depressed mood and subjective health symptoms as predictors of mortality in patients with congestive heart failure: a two-year follow-up study. *International Journal of Psychiatry in Medicine.* 1999; 29 (3), 311-326.

[40]   Blumenthal, JA; Sherwood, A. Mental stress and coronary disease: The smart-heart study. *NC Medical Journal,* 1999; 60(2): 95-99.

[41]   Wassertheil-Smoller, S; Shumaker, S. Depression and cardiovascular sequelae in postmenopausal women. *Archives of Internal Medicine.* 2004; 164: 289-298.

[42]   Agatisa, PK; Matthews, KA. Coronary and aortic calcification in women with a history of major depression. *Archives of Internal Medicine.* 2005; 165: 1229-1236.

[43]   DeSanctis, RW. Clinical manifestations of coronary artery disease: chest pain in women. In: Cardiovascular Health and Disease In Women, Wenger, NK, Speroff, L, Packard, B (Eds), Le Jacq Communications, Connecticut 1993. p.67.

[44]   Roger VL; Farkouh ME; Weston SA; Reeder GS; Jacobsen SJ; Zinsmeister AR; Yawn BP; Kopecky SL; Gabriel SE. Sex differences in evaluation and outcome of unstable angina. *JAMA* 2000;283:646-652.

[45]   Scirica BM; Moliterno DJ; Every NR et al.. Differences between men and women in the management of unstable angina pectoris (The GUARANTEE Registry). The GUARANTEE Investigators. *Am. J. Cardiol.* 1999;84:1145-1150.

[46]   D'Antono B; Dupuis G; Fortin C; Arsenault A; Burelle D. Angina symptoms in men and women with stable coronary artery disease and evidence of exercise-induced myocardial perfusion defects. *Am. Heart J.* 2006;151:813-819.

[47]   Orencia A; Bailey K; Yawn BP; Kottke TE. Effect of gender on long-term outcome of angina pectoris and myocardial infarction/sudden unexpected death. *JAMA* 1993;269:2392-7.

[48]   Lerner DJ; Kannel WB. Patterns of coronary heart disease morbidity and mortality in the sexes: a 26-year follow-up of the Framingham population. *Am. Heart J.* 1986;111:383-390.

[49]   Arnold AL, Milner KA, Vaccarino V. Sex and race differences in electrocardiogram use (the National Hospital Ambulatory Medical Care Survey). *Am. J. Cardiol.* 2001;88:1037-1040.

[50]   Lehmann J, Wehner PS, Lehmann CU, Savory LM. Gender bias in the evaluation of chest pain in the emergency department. *Am. J. Cardiol.* 1996;77:641-4

[51]   McSweeney JC; Cody M; O'Sullivan P, et al.. Women's early warning symptoms of acute myocardial infarction. *Circulation* 2003;108:2619-2623.

[52]   Goldberg RJ; O'Donnell C; Yarzebski J, et al.. Sex differences in symptom presentation associated with acute myocardial infarction: a population-based perspective. *Am. Heart J.* 1998;136:189-195.

[53]   Anand SS; Xie CC; Mehta S, et al. Differences in the management and prognosis of women and men who suffer from acute coronary syndromes. *J. Am. Coll Cardiol.* 2005;46:1845-1851.

[54]   Mosca L, Mochari H, Christian A, et al. National Study of Women's Awareness, Preventive Action and Barriers to Cardiovascular Health. *Circulation* 2006;113:525-34.

[55] Mosca L, Linfante AH, Benjamin EF, et al. National Study of Physicians Awareness and Adherence to Cardiovascular Disease Prevention Guidelines. *Circulation* 2005;111:499-510.

[56] Vidal, J. Updated review on the benefits of weight loss. *International Journal of Obesity* Related Metabolic Disorders. 2002 Dec;26 Suppl 4:S25-S28.

[57] Blair, SN; Kohl, HW 3rd; Paffenbarger, RS Jr; et. al. Physical fitness and all-cause mortality. A prospective study of healthy men and women. *Journal of the American Medical Association*. 1989 Nov 3; 262(17):2395-2401.

[58] Manson, JE; Hu, FB; Rich-Edwards, JW; et. al. A prospective study of walking as compared with vigorous exercise in the prevention of coronary heart disease in women. *New England Journal of Medicine*. 1999 Aug 26; 341(9):650-658.

[59] Anderson, JW; Konz, EC. Obesity and disease management: effects of weight loss on comorbid conditions. *Obesity Research*. 2001; 9: 326S-334S.

[60] Ades, PA; Waldmann, ML; Polk, DM; et. al. Referral patterns and exercise response in the rehabilitation of female coronary patients aged greater than or equal to 62 years. *American Journal of Cardiology*. 1992 Jun 1; 69(17):1422-1425.

[61] Verrill, D; Barton, C; Beasley, W; et al. Quality of life measures and gender comparisons in North Carolina cardiac rehabilitation programs. *Journal of Cardiopulmonary Rehabilitation and Prevention*. 2001; 21(1): 27-46.

[62] Lavie, CJ; Milani,RV; Cassidy, MM; et. al.Benefits of Cardiac Rehabilitation and Exercise Training in Older Persons. *American Journal of Geriatric Cardiology*. 1995 Jul;4(4):42-48.

[63] Lerner, D., Kannel, WB. Patterns of coronary heart disease morbidity and mortality in the sexes: a 26-year follow-up of the Framingham population. *American Heart Journal*. 1986; 111: 383-390.

[64] Becker, R., Corraro, J., Alpert, J. The decision to perform coronary bypass surgery in women. *American Heart Journal*, 1988; 116: 891-893.

[65] Cowley, MJ; Mullin, SM; Kelsey, SF; et. al. Sex differences in early and long-term results of coronary angioplasty in the NHLBI PTCA Registry. *Circulation*. 1985 Jan;71(1):90-97.

[66] Barber, K; Stommel, M; Kroll, J. et al. Cardiac rehabilitation for community-based patients with myocardial infarction: Factors predicting discharge recommendations and participation. *Journal of Clinical epidemiology*. 2001; 54: 1025-1030.

[67] Lerner, D; Kannel, W. Patterns of coronary heart disease morbidity and mortality in the sexes: a 26 year follow-up of the Framingham population. *American Heart Journal*. 1986; 111: 383-390.

[68] Caulin-Glaser, T., Blum, M., Schmeizl, R., et al. Gender differences in referral to cardiac rehabilitation programs after revascularization. *Journal of Cardiopulmonary Rehabilitation*. 2001; 21(1): 24-30.

[69] American Heart Association; Council on Clinical Cardiology (Subcommittee on Exercise, Cardiac Rehabilitation, and Prevention); Council on Nutrition, Physical Activity, and Metabolism (Subcommittee on Physical Activity); American Association of Cardiovascular and Pulmonary Rehabilitation. Cardiac rehabilitation and secondary prevention of coronary heart disease: an American Heart Association scientific

statement from the Council on Clinical Cardiology (Subcommittee on Exercise, Cardiac Rehabilitation, and Prevention) and the Council on Nutrition, Physical Activity, and Metabolism (Subcommittee on Physical Activity), in collaboration with the American Association of Cardiovascular and Pulmonary Rehabilitation. *Circulation.* 2005 Jan 25;111(3):369-376.

[70] Ades, PA; Balady, GJ; Berra, K. Transforming exercise-based cardiac rehabilitation programs into secondary prevention centers: a national imperative. *Journal of Cardiopulmonary Rehabilitation.* 2001; 21: 263-272.

[71] Williams, MA; Ades PA, Hamm LF, et al. Clinical evidence for a health benefit from cardiac rehabilitation: An Update. *American Heart Journal.* 2006; 152: 835-841.

[72] Shaw, DK; Heggestad-Hereford, JR.; et al. American Association of Cardiovascular and Pulmonary Rehabilitation Telemedicine Position Statement. *Journal of Cardiopulmonary Rehabilitation.* 2001; 21: 261-262.

[73] Suaya, JA; Shepard, DS. Use of cardiac rehabilitation by medicare beneficiaries after myocardial infarction or coronary artery bypass surgery. *Circulation.* 2007; 116: 1653-1662.

[74] Mochari, H; Lee, JR. Ethnic differences in the barriers and referral to cardiac rehabilitation among women hospitalized with coronary artery disease. *Preventive Cardiology.* 2006; 9: 8-13.

[75] Sanderson, BK; Bittner, V. Women in cardiac rehabilitation: outcomes and identifying risk for dropout. *American Heart Journal.* 2005; 150: 1052-1058.

[76] Allen, JK; Scott, LB. Disparities in women's referral to and enrollment in outpatient cardiac rehabilitation. *Journal of General Internal Medicine*, 2004; 19: 747-753.

[77] Thomas, RJ; Miller NH; Lamendola, C; et. al. National survey on Gender differences in Cardiac Rehabilitation: Patient characteristics and Enrollment Patterns. *Journal of Cardiopulmonary Rehabilitation.* 1996 Nov/Dec;16(6): 402-412.

[78] Chaoyang, L; Ford, E; McQuire, L; etal; Trends in hyperinsulinemia among nondiabetic adults in the U.S. Diabetes Care. Nov. 2006; 29(11): 2396-2402

[79] Flegal, KM; Carro,l MD; Ogden, CL; etal; Prevalence and trends in obesity among US adults, 1999-2000. *Journal of the American Medical Association.* 2002; 288:1723-1727.

[80] National Center for Health Statistics; Health, United States, 2006. 2006. DHHS publication number 2006-1232.

[81] Savage, PD; Brouchu, M; Ades, Philip. Gender Alters the High-density Lipoprotein cholesterol Respone to Cardiac Rehabilitation. *Journal of Cardiopulmonary Rehabilitation.* 2004; 24:248-256.

[82] Ades, PA; Savage, PD, Brawner, CA; et al. Aerobic Capacity in Patients Entering Cardiac Rehabilitation. *Circulation.* 2006; 113:2706-2712.

[83] Beckie, TM; Fletcher, GF; Beckstead, JW; et. al; Adverse Baseline Physiological and Psychosocial Profiles of Women Enrolled in a Cardiac Rehabilitation Clinical Trials. *Journal of Cardiopulmonary Rehabilitation and Prevention.* 2008; 28:52-60.

[84] Lavie, CJ; Milani, RV. Disparate Effects of Improving Aerobic Exercise Capacity and Quality of Life After Cardiac rehabilitation in Young and Elderly coronary Patients. *Journal of Cardiopulmonary Rehabilitation.* 2000; 20(4):235-240.

[85] Clark, AM; Hartling, L; Vandermeer, B; et. al. Meta-analysis: secondary prevention programs for patients with coronary artery disease. *Annals of Internal Medicine.* 2005;143:659-672.

[86] Taylor, RS; Brown, A; Ebrahim, S; et. al. Exercise-based rehabilitation for patients with coronary heart disease: systematic review and meta-analysis of randomized controlled trials. *American Journal of Medicine.* 2004; 116(10):682-692.

[87] Rosenson, R. Lipoprotein-altering therapies to prevent cardiovascular disease in patients with type 2 diabetes. *Cardiology Review.* 2003:1-9.

[88] Haffner, SM; Lehto, S; Ronnemma, T; et. al. Mortality from coronary heart disease in subjects with type 2 diabetes and in nondiabetic subjects with and without prior myocardial infarction. *New England Journal of Medicine.* 1998; 339:229-234.

[89] Hu, FB; Stampfer, MJ; Solomon, C; et. al. Physical activity and risk for cardiovascular events in diabetic women. Annals of Internal Medicine. 2001 Jan 16;134(2):96-105.

[90] Milani, RV; Lavie, CJ. Behavioral differences and effects of cardiac rehabilitation in diabetic patients following cardiac events. *American Journal of Medicine.* 1996;100:517-523.

[91] Lavie, CJ, Milani, RV. Cardiac rehabilitation and exercise training programs in metabolic syndrome and diabetes. Journal of Cardiopulmonary Rehab. 2005; 25:59-66.

[92] Banzer, JA; Maguire, TE; Kennedy, CM; et al. Results of cardiac rehabilitation in patients with diabetes mellitus. *American Journal of Cardiology.* 2004; 93:81-84.

[93] Verges, B ; Pastois-Verges, B ; Cohen, M ; et al. Effects of cardiac rehabilitation on exercise capacity in type 2 diabetic patients with coronary artery disease. *Diabetes Medicine.* 2004; 21:889-895.

[94] Hindman, L; Falko, JM; LaLonde, M; et. al. Clinical profile and outcome of diabetic and nondiabetic patients in cardiac rehabilitation. *American Heart Journal.* 2005 Nov; 150(5):1046-1051.

[95] Schuler, G ; Hambrecht, R ; Schlierf, G ; et al. Regular physical exercise and low-fat diet. Effects on progression of coronary artery disease. *Circulation.* 1992; 86:1-11.

[96] Sacks, FM; Tonkin, AM; Craven, T; et al. Coronary heart disease in patients with low LDL-cholesterol: benefit of pravastatin in diabetics and enhanced role for HDL-cholesterol and triglycerides as risk factors. *Circulation.* 2002; 105:1424-1428.

[97] Ades, PA; Coello, CE. Effects of exercise and cardiac rehabilitation on cardiovascular outcomes. *Med. Clin. North. Am.* 2000; 84:251-265.

[98] Jolliffe, JA; Rees, K; Taylor, RS; et al. Exercise-based rehabilitation for coronary heart disease (Cochrane review). The Cochrane Library. Chichester, UK: John Wiley sons; 2004:1.

[99] Niebauer, J; Hambrecht, R; Velich, T; et al. Attenuated progression of coronary artery disease after 6 years of multifactorial risk intervention: role of physical exercise. *Circulation.* 1997; 96:2534-2541.

[100] Heath, GW; Ehsani, AA; Hagberg, JM; et al. Exercise training improves lipoprotein lipid profiles in patients with coronary artery disease. *American Heart Journal.* 1983; 105; 889-895.

[101] Warner, JG Jr; Brubaker, PH; Zhu, Y; et al. Long-term (5 year) changes in HDL cholesterol in cardiac rehabilitation patients. Do sex differences exist? *Circulation.* 1995; 92: 773-777.

[102] Mendoza, SG; Carrasco, H; Zerpa, A; et al. Effects of physical training on lipids, lipoproteins, apolipoproteins, lipases, and endogenous sex hormones in men with premature myocardial infarction. Metabolism. 1991; 40:368-377.

[103] Sjostrom, CD; Lissner, L; Sjostrom, L. Relationships between changes in body composition and changes in cardiovascular risk factors: The SOS Intervention Study. Swedish Obese Subjects. Obesity Research. 1997; 5:519-530.

[104] Snow, R; La Londe, M; Hindman, L; Falko, J; Caulin-Glaser, T. Independent Effects of Cardiac Rehabilitation on Lipids in Coronary Artery Disease. Journal of Cardiopulmonary Rehabilitation. 2005 Sept/Oct. 25(5): 257-261.

[105] Expert panel on detection, evaluation, and treatment of high blood cholesterol in adults. Summary of the second report of the National Cholesterol Education Program (NCEP) expert panel on detection, evaluation, and treatment of high blood cholesterol in adults (Adult Treatment Panel II). Journal of the American Medical Association. 1993; 269:3015-3023.

[106] Gould, AL; Rossouw, JE; Santanello, NC; et. al. Cholesterol reduction yields clinical benefit: Impact of Statin Trials. *Circulation.* 1998; 97: 946-952.

[107] Sacks, FM; Pfeffer, MA; Moye, LA; et al. The effect of pravastatin on coronary events after myocardial infarction in patients with average cholesterol levels. Cholesterol and Recurrent Events Trial Investigators. *New England Journal of Medicine.* 1996; 335(14): 1001-1009.

[108] Velasco, JA; After 4S, CARE and LIPID: is evidence-based medicine being practiced? Atherosclerosis. 1999; 147:S39-S44.

[109] Boudoulas Meis, S; Snow, R; La Londe, M; et. al. A systematic Approach to Improve Lipids in Coronary Artery Disease Patients Participating in a Cardiac Rehabilitation Program. *Journal of Cardiopulmonary Rehabilitation.* 2006; 26: 355-360.

[110] Savage, PD; Lee, M. Weight reduction in the cardiac rehabilitation setting. *Journal of Cardiopulmonary Rehabilitation.* 2002; 22:154-160.

[111] Caulin-Glaser, T; Maciejewski, PK; Snow, R. et. al. Depressive symptoms and sex affect completion rates and clinical outcomes in cardiac rehabilitation. *Preventive Cardiology.* 2007 Winter; 10(1):15-21.

[112] Lavie, CJ; Milani, RV; Cassidy, MM; et. al. Benefits of cardiac rehabilitation and exercise training programs in women with depression. *American Journal of Cardiology.* 1999; 83:1480-1483.

[113] Hu, FB; Stampfer, M J; Solomon, C; et al. Physical activity and the risk for cardiovascular events in diabetic women. *Annals of Internal Medicine.* 2001:134:96-105.

[114] Yu, CM; Lau, CP; Cheung, B; et al. Clinical predictors of mortality and morbidity in patients with myocardial infarction or revascularization who underwent cardiac rehabilitation, and the Importance of diabetes and exercise capacity. *American Journal of Cardiology.* 2000; 85:344-349.

[115] Schmermund, A; Cardiorespiratory fitness importance of exercise for healthiness. Herz. 2004; 29(4) 365-372.

[116] Wessel, TR ; Arant, CB ; Olson, MB ; et al. Relationship of physical fitness vs body mass index with coronary artery disease and cardiovascular event in women. *Journal of the American Medical Association*. 2004; 292:1179-1187.

[117] Lesperance, F; Frasure-Smith, N; Talajic, M. Major depression before and after myocardial infarction: its nature and consequences. *Psychosomatic Medicine*, 1996; 58(2): 99-110.

[118] Frasure-Smith, N; Lesperance, F; Talajic, M. Depression and 18-month prognosis after myocardial infarction. *Circulation*. 1995; 91(4): 999-1005.

[119] Ziegelstein, RC. Depression in patients recovering from a myocardial infarction. *Journal of the American Medical Association*. 2001 Oct 3; 286(13):1621-1627.

[120] DiMatteo, MR; Lepper, HS; Croghn, TW. Depression is a risk factor for noncompliance with medical treatment: meta-analysis of the effects of anxiety and depression on patient adherence. *Archives of Internal Medicine*. 2000; 160:2101-2107.

[121] Wang, Y; Beydoun, MA. The Obesity Epidemic in the United States—Gender, Age, Socioeconomic, Racial/Ethnic, and Geographic Characteristics: A Systematic Review and Meta-Regression Analysis From the Center for Human Nutrition, Department of International Health, Johns Hopkins Bloomberg School of Public Health, Baltimore, MD. *Epidemiologic Reviews*. 2007; 29(1):6-28.

[122] Kip, KE; Marroquin, OC; Kelley, DE; et. al. Clinical Importance of Obesity Versus the Metabolic Syndrome in Cardiovascular Risk in Women: A Report From the Women's Ischemia Syndrome Evaluation (WISE) Study. *Circulation.* 2004; 109:706-713.

In: Heart Disease in Women
Editor: B. V. Larner and H. R. Pennelton

ISBN 978-1-60692-066-4
© 2009 Nova Science Publishers, Inc.

Chapter II

Effects of Estrogen and its Receptors on Myocardial Infarction

Jiang Hong[1], Chen Jing, He Bo, and Lu Zhi-bing

Department of Cardiology, Renmi Hospital, Wuhan University, Wuhan 430060 China

Abstract

The higher cardiovascular risk in men and post-menopausal women implies a protective action of estrogen. A large number of experimental studies have provided strong evidence indicating that estrogen has protective effect in the process of myocardial infarction (MI). Estrogen may prevent deterioration of cardiac function post-MI through improving heart failure of cadiocyte biology and also through mediating arrhythmia. The alternations by estrogen in immune function, apoptosis and endothelial progenitor cells after MI may be the most important mechanisms for cadiocyte survival. For the control of cardiac hypertrophy, estrogen acts as both a potent vasodilator and a direct mediator for cadiocyte. The major mechanisms underlying arrhythmia effect may involve affecting neural remodeling, electrical remodeling and structural remodeling. In this article, we mainly focus on the current mechanisms underlying the estrogen effects after MI through genomic pathway and non-genomic pathway. A further understanding of estrogen and estrogen receptors function and regulation may lead to the development of highly specific prevention and treatment of cardiovascular diseases.

Key words: estrogen, myocardial infarction, women

Sex-related differences in cardiovascular morbidity and mortality have long been recognized [1]. The incidence of cardiovascular disease in premenopausal women is lower

---

[1]Address correspondence to: JIANG Hong, Department of Cardiology, Renmin Hospital, Wuhan University, Wuhan, China, Email: pyh_hongj@163.com.

compared with age-matched men but increases rapidly after menopause up to a level close to that in men [2-4]. Previous studies have demonstrated that gender specific differences in myocardial infarction (MI) are largely mediated by sex hormones, especially, estrogen [5-8]. Estrogen may play important roles in MI through its effect on heart failure and arrhythmia. In this chapter, molecular and signaling mechanisms of estrogen underlying these processes in MI will be discussed in detail.

1. Estrogen and Heart Failure Post-MI

Data from several clinical heart failure trials show that women with heart failure after MI have a better prognosis than men [9-12]. It is now recognized that gender plays a crucial role in ischemia/reperfusion (I/R) and MI-induced cardiac dysfunction [13-15]. Patten et al. suggest that female sex and estrogen may favorably affect heart failure prognosis [16], but the mechanisms underlying these effects are not known. We will mainly focus on the effect of estrogen on cadiocyte protection process that is related to heart failure post-MI.

1.1. Estrogen and Inflammation

The myocardium itself intensely generates inflammatory mediators, such as TNF-α [17], IL-1β [18], and IL-6 [19], in response to MI injury. These inflammatory mediators contribute to myocardial functional depression. Several studies [20-21] indicate that female rats experiencing I/R have better functional recovery and decreased expression of inflammatory mediators than male rats. Sex hormones, especially estrogen [22-23], are important modifiers of the acute inflammatory response to injury.

The mechanisms by which estrogen affects proinflammatory cytokine expression and immune function after MI are being actively investigated. Myocardial inflammation plays a critical role in I/R injury and is characterized by the expression of inflammatory cytokines and the activation of the mitogen-activated protein kinase (MAPK) family −− p38 MAPK, c-Jun N-terminal kinase (JNK) and extracellular signal-regulated kinase (ERK) p42/p44 [24]. It has been shown that the critical component of the signal transduction pathways leading to myocardial inflammation and dysfunction is the activation of p38 MAPK and JNK [24]. Both enzymes activation can lead to increased expression of proinlammatory cytokines, which may negatively affect myocardial function; however, activation of ERK is observed to improve cardiac functional recovery [25]. It appears that gender differences exist in the MAPK signaling pathways in the MI-induced injury. Observations of decreased activation of p38 MAPK pathway in females after I/R have been correlated with decreased myocardial TNF-α, IL-1β, and IL-6 expression [26]. In addition, there are no sex differences in I/R-induced myocardial IL-10 levels which acts as a negative regulator of inflammatory cytokine synthesis [26]. JNK activation, another member of MAPK family, is partly responsible for the expression of proinflammatory cytokine after I/R injury. Previous studies demonstrated that a significant reduction in JNK and its downstream targets activation occurred in cadiocytes and animal hearts treated with 17β-estradiol, followed by decreased expression of proinflammatory cytokine [27].

Recently, there are several studies focusing on the role of estrogen receptors (ERs) in MAPK signaling. Migliacciio et al. determine that activation of MAPK pathway by estrogen requires the ligand occupancy of the ERs [28]. In the ER-α knockout mouse hearts models, Meldrum et al. indicate that ER-α is responsible for increasing protective ERK1/2 activation and decreasing JNK activation during myocardial ischemia in females, and no significant differences between what and what were found in p38 MAPK activation [29]. This differential activation confirms that estrogen induced a rapid activation of ERK and JNK but had only a minor effect on p38 MAPK activation [29]. Therefore, these findings suggest that ER-α may mediate inflammation via differential activation of the MAPK family. However, Expression of ER-α and ER-β varies in different tissues and species [30-32]. In human myocardial tissue, the presence of ER-α is well established. In contrast, some investigators have questioned whether heart express ER-β or not [33-34]. This uncertainty regarding the expression of the ERs in myocardium highlights the need to delineate the role of ER-α and ER-β in myocardial I/R injury. Until now, there are still few studies to elucidate the effect of ER-β on the inflammation in the MI-induced injury.

1.2. Estrogen and Apoptosis

Animal and human studies have demonstrated that the presence of cadiocytes apoptosis within both the infarct and peri-infarct zones after coronary occlusion [35-37]. Cadiocyte apoptosis participates in the wall and chamber dilation of the post infracted heart. The degree of cadiocyte apoptosis plays an important role in the initiation of ventricular dysfunction and its progression to severe cardiac decompensation [38]. Interference with cell apoptosis in the surviving myocardium after infarction decreases ventricular loading, chamber dilation and hypertrophy [38]. The results in current studies indicate that the magnitude of cadiocyte apoptosis differed significantly in women and men [39]. The male heart loses 64×106 cadiocytes per year during adulthood and senescence, while the losing degree cadiocytes of female heart is lower than that in men [40]. Autopsy studies have shown that female gender is associated with less cadiocyte apoptosis in heart failure after MI [40]. These observed gender differences in cadiocyte survival provide a plausible explanation for the beneficial effect of female on heart failure progression. A relevant question is whether the women heart protected from estrogen is less susceptible to death signals and possesses an inherent ability to counteract the activation of the endogenous cell death pathway. It appears that estrogen may mediate both the anti-apoptosis and apoptosis system simultaneously (Figure 1).

1.2.1. The Effect of Estrogen on Anti-Apoptosis System
Physiological estrogen replacement reduces cadiocyte apoptosis after MI in ovariectomized female mice. Estrogen treatment has been shown to result in activation of the prosurvival serine-threonine kinases Akt in a PI3kinase (PI3K) -depedent manner, which results in the reduction in cadiocyte apoptosis at 24 h and 72 h post-MI [41].

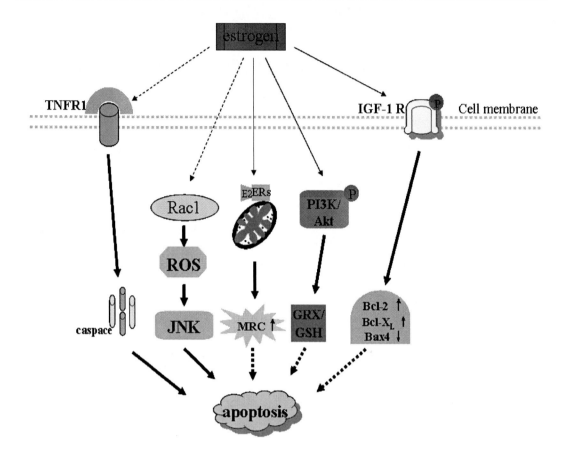

Figure 1. The effect of estrogen on apoptosis post-MI. Estrogen activates the anti-apoptotic system (PI3K/Akt, IGF-1R and mitochondrion) to inhibit cadiocyte apoptosis. In the apoptotic system, estrogen decreases the activity of TNFR1 and JNK pathway and exerts the negative effect on apoptosis. The solid line indicates the positive effect; the dash line indicates the negative effect.

The role of the ER-β -mediated pathway in this cytoprotection has been demonstrated. In the myocardiac H9c2 cells protected with estrogen , inhibition of ER-β activity abolished the protective effect of estrogen on cell survival as well as the activity of Akt concomitant with a decrease of glutaredoxin (GRX) and gamma-glutamylcysteine synthetase, a rate-limiting enzyme for the synthesis of GSH [42]. These results suggested that the cytoprotective effects of estrogen through GRX/GSH system acrivated by Akt, a pathway that is mediated, at least in part, by ER-β. The mechanisms by which whether estrogen activates PI3K/Akt signaling in cadiocytes through ER-α manner are not clear. It is very likely that ER-α specifically mediates this estrogen effect, which is consistent with the results shown in vascular endothelial cells where estrogen rapidly stimulates endothelial nitric oxide synthase activity, in part, via activation of PI3K/Akt pathways through a nongenomic mechanism of ER-α [43].

In addition, depressed mtDNA-encoded genes required for mitochondrial respiratory complex (MRC) activity have been reported to promote the release of cytochrome *c* from mitochondria into the cytosol and induce myocardial cell apoptosis [44]. Although ERs are generally perceived to be nuclear-located ligand-dependent transcription factors or rapidly mobilizing signals at the plasma membrane [45], some ERs have also been shown to be localized in mitochondria and they directly enhance the levels of mitochondrial DNA (mtDNA)-encoded transcripts [46]. Studies have also been reported that human mtDNA contains putative ERE [46]. Recent studies have demonstrated that estrogen enhances the mitochondrial levels of ERs and increases the transcript levels of several MRC proteins and MRC activity. These observations suggest that mtDNA-encoded MRC could be the substrate for effect of estrogen on the mitochondrial ERs. Other studies confirmed the mechanism of mitochondrial ER-β effects. Estrogen treatment normalized cardiac mitochondrial ER-β expression and increased mitochondrial ER-β DNA-binding activity. This was accompanied by an increase in MRC-IV gene expressions and activity, while MRC-I gene expression remained unchanged. Inhibition of MRC-IV abolished the estrogen-mediated cardioprotection, ATP production, mitochondrial cytochrome c release, caspase-3 cleavage, and apoptosis [47]. Thus estrogen and ER-β-mediated cardioprotection appear to be mediated via mitochondrial ER-β-dependent MRC-IV activity and inhibition of mitochondrial apoptotic signaling pathways [47]. However, this conclusion is obtained in the rat trauma-hemorrhage models. Although the similar mechanism exists between trauma-hemorrhage and MI, it is necessary to further prove this mechanism in the post-MI.

Furthermore, stimulation of the insulin-like growth factor-1 (IGF-1) /IGF-1 receptor system enhances the expression of antiapoptotic gene products, such as Bcl-2 and Bcl-XL[48], and decreased the induction of proapoptotic proteins, such as Bax4 [49]. This process may counter-act cell death signals. Much evidence indicates that estrogen improves cell survival through phosphorylation of IGF-1 receptors and mediation of apoptosis-related proteins [14].

1.2.2. The Effect of Estrogen on Apoptosis System

JNK has been found to be activated during ischemia-reperfusion in the heart [50]. The specific molecular targets of JNK include transcription factor AP-1 (mainly c-Jun, JunB, and ATF-2), p53, and c-Myc, as well as many other nontranscription factors such as Bcl-2 family members [51-52], which are related to apoptotic cell death factors. It is generally thought that JNK activation is particularly important for apoptosis induced oxidative stress [53]. Signaling pathways of JNK activation are mediated by reactive oxygen species (ROS) from either exogenous or endogenous sources. One of the main routes involving ASK1 is via the ASK1–MKK4/MKK7–JNK module [54]. In addition, many other ASK1-independent pathways have been identified, including the Src–Gab1 pathway, the GSTk pathway, and the RIP–TRAF2 and membrane lipid raft pathway [53]. In animal study, estrogen treatment attenuates nicotinamide adenine dinucleotide phosphate oxidase activity and superoxide anion production via downregulation of Rac1, followed by reducing the activation of apoptosis signal-regulating kinase 1 and its downstream effecter JNK [55]. This correlates with reduced apoptosis in cadiocytes. These findings indicate that estrogen treatment participates in antioxidative mechanisms and JNK-mediated apoptosis.

Tumor necrosis factor-α (TNF) is increased in myocardial tissue after ischemia and reperfusion (I/R). TNF contributes to postischemic myocardial apoptosis [56-57], which may be mediated by the 55-kDa TNF receptor 1 (TNFR1). Although decreasing the TNF level in animals is beneficial after myocardial ischemia, simply decreasing the bioavailability of TNF in humans with heart failure was not beneficial [58]. This leads to the important appreciation that TNF may have different effects in the heart, depending on which receptors are activated. Females have a lower incidence of heart failure and a higher heart failure survival than males, but there are no sex-related differences in the expression of TNFR1 protein and TNF in the myocardium [59]. Recent studies have shown that females have improved myocardial functional recovery through TNFR1 signaling resistance, following acute I/R compared with males. In the TNFR1-knockout mice, TNFR1 ablation improves postischemic myocardial function through decreased activation of p38 MAPK and reduced expression of IL-1β and IL-6 in males but not in females. Furthermore, wide-type females expresse more suppressor of cytokine signaling protein 3 after I/R, which may in part explain TNFR1 signaling resistance in the female myocardium [59]. However, until now, the accurate mechanism by which estrogen and its receptors mediated this signaling resistance, is still not fully understood.

1.3. Estrogen and EPCs

Extensive experimental and clinical evidence indicates that the infarcted heart can be repaired by endogenous as well as exogenous EPCs [60-63]. Experimental studies have reported that EPCs are mobilized after MI, home to the infracted myocardium, and improve left ventricular perfusion and function [62]. Although EPCs have the ability to differentiate into a cardiomyocytic phenotype in vitro, EPC-induced beneficial effects appear to stem primarily from myocardial neovascularization [64]. Previous findings have proved that the potential role of estrogen in EPC recruitment for myocardial microvascular repair [65-66]. As measured in the healthy subjects, EPCs are higher in fertile women than in men, but are not different between postmenopausal women and age-matched men [67]. Moreover, EPCs and soluble c-kit ligand vary in phase with menstrual cycle in ovulatory women, suggesting cyclic bone marrow mobilization [67]. EPCs cultured from females are more clonogenic, adherent and proangiogenic potential than male EPCs [155]. Under the physiological concentrations of estrogen, proliferation and migration are stimulated, whereas apoptosis is inhibited on day 7 cultured EPCs [68].

Recent studies have demonstrated that aging or senescence constitutes a potential limitation to the ability of EPCs to sustain ischemic tissue and repair. Conversely, estrogens have been shown to be able to prevent senescence of EPCs. In vitro, 17beta-estradiol dose-dependently inhibited the onset of human EPCs senescence in culture through the increase of telomerase activity. The mechanisms involve that 17beta-estradiol dose-dependently lead to phosphorylation and activation of Akt in EPCs, followed by increasing the catalytic subunit, telomerase reverse transcriptase [69]. In addition, previous studies have shown that SDF-1 and VEGF participate in EPCs homing via PI3K/Akt activation [70-71]. Our previous studies also have demonstrated that SDF-1/CXCR4 plays an important role in EPCs homing. The specific antagonists against Akt or CXCR4 blocked EPCs homing after MI. Zheng H et al. indicate that SDF-1 stimulates EPCs homing through eNOS activation under the PI3K/Akt signal transduction [72]. In addition, our group also has observed that EPCs modified with VEGF-gene plasmid enhance EPCs homing [73]. The major mechanism may involve the up-regulation of VCAM-1, ICAM-1 and E-selectin, which exert great impact on EPCs homing, stimulated by PI3K/Akt activation [74]. Several studies have showed that EPCs treated with both 17beta-estradiol and VEGF are more likely to integrate into the network formation than those treated with VEGF alone [69]. Since estrogen has the capacity to activate the PI3K/Akt signaling, we postulated that estrogen may induce EPCs homing after MI via PI3K/Akt activation. Further studies are needed to explore the effect of estrogen on the Akt subtype, such as Akt1 and Akt2 and to determine which subtype plays a predominant role in estrogen-induced EPCs homing.

It seems that estrogen modulates the kinetics of circulating EPCs in the ERs-manner and favorably affects neovascularization after ischemic injury. At present, the specific roles of ER-α and ER-β in the cardiovascular system remain incompletely understood. Hamada et al. have identified a different role of the two ERs in cardiac repair. In vitro, the effects of estrogen on EPCs function are severely impaired in ER-α deficient (ER-α -/-) mice, whereas they are moderately attenuated in EPCs from ER-β deficient (ER-β-/-) mice. In vivo, both the mobilization of endogenous EPCs after MI and the homing of exogenous EPCs to the infarct border zone after estrogen treatment are significantly lower in wild-type mice recipients of ER-α -/- or ER-β-/- marrow. The absence of ER-α has a consistently greater impact on the EPCs function than the absence of ER-β does [75]. Interestingly, cultured human EPCs from peripheral blood mononuclear cells discloses consistent gene expression of ER-α as well as downregulated gene expressions of ER-β [68]. These data demonstrate that although both ERs participate in estrogen-induced cardiac repair via EPCs, ER-α signaling is considerably more important in mediating these processes.

1.4. Estrogen and Cardiac Hypertrophy

The Results from recent studies suggest that a multilevel gender difference in post-infarction remodeling [76]. Estrogen is detrimental at the time of MI or early post-MI [77]. The reason may be related to the role of estrogen in scar formation. The process of scar formation takes 3 weeks in the rat and involves the deposition of extracellular matrix which serves to limit infarct expansion. The suppressive effect of estrogen on fibroblast growth and collagen synthesis may be in part responsible for the increased scar size [78-79]. In addition to its direct effect on collagen synthesis, estrogen may inhibit the response to other factors that are normally upregulated after MI and increase extracellular matrix formation [80]. Chronically, estrogen can normalize wall tension and inhibit LV dilatation. The cellular morphology study by Crabbe et al. have found that the degree of post-infarction cellular hypertrophy in men is nearly twice than that observed in women on the basis of cell volume analysis [76].

There are numerous potential mechanisms by which estrogen may prevent the adverse LV remodeling after MI. An effect of vascular function can attenuate cardiac remodeling as a result of a decrease in myocardial wall stress. Estrogen acts as a potent vasodilator by increasing NO production via stimulation of eNOS and via a decrease of endothelin-1 levels [1]. Furthermore, estrogen is an inhibitor of vascular smooth muscle cells proliferation and migration [81]. Estrogen can also cause interference with rennin-angiotensin system by decreasing aortic wall angiotensin-converting enzyme activity [82] and by down-regulating angiotensin II receptor subtype1 expression in VSMCs [83]. Additional protective mechanisms of estrogens, which are more important, involve the direct anti-hypertrophy impact on cadiocytes in the process of remodeling.

1.4.1. Role of ERs in Cadiocyte Hypertrophy

Several studies suggests that cardiac hypertrophy is attenuated by ER-α and ER-β selective agonists. Treatment with the ER-α agonist,   the ER-β agonist, or the nonselective ER alters the expression levels of specific proteins involved in cardiac contractility (α-myosin heavy chain), signal transduction (neurabin II), energy metabolism (ATP-synthase α-chain), cellular stress response, and extracellular matrix formation (fibromodulin) [84]. These results indicate that activation of either ER-α or ER-β specifically contributes to attenuate cardiovascular remodeling with the alteration of the cardiac protein expression [84]. Other studies have found that systemic deletion of ER-β in female mice increases mortality, aggravates clinical and biochemical markers of heart failure, and contributes to impaired expression of Ca2+-handling proteins in chronic heart failure after MI [85]. However, Doevendans et al. demonstrated that estrogen treatment reduced cardiac hypertrophy significantly in wild-type and ER-α-deficient mice but not in ER-β-deficient mice [86]. This finding suggests that estrogen, through ER-β-mediated mechanisms, protects the heart against left ventricular hypertrophy [86]. However, post-infarction remodeling is a clinical syndrome that involves multiple levels and systems. Systemic deletion of ER-α and ER-β in the mice does not enable differentiation of cardiac from systemic effects of ERs. Thus, with the recent development of selective ER-α and ER-β agonists, it is no longer that the investigators are limited exclusively in system-genetic mouse models, but to explore extensive ER-α and ER-β function only in heart.

1.4.2. Anti-Hypertrophy Pathway Induced by Estrogen

In general, the actions of estrogen may be mediated through ERs by transcribing expression of cardiac-specific genes leading to the anti-hypertrophy effects.

Atrial natriuretic factor (ANF) gene expression in the heart is up-regulated by diverse hypertrophic stimuli in humans [87]. Previous studies have already provided evidence for an anti-hypertrophic role of ANF on the development of cardiac enlargement [88]. ANF accumulation in the myocyte most likely enhances ANF receptor activation, then evokes cytoplasmic cGMP signaling downstream of the GC-A receptor, which has the potential antagonistic effects on cadiocyte hypertrophy [89]. De Jager et al. have showed that estrogen modulates transactivation of the ANF gene through a genomic, ERs-dependent pathway [90]. Since no consensus ER-binding element in the proximal ANF promoter, it is probable that ERs may influence ANF promoter activity indirectly through interactions with other cofactors, such as Sp-1, which can recognize the multiple important *cis*-acting element in the ANF promoter [90]. Another study provided evidence that estrogen inhibits hypertrophic signaling ERK and PKC pathway dependent upon the ability of the sex steroid to up-regulate ANF production and secretion [91].

Another important pathway that is utilized by multiple hypertrophic stimuli involves the activation of the tyrosine phosphatase, calcineurin. When calcineurin is induced, it dephosphorylates and promotes the translocation of the transcription factor NF-ATc3 to the nucleus. In the nucleus, NF-AT cooperates with the transcription factor GATA-4 to up-regulate hypertrophic genes [92]. The mechanism of estrogen reducing calcineurin activity may depend on stimulation of the potent calcineurin inhibitor MCIP1 [91]. It seems that estrogen up-regulation of MCIP occurs through PI3K-dependent signaling from plasma membrane-localized ER [91].

Nitrogen monoxidum (NO) has been shown to attenuate cardiac myocyte hypertrophy. Recent studies have focused on the molecular link between NO and a component of the cardiac myocyte cytoskeleton. cDNA expression array analysis identified that muscle LIM protein (MLP) gene, functionally important in the context of cardiac hypertrophy and failure, is down-regulated by NO in cardiac cadiocyte [93]. Thus MLP downregulation may inhibit hypertrophic growth in the pathophysiological conditions with increased cardiac NO production [93]. In chronic heart failure, increased systemic NO production and enhanced enzymatic activity of myocardial inducible NOS (NOSII) have been reported [94-96]. Currently, several studies have shown that the estrogen is capable of increasing NO production and stimulating eNOS. However, whether estrogen participates in NOSII activity is not clearly demonstrated. Further experiments are required to determine the effect of estrogen on ventricular hypertrophy through NO-induced partial cardiac myocyte cytoskeleton deficiency in MI.

Despite many researches have regarded the cardioprotective effects of estrogen-replacement therapy, more recent double-blind and randomized clinical trials, such as Heart and Estrogen/progestin Replacement Study (HERS) and the Terminated Women's Health Initiative (WHI) Trial, have reported that therapy with conjugated equine estrogens and progesterone or with conjugated equine estrogens alone has no beneficial impact on the primary or secondary prevention of coronary artery disease in postmenpausal women [97]. These results may be associated with profound alteration in cardiac ERs expression and estradiol metabolism. A common variation in genes associated with ER-α was associated with an increased risk of MI and ischemic heart disease in patients from the study involved 2617 men and 3791 postmenopausal women from The Rotterdam Study [98]. These findings support the importance of ERs in cardiovascular disease susceptibility. ERs variation also could explain recent conflicting data regarding the effects of hormone therapy on cardiovascular disease in women. Furthermore, in humans and experimental animals, testosterone has been related with an increased risk of coronary artery disease by adversely affecting the plasma lipid and lipoprotein profile, thrombosis, inflammation and cardiac hypertrophy [5, 99]. Perhaps the gender differences are not entirely due to decreased estrogen, but also associated with significant amounts of circulating testosterone produced and secreted by postmenopausal ovaries. Therefore, the controvertible results above mentioned may partly root in the individual difference of testosterone in postmenopausal women.

2. Estrogen and Arrhythmia Post-MI

Ventricular arrhythmias after MI are relatively common, especially in those persons with more severe MI and no prior history of coronary disease [100]. Epidemiological studies have showed that gender difference exists in arrhythmia and sudden cardiac death between women and men [101]. Experimental animal studies have demonstrated that estrogen may mediate arrhythmic effect in MI [102-105], however the exact mechanisms of which are not clearly understood. The effects of estrogen on neural, electrophysiological and structural remodeling may contribute to the effect in cardiac arrhythmias.

2.1. Estrogen and Neural Remodeling

Previous studies have showed that increased sympathetic nerve activity plays an important role in the genesis of ventricular arrhythmias and sudden cardiac death during a chronic stage of MI [106-110]. It is known that MI results in cardiac nerve injury [111-112] and followed by nerve sprouting [113]. Abnormal patterns of neurilemma proliferation have been documented in infarcted human hearts [114] and sympathetic scintigraphy has demonstrated both denervation and reinnervation after MI [111]. Our lab research [115] has also indicated the relationship between neural remodeling and ventricular arrhythmias after MI.

Estrogen has been shown to exert antiarrhythmic effect after myocardial infarction. Chronic administration of 17beta-estradiol after infarction may attenuate the arrhythmogenic response to programmed electrical stimulation [116]. There is evidence that cardiovascular protection by estrogen is partly mediated through modulation of autonomic nervous system function [117]. The regeneration effort of sympathetic nerve is triggered by the reexpression of nerve growth factor (NGF) or other neurotrophic factor genes in the non-neural cells around the site of injury [118]. NGF is critical for the survival, differentiation, and synaptic activity of the peripheral sympathetic nervous systems [119]. Overexpression of NGF in the heart results in cardiac hyperinnervation [120] and sympathetic nerve regeneration after MI [121]. Kaur et al. have indicated that estrogen decreased expression levels of NGF protein in the superior cervical ganglion and its vascular targets, indicating reduced sympathetic nervous system activation [122]. In addition, estrogen has a role in inhibiting sympathetic hyperinnervation after infarction, probably through an endothelin-1-depedent pathway which is a key regulator of NGF induction in the heart [116].

2.2. Estrogen and Electrical Remodeling

The essence of arrhythmia seems to be an electrical activity disturbance in cardiac cadiocyte. The abnormalities of electrical activity have a great contribution to arrhythmogenesis. Experimental studies have documented that electrical remodeling occurs in both infarcted and noninfarcted cardiac cadiocyte after MI that plays an essential role in arrhythmia [107-108]. It is shown by several studies that estrogen may mediated arrhythmias by directly affecting electrophysiological alterations [102-105]. The mechanisms may include activating ATP-sensitive potassium (KATP) channels [104-105], inhibiting calcium channels [103], downregulating Kv4.3 expression [102]. All of the above ionic channels are important for the induction of abnormal automaticity and reentrant arrhythmias.

2.2.1. Activating ATP-sensitive Potassium (KATP) Channels

The KATP channel is an ionic channel modulated by intracellular ATP concentration. The KATP will be activated when intracellular ATP concentration is lower than normal level, resulting in an increasing outward K+ flow. This outward K+ current has been shown to contribute to repolarization phase of myocardial action potential [104]. One consequence of KATP channels opening is enhancing the shortening of the action potential duration by accelerating repolarization by increasing outward K+ current and inhibiting calcium entering into the cells [123]. It has been observed in experimental study [105] that KATP channel activation is involved in the mechanism modulating estrogen-induced reduction of arrhythmias after MI. Furthermore, there are variable amounts of myocardial ATP-sensitive K+ channels in different species. The different amount of KATP channels explains, at least in part, the reason by which estrogen only produces an antiarrhythmic effect at 10-fold the physiological doses in rats compared with that in dogs at physiological doses[124]. However, how estradiol activates KATP channel is not fully defined.

2.2.2. Inhibiting Calcium Channels

L-type Ca2+ current (ICa,L) is one of the predominant currents contributing to ventricular cadiocyte repolarization. The ICa,L is activated initially during the action potential upstroke providing Ca2+-entry for excitation-contraction coupling [125-126]. It also exhibits a maintained ingredient making a major contribution to the depolarized plateau phase (phase 2) [125-126]. As a main inward current during repolarization, ICa,L abnormalities may contribute to the abnormalities of effective refractoestrobeneriod (ERP), dispersion of repolarization (DOR) and early after depolarizations (EADs) ,all of which are currently thought to be principal way leading to arrhythmias. After MI, the infarcted cadiocyte have a shorter ERP and increased DOR facilitating the formation of circultous pathway for reentrant. The increase in intracellular calcium concentrations of the infarcted cardiocytes may exacerbate this process and can also produce triggered arrhythmias [127]. It has been known that estrogen can rapidly inhibit ICa,L [128] and attenuate calcium influx to avoid calcium overload so that the incidence of triggered arrhythmias will be signifcantly decreased. However, signaling pathways for modulation of ICa,L by estrogen are not completely known. Both genomic pathway and non-genomic pathway may participate in this process.

In the genomic signaling pathway, estrogen binds to cytosolic estrogen receptors. Ligand-bound estrogen receptors translocate into nucleus, dimerize, and bind to the genes containing hormone responsive element (HRE) in the promoter region, leading to trans-repression of calcium channels [129].

In addition to genomic pathway, the ICa,L channels are phosphorylated and activated via a PKA-dependent mechanism [130]. NO released by estrogen stimulation antagonized PKA-dependent activation of the ICa,L channels via a cGMP-dependent mechanism [130]. NO exhibits its actions probably through two distinct mechanisms (Figure 2). One is that NO binds to the haem iron of soluble guanylate cyclase (sGC), and an NO-bound actived sGC converts GTP to cGMP [131]. The increasing intracellular concentration of cGMP inhibits ICa,L channel protein phosphorylation to attenuate ICa,L. The other one is that NO modifies the cystine residues in proteins by S-nitrosylation [132-134]. There are three main targets of cGMP in cadiocyte, including protein kinaseG (PKG), phosphodiesterase 2 (PDE2), and phosphodiesterase 3 (PDE3). In human, low concentrations of cGMP may stimulate ICa,L through PDE3 inhibition, and high concentrations may inhibit ICa,L by stimulation of PDE2 (Figure 3) [135].

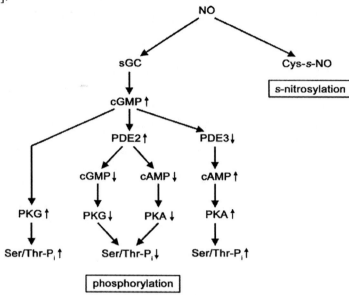

Figure 2. Two major mechanisms of NO actions. NO binds to the haem iron in the sGC, and releases cGMP. cGMP then activates PKG or PDE2, or inhibits PDE3. NO also exhibits its actions by directly nitrosylating the thiol of Cys residue in target proteins.

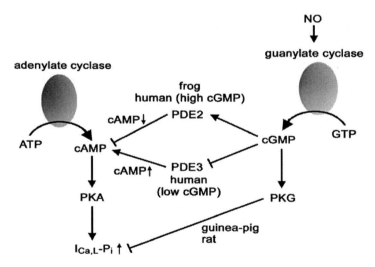

Figure 3. Cross-talk regulation of ICa,L by cAMP and cGMP. cAMP phosphorylates the ICa,L channel via a PKA-dependent mechanism, and activates its function. In guinea-pig and rat, cGMP induces phosphorylation of the ICa,L channel by PKG, which inhibits cAMP-enhanced ICa,L. In frog, cGMP activates PDE2 which hydrolyses cAMP and thereby exhibits antagonistic effects of cAMP. In human, low concentrations of cGMP stimulate ICa,L through PDE3 inhibition, and highconcentrations inhibit ICa,L by stimulation of PDE2.

In addition, estrogen exhibits rapid actions against calcium approximately via activation of PI3K-Akt signaling cascade [136] and mitogen-activated protein kinase (MAPK) signaling cascade [137-138]. Estrogen may exhibit calcium channel inhibition during ischemia–reperfusion injury via PI3K-Akt-dependent activation of eNOS and NO release [139-140]. Estrogen may elicit rapid phosphorylation of an adaptor protein, Shc, in an ER-α manner [141-142]. This leads to subsequent activation of Raf and ERK-1/2 [143-144], and then regulates calcium channels ultimately.

2.2.3. Down-regulating Kv4.3 Expression

The Kv4.3 channel activity gives rise to the transient outward potassium current (Ito), and plays an important role in pacing electrical activity of cadiocyte. It appears that Kv4.3 coassembles with KChIP2 (one β-subunits of Kv4.3 channels) to form Ito currents of cadiocyte in the rodent ventricles [145]. Antisense oligonucleotides directed against Kv4.3 attenuate ventricular Ito of the mouse [145-146]. Ito participates in the early repolarization phase of the action potential and its modulation has been known to affect notably the shape of cardiac action potential [147]. In human, Kv4.3 is most likely to encode all of the native cardiac Ito [148]. Thus, the alteration of Ito caused by Kv4.3 abnormality may lead to inhomogeneity of electrophysiological properties of cadiocyte.

Estrogen has been shown to downregulate Kv4.3 expression in cadiocyte after MI, which will decrease the number of Kv4.3 channel protein synthesis and attenuate Ito [102]. As Ito plays a role in repolarization of the action potential, a decrease in K+ currents that underlie Ito may prolong the action potential duration (APD) and effective refractory period (ERP). Two mechanisms by which estrogen controlling the number of Kv4.3 channels at the plasma membrane are: 1) direct inhibition at the transcriptional level, and 2) indirect inhibition via the reduced or enhanced synthesis of chaperon proteins that favor or inhibit intracellular trafficking, respectively[149].

Transcriptional regulation by estrogen may be a significant factor modulating molecular remodeling of Kv4 genes. Both subtypes of ER, ER-α and ER-β, are members of the nuclear receptor superfamily [150-151]. Classically, ERs regulates gene expression in target tissues in a ligand-dependent manner [152-154]. The ligand-receptor complex then binds to an estrogen response element (ERE) localized in the promoter region of target genes activating gene transcription of Kv4.3. The coordinated actions of the ligand-independent activation function domain (AF-1) in the N terminus and the ligand-dependent AF-2 region in the hormone-binding domain [15-156] may lead to a decreasing of Kv4.3 mRNA expression, resulting in reduction of Kv4.3 channel protein synthesis and attenuation of Ito current.

Another mechanism by which estrogen regulates surface expression of Kv4.3 channels may be altering intracellular trafficking [149], since an intriguing finding shows that, at late pregnancy, the Kv4.3 channel protein is preferentially located in perinuclear organelles. "Chaperon" or "escort" proteins, namely KChAP and KChIP, have been recently shown to favor the expression level of Kv4.3 channels [157-158]. In rat myometrium, decreased channel protein and surface expression of MaxiK channels at the end of pregnancy are also accompanied by perinuclear localization [159]. These findings strongly indicate that, in addition to a direct transcriptional regulation of Kv4.3 protein synthesis, altered intracellular trafficking may be an additional mechanism for Kv4.3 downregulation. It is supposed that estrogen could inhibit "Chaperon" proteins synthesis via a genomic pathway to decrease chaperon protein trafficking towards plasma membrane. As "Chaperon" proteins play an important role in membrane surface expression of Kv4.3 channels, the decrease of chaperon proteins would reduce the number of Kv4.3 channels in the membrane surface. Although the above findings are observed basically in myometrium, the deduction and conclusion might also be applicable in cadiocyte.

2.3. Estrogen and Structural Remodeling

In the heart, gap junctions (GJs), constructed from connexins (Cx), provide a pathway of intercellular current flow, enabling concerted action potential propagation and contraction. Connexin43 (Cx43) is the most abundant and ubiquitous Cx in the mammalian heart. It has been demonstrated that deranged expression and organization of Cx43 GJs, which is called GJs remodeling, appears in the ventricular muscles in MI [160]. The Cx43 level are markedly reduced in MI hearts [161]. Such GJs remodeling may create arrhythmogenic substrates by modulating the propagation of excitation. Estrogen may ameliorate this process by up-regulating Cx43 through activation of PKC pathway [162], to improve the electrical coupling of cardiac cadiocyte, resulting in a smoother propagation of excitation and homogeneous repolarization in the ventricle after MI.

In addition, the increase of cardiac fibroblast proliferation and collagen synthesis after MI, the so-called matrix remodeling, also participate in the initiation of reentrant arrhythmias. Previous studies showed that Estrogen may take inhibitive effects on cardiac fibroblast proliferation and collagen synthesis process [163-166]. It has been known that most estrogen effects on cardiac fibroblasts are mediated by ERs [163-164]. Upon binding to ERs, estrogen has been showed to regulate intracellular signal transduction, including ERK activation in the MAPK pathway and cyclin-dependent kinase inhibition of the cell-cycling pathway [156]. Furthermore, estrogen can also influence cardiac fibroblast growth and function in an ERs-independent manner. Cardiac Fibroblasts express cytochrome p450 enzymes that convert estradiol to various bioactive metabolites [166], such as hydroxyestradiols and methoxyestradiols, which are more potent than estradiol in inhibiting fibroblast growth [167-169]. These observations indicate that cardiac metabolism of estradiol may be important in regulating matrix remodeling of the heart through a ERs-independent mechanism. The inhibition of the fibroblast proliferation collagen formation by estrogen in myocardial cells may finally reduce the risk of reentrant arrhythmias in MI heart.

In this chapter, we mainly focus on the cardioprotective role of estrogen in MI. Although the overwhelming evidence from experimental studies suggest a cardioprotective role of estrogen in MI, the contradictory outcomes from animal studies and clinical trials on hormone replacement therapy make clinicians and research scientists fall into a dilemma. In the future, several important factors need more consideration. (1) Genomic and non-genomic actions of estrogen in MI: Although several possible signaling pathways have been described in this chapter, the exact mechanism of each pathway for cardioprotective effect needs further investigation to confirm. (2) Estrogen sensitivity in cardiac myocytes: The lack of cardiovascular protection of estrogen by hormone replacement therapy in some clinical trials may be due to impaired ERs expression and/or blunted responsiveness to estradiol. It is necessary to confirm the estrogen sensitivity so that more specific therapy can be taken. (3) GPR-30—a new estrogen binding receptor: GPR-30 has been demonstrated in cancer cell lines and fibroblasts. Whether GPR-30 is present in cardiovascular cells, expression levels and its function under various conditions need to determine. Taken together, a further understanding of estrogen and estrogen receptors function and regulation may lead to the development of highly specific prevention and treatment of cardiovascular diseases.

References

[1]   Hügel S, Reincke M, Strömer H, et al. Evidence against a role of physiological concentrations of estrogen in post-myocardial infarction remodeling. *J Am Coll Cardiol*, 1999, 34:1427-1434.

[2]   Karlson BW, Herlitz J, Hartford M. Prognosis in myocardial infarction in relation to gender. *Am Heart J,* 1994, 128: 477– 483.

[3]   Demirovic J, Blackburn H, McGovern PG, et al. Sex differences in early mortality after acute myocardial infarction (The Minnesota Heart Survey). *Am J Cardiol*, 1995, 75:1096 –1101.

[4]   Brett KM, Madans JH. Long-term survival after coronary heart disease. Comparisons between men and women in a national sample. *Ann Epidemiol*, 1995, 5: 25–32.

[5]   Cavasin MA, Sankey SS, Yu AL, et al. Estrogen and testosterone have opposing effects on chronic cardiac remodeling and function in mice with myocardial infarction. *Am J Physiol Heart Circ Physiol*, 2003, 284:H1560– H1569.

[6]   Cavasin MA, Tao Z, Menon S, et al. Gender differences in cardiac function during early remodeling after acute myocardial infarction in mice. *Life Sci*, 2004, 75: 2181– 2192.

[7]   Wakatsuki A, Ikenoue N, Shinohara K, et al. Effect of lower dosage of oral conjugated equine estrogen on inflammatory markers and endothelial function in healthy postmenopausal women. *Arterioscler Thromb Vasc Biol*, 2004, 24: 571–576.

[8]   Wu JC, Nasseri BA, Bloch KD, et al. Influence of sex on ventricular remodeling after myocardial infarction in mice. *J Am Soc Echocardiogr*, 2003, 16: 1158– 1162.

[9]   Ghali JK, Pina IL, Gottlieb SS, et al. Metoprolol CR/XL in female patients with heart failure: analysis of the experience in Metoprolol Extended-Release Randomized Intervention Trial in Heart Failure (MERIT-HF). *Circulation*, 2002, 105:1585–1591.

[10]   Ho KK, Pinsky JL, Kannel WB, et al. The epidemiology of heart failure: the Framingham Study. *J Am Coll Cardiol*, 1993, 22: 6A–13A.

[11]   Levy D, Kenchaiah S, Larson MG, et al. Long-term trends in the incidence of and survival with heart failure. *N Engl J Med*, 2002, 347: 1397–1402.

[12]   Simon T, Mary-Krause M, Funck-Brentano C, et al. Sex differences in the prognosis of congestive heart failure: results from the Cardiac Insufficiency Bisoprolol Study (CIBIS II), *Circulation*, 2001, 103: 375–380.

[13]   Angele MK, Xu YX, Ayala A, et al. Gender dimorphism in trauma-hemorrhage induced thymocyte apoptosis. *Shock*, 1999, 12: 316-322.

[14]   Guerra S, Leri A, Wang X, et al. Myocyte death in the failing human heart is gender dependent. *Circ Res*, 1999, 85: 856-866.

[15]   Wang M, Baker L, Tsai BM, et al. Sex differences in the myocardial inflammatory response to ischemia/reperfusion injury. *Am J Physiol Endocrinol Metab*, 2005, 288: E321-E326.

[16]   Patten RD, Karas RH. Estrogen replacement and cardiomyocyte protection. *Trends Cardiovasc Med*, 2006, 16: 69-75.

[17]   Cain BS, Meldrum DR, Meng X, et al. p38 MAPK inhibition decreases TNF-α production and enhances postischemic human myocardial function. *J Surg Res*, 1999, 83: 7-12.

[18]   Maass DL, White J, Horton JW. IL-1β and IL-6 act synergistically with TNF-α to alter cardiac contractile function after burn trauma. *Shock*, 2002, 18: 360-366.

[19]   Wang M, Sankula R, Tsai BM, et al. P38 MAPK mediates myocardial proinflammatory cytokine production and endotoxin-induced contractile suppression. *Shock*, 2004, 21: 170-174.

[20]   Wichmann MW, Zellweger R, DeMaso CM, et al. Enhanced immune responses in females, as opposed to decreased responses in males following haemorrhagic shock and resuscitation. *Cytokine*, 1996, 8: 853-863.

[21]   Yokoyama Y, Schwacha MG, Samy TS, et al. Gender dimorphism in immune responses following trauma and hemorrhage. *Immunol Res*, 2002, 26: 63-76.

[22]   Samy TS, Zheng R, Matsutani T, et al. Mechanism for normal splenic T lymphocyte functions in proestrus females after trauma: enhanced local synthesis of 17β-estradiol. *Am J Physiol Cell Physiol*, 2003, 285: C139-C149.

[23]   Mizushima Y, Wang P, Jarrar D, et al. Estradiol administration after trauma-hemorrhage improves cardiovascular and hepatocellular functions in male animals. *Ann Surg*, 2000, 232: 673-679.

[24]   Pitcher JM, Wang M, Tsai BM, et al. Endogenous estrogen mediates a higher threshold for endotoxin-induced myocardial protection in females. *Am J Physiol Regul Integr Comp Physiol*, 2006, 290: R27-33.

[25]   Khan TA, Bianchi C, Ruel M, et al. Mitogenactivated protein kinase pathways and cardiac surgery. *J Thorac Cardiovasc Surg*, 2004, 127: 806-811.

[26]   Wang M, Baker L, Tsai BM, et al. Sex differences in the myocardial inflammatory response to ischemia-reperfusion injury. *Am J Physiol Endocrinol Metab*, 2005, 288: E321-326.

[27]   Eckhoff DE, Smyth CA, Eckstein C, et al. Suppression of the c-Jun N-terminal kinase pathway by 17beta-estradiol can preserve human islet functional mass from proinflammatory cytokine-induced destruction. *Surgery,* 2003, 134: 69-79.

[28]   Migliaccio A, Di Domenico M, Castoria G, et al. Tyrosine kinase/p21ras/MAP-kinase pathway activation by estradiol-receptor complex in MCF-7 cells. *EMBO J*, 1996, 15: 1292-1300.

[29]   Wang M, Crisostomo P, Wairiuko GM, et al. Estrogen receptor-alpha mediates acute myocardial protection in females. *Am J Physiol Heart Circ Physiol,* 2006, 290: H2204-2209.

[30] Gudino-Cabrera G, Nieto-Sampedro M. Estrogen receptor immunoreactivity in Schwann-like brain macroglia. *J Neurobiol*, 1999, 40: 458-470.

[31] Beato, M., Herrlich, P., and Schutz, G. Steroid hormone receptors: Many actors in search of a plot. *Cell*, 1995, 83: 851-857.

[32] Couse, J.F. and Korach, K.S. Estrogen receptor null mice: What have we learned and where will they lead us? *Endocr Rev*, 1999, 20: 358-417.

[33] Forster C, Kietz S, Hultenby K, et al. Characterization of the ERβ-/- mouse heart. *Proc Natl Acad Sci*, 2004, 101: 14234-14239.

[34] Kuiper GG, Carlsson B, Grandien K, et al. Comparison of the ligand binding specificity and transcript tissue distribution of estrogen receptors α and β. *Endocrinology*, 1997, 138: 863-870.

[35] Abbate A, Bussani R, Biondi-Zoccai GG, et al. Infarct-related artery occlusion, tissue markers of ischaemia, and increased apoptosis in the peri-infarct viable myocardium. *Eur Heart J*, 2005, 26: 2039-2045.

[36] Gomez L, Chavanis N, Argaud L, et al. Fas-independent mitochondrial damage triggers cardiomyocyte death after ischemia-reperfusion. *Am J Physiol Heart Circ Physio*, 2005, 289: H2153-2158.

[37] Townsend PA, Scarabelli TM, Pasini E, et al. Epigallocatechin-3-gallate inhibits STAT-1 activation and protects cardiac myocytes from ischemia/reperfusion induced apoptosis. *FASEB J*, 2004, 18: 1621-1623.

[38] Goussev A, Sharov VG, Shimoyama H, et al. Effects of ACE inhibition on cardiomyocyte apoptosis in dogs with heart failure. *Am J Physiol*, 1998, 275: H626-631.

[39] Adams KF, Sueta CA, Gheorghiade M, et al. Gender differences in survival in advanced heart failure: insights from the FIRST study. *Circulation*, 1999, 99: 1816-1821.

[40] Guerra S, Leri A, Wang X, et al. Myocyte death in the failing human heart is gender dependent. *Circ Res*, 1999, 85: 856-866.

[41] Patten RD, Pourati I, Aronovitz MJ, et al. 17beta-estradiol reduces cardiomyocyte apoptosis in vivo and in vitro via activation of phospho-inositide-3 kinase/Akt signaling. *Circ Res*, 2004, 95: 692-699.

[42] Urata Y, Ihara Y, Murata H, et al. 17Beta-estradiol protects against oxidative stress induced cell death through the glutathione/glutaredoxin-dependent redox regulation of Akt in myocardiac H9c2 cells. *J Biol Chem*, 2006, 281: 13092-13102.

[43] Haynes MP, Sinha D, Russell KS, et al. Membrane estrogen receptor engagement activates endothelial nitric oxide synthase via the PI3-kinase-Akt pathway in human endothelial cells. *Circ Res*, 2000, 87: 677-682.

[44] Chan SH, Wu KL, Wang LL, et al. Nitric oxide- and superoxi-dedependent mitochondrial signaling in endotoxin-induced apoptosis in the rostral ventrolateral medulla of rats. *Free Radical Biol Med*, 2005, 39: 603–618.

[45] Chung TH, Wang SM, and Wu JC. 17beta-estradiol reduces the effect of metabolic inhibition on gap junction intercellular communication in rat cardiomyocytes via the estrogen receptor. *J Mol Cell Cardiol*, 2004, 37: 1013-1022.

[46] Chen JQ, Eshete M, Alworth WL, et al. Binding of MCF-7 cell mitochondrial proteins and recombinant human estrogen receptors alpha and beta to human mitochondrial DNA estrogen response elements. *J Cell Biochem*, 2004, 93: 358-373.

[47] Hsieh YC, Yu HP, Suzuki T, et al. Upregulation of mitochondrial respiratory complex IV by estrogen receptor-beta is critical for inhibiting mitochondrial apoptotic signaling and restoring cardiac functions following trauma-hemorrhage. *J Mol Cell Cardiol*, 2006, 41: 511-21.

[48] Toms SA, Hercbergs A, Liu J, et al. Antagonist effects of insulin-like growth factor 1 on protein kinase inhibitor-mediated apoptosis in human glioblastoma cells in association with bcl-2 and bcl-xL. *J Neurosurg*, 1998, 88: 884-889.

[49] Wang L, Ma W, Markovich R, et al. Insulin-like growth factor 1 modulates induction of apoptotic signaling in H9C2 cardiac muscle cells. *Endocrinology*, 1998, 139: 1354-1364.

[50] Cao JM, Chen LS, KenKnight BH, et al. Nerve sprouting and sudden cardiac death. *Circ Res*, 2000, 96: 816-821.

[51] Davis, R. J. Signal transduction by the JNK group of MAP kinases. *Cell*, 2000, 103: 239-252.

[52] Minden, A., Karin, M. Regulation and function of the JNK subgroup of MAP kinases. *Biochim Biophys Acta*, 1997, 1333: F85-104.

[53] Shen HM, Liu ZG. JNK signaling pathway is a key modulator in cell death mediated by reactive oxygen and nitrogen species. *Free Radic Biol Med*, 2006, 40: 928-39.

[54] Song, J. J., Lee, Y. J. Differential role of glutaredoxin and thioredoxin in metabolic oxidative stress-induced activation of apoptosis signalregulating kinase 1. *Biochem J*, 2003, 373: 845-853.

[55] Satoh M, Matter CM, Ogita H, et al. Inhibition of apoptosis-regulated signaling kinase-1 and prevention of congestive heart failure by estrogen. *Circulation*, 2007, 115: 3197-3204.

[56] Oral H, Dorn GW 2nd, Mann DL. Sphingosine mediates the immediate negative inotropic effects of tumor necrosis factor-αin the adult mammalian cardiac myocyte. *J Biol Chem*, 1997, 272: 4836-4842.

[57] Krown KA, Page MT, Nguyen C, et al. Tumor necrosis factor α-induced apoptosis in cardiac myocytes: involvement of the sphingolipid signaling cascade in cardiac cell death. *J Clin Invest*, 1996, 98: 2854-2865.

[58] Mann DL, McMurray JJ, Packer M, et al. Targeted anticytokine therapy in patients with chronic heart failure: results of the Randomized Etanercept Worldwide Evaluation (RENEWAL). *Circulation*, 2004, 109:1594-1602.

[59] Wang M, Tsai BM, Crisostomo PR, et al. Tumor necrosis factor receptor 1 signaling resistance in the female myocardium during ischemia. *Circulation*, 2006, 114(1 Suppl): I282-289.

[60] Wang X, Hu Q, Nakamura Y, et al. The role of the sca-1+/CD31- cardiac progenitor cell population in postinfarction left ventricular remodeling. *Stem Cells*, 2006, 24: 1779-1788.

[61]   Zaruba MM, Huber BC, Brunner S, et al. Parathyroid hormone treatment after myocardial infarction promotes cardiac repair by enhanced neovascularization and cell survival. *Cardiovasc Res*, 2008, [Epub ahead of print].

[62]   Wu Y, Ip JE, Huang J, et al. Essential role of ICAM-1/CD18 in mediating EPC recruitment, angiogenesis, and repair to the infarcted myocardium. *Circ Res*, 2006, 99: 315-322.

[63]   Li Z, Wu JC, Sheikh AY, et al. Differentiation, survival, and function of embryonic stem cell derived endothelial cells for ischemic heart disease. *Circulation*, 2007, 116(11 Suppl): I46-54.

[64]   Dawn B, Bolli R. Increasing evidence that estrogen is an important modulator of bone marrow-mediated cardiac repair after acute infarction. *Circulation*, 2006, 114: 2203-2205.

[65]   Iwakura A, Shastry S, Luedemann C, et al. Estradiol enhances recovery after myocardial infarction by augmenting incorporation of bone marrow–derived endothelial progenitor cells into sites of ischemia-induced neovascularization via endothelial nitric oxide synthase–mediated activation of matrix metalloproteinase-9. *Circulation*, 2006, 113: 1605–1614.

[66]   Hamada H, Kim MK, Iwakura A, et al. Estrogen receptors alpha and beta mediate contribution of bone marrow-derived endothelial progenitor cells to functional recovery after myocardial infarction. *Circulation*, 2006, 114: 2261-2270.

[67]   Fadini GP, de Kreutzenberg S, Albiero M, et al.Gender Differences in Endothelial Progenitor Cells and Cardiovascular Risk Profile: The Role of Female Estrogens. *Arterioscler Thromb Vasc Biol*, 2008, [Epub ahead of print].

[68]   Masuda H, Kalka C, Takahashi T, et al. Estrogen-mediated endothelial progenitor cell biology and kinetics for physiological postnatal vasculogenesis. *Circ Res*, 2007, 101: 598-606.

[69]   Imanishi T, Hano T, Nishio I. Estrogen reduces endothelial progenitor cell senescence through augmentation of telomerase activity. *J Hypertens*, 2005, 23: 1699-1706.

[70]   Li B, Sharpe EE, Maupin AB, et al. VEGF and PlGF promote adult vasculogenesis by enhancing EPC recruitment and vessel formation at the site of tumor neovascularization. *FASEB J*, 2006, 20: 1495-1497.

[71]   Carr AN, Howard BW, Yang HT, et al. Efficacy of systemic administration of SDF-1 in a model of vascular insufficiency: support for an endothelium-dependent mechanism. *Cardiovasc Res*, 2006, 69: 925-35.

[72]   Zheng H, Fu G, Dai T, et al. Migration of endothelial progenitor cells mediated by stromal cell-derived factor-1alpha/CXCR4 via PI3K/Akt/eNOS signal transduction pathway. *J Cardiovasc Pharmacol*, 2007, 50: 274-280.

[73]   Zhu LH, Jiang H, Chen J, et al. The effect of intravenous infusion of rabbit bone marrow-derived endothelial cells transfected with vascular endothelial growth factor gene on carotid restenosis prevention. *Chinese Journal of Geriatrics*, 2007, 26: 383-386.

[74]   Kim W, Moon SO, Lee S,et al. Adrenomedullin reduces VEGF-induced Endothelial adhesion molecules and adhesiveness through a phosphatidylinositol 3'-kinase pathway. *Arterioscler Thromb Vasc Biol*, 2003, 23:1377-1383.

[75] Hamada H, Kim MK, Iwakura A, et al. Estrogen receptors alpha and beta mediate contribution of bone marrow-derived endothelial progenitor cells to functional recovery after myocardial infarction. *Circulation*, 2006, 114: 2261-2270.

[76] Crabbe DL, Dipla K, Ambati S, et al. Gender differences in post-infarction hypertrophy in end-stage failing hearts. *J Am Coll Cardiol*, 2003, 41: 300-306.

[77] Smith PJ, Ornatsky O, Stewart DJ, et al. Effects of estrogen replacement on infarct size, cardiac remodeling, and the endothelin system after myocardial infarction in ovariectomized rats. *Circulation*, 2000, 102: 2983-2989.

[78] Pfeffer JM, Pfeffer MA, Fletcher PJ, et al. Progressive ventricular remodeling in rat with myocardial infarction. *Am J Physiol*, 1991, 260: H1406-1414.

[79] Kwan G, Neugarten J, Sherman M, et al. Effects of sex hormones on mesangial cell proliferation and collagen synthesis. *Kidney Int*, 1996, 50: 1173-1179.

[80] Dubey RK, Gillespie DG., Jackson EK, et al. 17b-Estradiol, its metabolites, and progesterone inhibit cardiac fibroblast growth. *Hypertension*, 1998, 31: 522-528.

[81] Dai-Do D, Espinosa E, Liu G, et al. 17 beta-estradiol inhibits proliferation and migration of human vascular smooth muscle cells: similar effects in cells from postmenopausal females and in males. *Cardiovasc Res*, 1996, 32: 980-985.

[82] Tanaka M, Nakaya S, Watanabe M, et al. Effects of ovariectomy and estrogen replacement on aorta angiotensin-converting enzyme activity in rats. *Jpn J Pharmaco*, 1997, 73: 361-363.

[83] Nickenig G, Ba¨umer AT, Grohe` C, et al. Estrogen modulated AT1 receptor gene expression in vitro and in vivo. *Circulation*, 1998, 97: 2197-2201.

[84] Arias-Loza PA, Hu K, Dienesch C, et al. Both estrogen receptor subtypes, alpha and beta, attenuate cardiovascular remodeling in aldosterone salt-treated rats. *Hypertension*, 2007, 50: 432-438.

[85] Pelzer T, Loza PA, Hu K, et al. Increased mortality and aggravation of heart failure in estrogen receptor-beta knockout mice after myocardial infarction. *Circulation*, 2005, 111: 1492-1498.

[86] Babiker FA, Lips D, Meyer R, et al. Estrogen receptor beta protects the murine heart against left ventricular hypertrophy. *Arterioscler Thromb Vasc Biol*, 2006, 26: 1524-1530.

[87] Silberbach M, Gorenc T, Hershberger RE, et al. Extracellular signalregulated protein kinase activation is required for the antihypertrophic effect of atrial natriuretic factor in neonatal rat ventricular myocytes. *J Biol Chem*, 1999, 274: 24858-24864.

[88] Deschepper CF, Masciotra S, Zahabi A, et al. Functional alterations of the Nppa promoter are linked to cardiac ventricular hypertrophy in WKY/WKHA rat crosses. *Circ Res*, 2001, 88: 223–228.

[89] Babiker FA, De Windt LJ, van Eickels M, et al. 17beta-estradiol antagonizes cardiomyocyte hypertrophy by autocrine/paracrine stimulation of a guanylyl cyclase A receptor-cyclic guanosine monophosphate-dependent protein kinase pathway. *Circulation*, 2004, 109: 269-276.

[90] De Jager T, Pelzer T, Muller-Botz S, et al. Mechanisms of estrogen receptor action in the myocardium: rapid gene activation via the ERK1/2 pathway and serum response elements. *J Biol Chem*, 2001, 276: 27873–27880.

[91]   Pedram A, Razandi M, Aitkenhead M, et al. Estrogen inhibits cardiomyocyte hypertrophy in vitro. Antagonism of calcineurin-related hypertrophy through induction of MCIP1. *J Biol Chem*, 2005, 280: 26339-26348.

[92]   Wu CH, Liu JY, Wu JP, et al. 17beta-estradiol reduces cardiac hypertrophy mediated through the up-regulation of PI3K/Akt and the suppression of calcineurin/NF-AT3 signaling pathways in rats. Life Sci, 2005, 78: 347-356.

[93]   Heineke J, Kempf T, Kraft T, et al. Downregulation of cytoskeletal muscle LIM protein by nitric oxide: impact on cardiac myocyte hypertrophy. *Circulation*, 2003, 107: 1424-32.

[94]   Haywood GA, Tsao PS, von der Leyen HE, et al. Expression of inducible nitric oxide synthase in human heart failure. *Circulation*, 1996, 93: 1087-1094.

[95]   Drexler H, Kastner S, Strobel A, et al. Expression, activity and functional significance of inducible nitric oxide synthase in the failing human heart. *J Am Coll Cardiol*, 1998, 32: 955-963.

[96]   Vejlstrup NG, Bouloumie A, Boesgaard S, et al. Inducible nitric oxide synthase (iNOS) in the human heart: expression and localization in congestive heart failure. *J Mol Cell Cardiol*, 1998, 30: 1215-1223.

[97]   Jazbutyte V, Hu K, Kruchten P, et al. Aging reduces the efficacy of estrogen substitution to attenuate cardiac hypertrophy in female spontaneously hypertensive rats. *Hypertension*, 2006, 48: 579-586.

[98]   Schuit SC, Oei HH, Witteman JC et al. Estrogen receptor alpha gene polymorphisms and risk of myocardial infarction. *JAMA*, 2004, 291:2969-2977.

[99]   Cavasin MA, Tao ZY, Yu AL,et al. Testosterone enhances early cardiac remodeling after myocardial infarction, causing rupture and degrading cardiac function. *Am J Physiol Heart Circ Physiol*, 2006, 290: H2043-2050.

[100]   Danielle M, Brandi J, Bernard J, et al. Ventricular arrhythmias after acute myocardial infarction: A 20-year community study. *Am Heart J*, 2006, 4: 806-812.

[101]   Kannel WB, Wilson PWF, D'Agostino RB, et al. Sudden coronary death in women. *Am Heart J*, 1998, 136: 205-212.

[102]   Korte T, Fuchs M, Arkudas A, et al. Female mice lacking estrogen receptor beta display prolonged ventricular repolarization and reduced ventricular automaticity after myocardial infarction. *Circulation*, 2005, 111: 2282-2290.

[103]   Nakajima T, Iwasawa K, Oonuma H, at al. Antiarrhythmic effect and its underlying ionic mechanism of 17beta-estradiol in cardiac myocytes. *Br J Pharmacol*, 1999, 127: 429-440.

[104]   Lee TM, Su SF, Tsai CC, et al. Cardioprotective effects of 17β-estradiol produced by activation of mitochondrial ATP-Sensitive K+ Channels in canine hearts. *J Mol Cell Cardiol*, 2000, 32: 1147-1158.

[105]   Tsai CH, Su SF, Chou TF, et al. Differential effects of sarcolemmal and mitochondrial KATP channels activated by 17β-estradiol on reperfusion arrhythmias and infarct sizes in canine hearts. *J Pharmacol Exp Therap*, 2002, 301: 234-240.

[106]   Cao JM, Fishbein MC, Han JB, et al. Relationship between regional cardiac hyperinnervation and ventricular arrhythmia. *Circulation*, 2000, 101: 1960-1969.

[107] Chen PS, Chen LS, Cao JM, et al. Sympathetic nerve sprouting, electrical remodeling and the mechanisms of sudden cardiac death. *Cardiovascular Research*, 2001, 50: 409-416.

[108] Cao JM, Chen LS, KenKnight BH, et al. Nerve sprouting and sudden cardiac death. *Circ Res*, 2000, 96: 816-821.

[109] Lai AC, Wallner K, Cao JM, et al. Colocalization of tenascin and sympathetic nerves in a canine model of nerve sprouting and sudden cardiac death. *J Cardiovasc Electrophysiol*, 2000, 11, 1345-1351.

[110] Zipes DP, Barber MJ, Takahashi N, et al. Influence of the autonomic nervous system on the genesis of cardiac arrhythmias. *PACE*, 1983, 6: 1210-1220.

[111] Zipes DP. Influence of myocardial ischemia and infarction on autonomic innervation of heart. *Circulation*, 1990, 82:1095–1104.

[112] Barber MJ, Mueller TM, Henry D, et al. Transmural myocardial infarction in the dog produces sympathectomy in noninfarcted myocardium. *Circulation*, 1983, 67: 787–796.

[113] Nori SL, Gaudino M, Alessandrini F, Bronzetti E, Santarelli P. Immunohistochemical evidence for sympathetic denervation and reinnervation after necrotic injury in rat myocardium. *Cell Mol Biol*, 1995, 41:799–807.

[114] Vracko R, Thorning D, Frederickson RG. Nerve fibers in human myocardial scars. *Hum Pathol*, 1991, 22:138–146.

[115] Lu ZB, Jiang H, Yu Y, et al. Relation ship between sympathetic remodeling and electrical remodeling a t infracted border zone of rabbit with chronic myocardial infarction. *Chin J Cardiol*, 2006, 34, 1016-1020.

[116] Tsung-Ming L, Mei-Shu L, Nen-Chung C. Physiological concentration of 17β-Estradiol on Sympathetic Reinnervation in Ovariectomized Infarcted Rats. *Endocrinology*, 2007, 859: 1-25.

[117] Du XJ, Riemersma RA, Dart AM. Cardiovascular protection by oestrogen is partly mediated through modulation of autonomic nervous function. *Cardiovasc Res*, 1995, 30: 161–165.

[118] Levi-Montalcini R. Growth control of nerve cells by a protein factor and its antiserum. *Science*, 1964, 143:105–110.

[119] Snider WD. Functions of the neurotrophins during nervous system development: what the knockouts areteaching us. *Cell*, 1994, 77: 627-638.

[120] Hassankhani A, Steinhelper ME, Soonpaa MH, et al. Overexpression of NGF within the heart of transgenic mice causes hyperinnervation, cardiac enlargement, and hyperplasia of ectopic cells. *Dev Biol*, 1995, 169: 309-321.

[121] Zhou S, Chen LS, Miyauchi Y, et al. Mechanisms of cardiac nerve sprouting after myocardial infarction in dogs. *Circ Res*, 2004, 95: 76-83.

[122] Kaur G, Janik J, Isaacson LG, Callahan P. Estrogen regulation of neurotrophin expression in sympathetic neurons and vascular targets. *Brain Res*. 2007, 30; 1139:6-14.

[123] Jovanovic N, Jovanovic S, Jovanovic A, et al. Gene delivery of Kir6.2/SUR2A in conjunction with pinacidil handles intracellular Ca2+ homeostasis under metabolic stress. *FASEB J*, 1999, 13: 923-929.

[124] Li HY, Bian JS, Kwan YW, et al. Enhanced responses to 17β-estradiol in rat heart treated with isoproterenol: involvement of a cyclic AMPdependent pathway. *J Pharmacol Exp Ther*, 2000, 293: 592-598.

[125] Linz KW, Meyer R. Control of L-type calcium current during the action potential of guinea-pig ventricular myocytes. *J Physiol (Lond)*, 1998, 513: 425-442.

[126] Linz KW, Meyer R. Profile and kinetics of L-type calcium current during the cardiac ventricular action potential compared in guinea-pig, rats and rabbits. *Pflugers Arch*, 2000, 439: 588-599.

[127] Li GR, Ferrier GR. Verapamil prevents slowing of transmural conduction and suppresses arrhythmias in an isolated guinea pig ventricular model of ischemia and reperfusion. *Circ Res*, 1992, 70: 651-659.

[128] Gupte SA, Tateyama M, Okada T, Oka, et al. Epiandrosterone, a metabolite of testosterone precursor, blocks L-type calcium channels of ventricular myocytes and inhibits myocardial contractility. *J Mol Cell Cardiol*, 2002, 34: 679-688.

[129] Weber K, Erben RG, Rump A, Adamski J. Gene structure and regulation of the murine epithelial calcium channels ECaC1 and 2. *Biochem Biophys Res Commun*, 2001, 289:1287-94.

[130] Furukawa T, Kurokawa J. Regulation of cardiac ion channels via non-genomic action of sex steroid hormones: Implication for the gender difference in cardiac arrhythmias. *Pharmacol Ther*, 2007, 115:106-115.

[131] Murad F. Shattuck Lecture. Nitric oxide and cyclic GMP in cell signaling and drug development. *N Engl J Med*, 2006, 355: 2003-2011.

[132] Jaffrey SR, Erdjument-Bromage H, Ferris CD, et al. Protein S-nitrosylation: a physiological signal for neuronal nitric oxide. *Nat Cell Biol*, 2001, 3: 193-197.

[133] Hess DT, Matsumoto A, Kim SO, et al. Protein S-nitrosylation: purview and parameters. *Nat Rev*, 2005, 6: 150-166.

[134] Saraiva RM, Hare JM. Nitric oxide signaling in the cardiovascular system: Implications for heart failure. *Curr Opin Cardiol*, 2006, 21: 221-228.

[135] Vandecasteele G., Verde I, Rucker-Martin C, et al. Cyclic GMP regulation of the L-type Ca2+ channel current in human atrial myocytes. *J Physiol*, 2001, 33: 329-340.

[136] Haynes MP, Li L, Sinha D, et al. Src kinase mediates phosphatidylinositol 3-kinase/Akt-dependent rapid endothelial nitric-oxide synthase activation by estrogen. *J Biol Chem*, 2003, 278: 2118-2123.

[137] Endoh H, Sasaki H, Maruyama K, et al. Rapid activation of MAP kinase by estrogen in the bone cell line. *Biochem Biophys Res Commun*, 1997, 235: 99-102.

[138] Watters JJ, Campbell JS, Cunningham MJ, et al. Rapid membrane effects of steroids in neuroblastoma cells: effects of estrogen on mitogen activated protein kinase signalling cascade and c-fos immediate early gene transcription. *Endocrinology*, 1997, 138: 4030-4033.

[139] Fraser H, Davidge ST, Clanachan AS. Activation of Ca2+- independent nitric oxide synthase by 17b-estradiol in post-ischemic rat heart. *Cardiovasc Res*, 2000, 46: 111-118.

[140] Wang, X, Abdel-Rahman AA. Estrogen modulation of eNOS activity and its association with caveolin-3 and calmodulin in rat hearts. *Am J Physiol*, 2002, 282: H2309-2315.

[141] Migliaccio E, Giorgio M, Mele S, et al. The p66shc adaptor protein controls oxidative stress response and life span in mammals. *Nature*, 1999, 402: 309-313.

[142] Song RXD, McPherson RA, Adam L, et al. Linkage of rapid estrogen action to MAPK activation by ERa-Shc association and Shc pathway activation. *Mol Endocrinol*, 2002, 16: 116-127.

[143] Pelicci G, Lanfrancone L, Salcini AE, et al. Constitutive phosphorylation of Shc proteins in human tumors. *Oncogene*, 1995, 11: 899-907.

[144] Boney CM, Gruppuso PA, Faris RA, et al. The critical role of Shc in insulin-like growth factor-I-mediated mitogenesis and differentiation in 3T3-L1 preadipocytes. *Mol Endocrinol*, 2000, 14: 805-813.

[145] Fiset C, Clark RB, Shimoni Y, et al. Shal-type channels contribute to the Ca2+-independent transient outward K+ current in rat ventricle. *J Physiol*, 1997, 500: 51-64.

[146] Guo W, Li H, Aimond F, et al. Role of heteromultimers in the generation of myocardial transient outward K+ currents. *Circ Res*, 2002, 90: 586-593.

[147] Hoppe UC, Marban E, Johns DC. Molecular dissection of cardiac repolarization by in vivo Kv4.3 gene transfer. *J Clin Invest*, 2000, 105: 1077-1084.

[148] Ka¨a¨b, S., Dixon, J., Duc, J., et al. Molecular Basis of Transient Outward Potassium Current Downregulation in Human Heart Failure: A Decrease in Kv4.3 mRNA Correlates With a Reduction in Current Density. *Circulation*, 1998, 98: 1383-1393.

[149] Min S, Gustavo H, Mansoureh E, et al. Remodeling of Kv4.3 Potassium Channel Gene Expression under the Control of Sex Hormones. *J Biol Chem*, 2001, 34: 31883-31890.

[150] Mangelsdorf DJ, Thummel C, Beato M, et al. The nuclear receptor superfamily: The second decade. *Cell*, 1995, 83: 835-839.

[151] Beato M, Herrlich P, Schutz G. Steroid hormone receptors: Many actors in search of a plot. *Cell*, 1995, 83: 851-857.

[152] Mendelsohn ME, Karas RH. The protective effects of estrogen on the cardiovascular system. *N Engl J Med*, 1999, 340: 1801-1811.

[153] Babiker FA, De Windt LJ, van Eickels M, et al. Estrogenic hormone action in the heart: Regulatory network and function. *Cardiovasc Res*, 2002, 53: 709-719.

[154] Hall JM, Couse JF, Korach KS. The multifaceted mechanisms of estradiol and estrogen receptor signaling. *J Biol Chem*, 2001, 276: 36869-36872.

[155] Rosenfeld MG, Glass CK. Coregulator codes of transcriptional regulation by nuclear receptors. *J Biol Chem*, 2001, 276: 36865-36868.

[156] McDonnell DP, Norris JD. Connections and regulation of the human estrogen receptor. *Science*, 2002, 296: 1642-1644.

[157] Wible, B. A., Kuryshev, Y. A., and Brown, A. M. Cloning and Expression of a Novel K+ Channel Regulatory Protein, KChAP. *J Biol Chem*, 199, 273: 11745–11751.

[158] An, W. F., Bowlby, M. R., Betty, M., et al. Modulation of A-type potassium channels by a family of calcium sensors. *Nature*, 2000, 403: 553-556.

[159]   Song M., B. Barila, R. Olcese, et al. Hormonal control of protein expression and mRNA levels of the MaxiK channel a subunit in myometrium. *FEBS Letters*, 1999, 460: 427-432.

[160]   Severs NJ, Coppen SR, Dupont E, et al. Gap junction alterations in human cardiac disease. *Cardiovasc Res*, 2004, 62: 368-377.

[161]   Mari Amino, Koichiro Yoshioka, Teruhisa Tanabe,et al. Heavy ion radiation up-regulates Cx43 and ameliorates arrhythmogenic substrates in hearts after myocardial infarction. *Cardiovasc Res*, 2006, 72: 412-421.

[162]   Chung TH, Wang SM, Wu JC. 17h-estradiol reduces the effect of metabolic inhibition on gap junction intercellular communication in rat cardiomyocytes via the estrogen receptor. *J Mol Cell Cardiol*, 2004, 37: 1013-1022.

[163]   Lee HW, Eghbali-Webb M. Estrogen enhances proliferative capacity of cardiac fibroblasts by estrogen receptor- and mitogen-activated protein kinase-dependent pathways. *J Mol Cell Cardiol*, 1998, 30: 1359-1368.

[164]   Watanabe T, Akishita M, He H, et al. 17h-estradiol inhibits cardiac fibroblast growth through both subtypes of estrogen receptor. *Biochem Biophys Res Commun*, 2003, 311: 454-459.

[165]   Mercier I, Colombo F, Mader S, et al.Ovarian hormones induce TGF-h3 and fibronectin mRNAs but exhibit a disparate action on cardiac fibroblast proliferation. *Cardiovasc Res*, 2002, 53: 728-739.

[166]   Dubey RK, Jackson EK. Cardiovascular protective effects of 17a-estradiol metabolites. *J Appl Physiol*, 2001, 91: 1868-1883.

[167]   Dubey RK, Gillespie DG., Jackson EK, et al. 17hestradiol, its metabolites, and progesterone inhibit cardiac fibroblast growth. *Hypertension*, 1998, 31: 522-528.

[168]   Dubey RK, Gillespie DG., Zacharia LC, et al. Methoxyestradiols mediate the antimitogenic effects of locally applied estradiol on cardiac fibroblast growth. *Hypertension*, 2002, 39: 412-417.

[169]   Dubey RK, Jackson EK, Gillespie DG., et al. Cytochromes 1A1/1B1- and catechol-Omethyltransferase-derived metabolites mediate estradiol induced antimitogenesis in human cardiac fibroblast. *J Clin Endocrinol Metab*, 2005, 90: 247-255.

In: Heart Disease in Women
Editor: B. V. Larner and H. R. Pennelton

ISBN 978-1-60692-066-4
© 2009 Nova Science Publishers, Inc.

Chapter III

Preeclampsia and Risk of Cardiovascular Disease: Epidemiology and Pathophysiology

Giovanna Oggè, Simona Cardaropoli and Tullia Todros
Department of Obstetrics and Gynecology, University of Turin, Italy

Preeclampsia: Definition and Epidemiology

Preeclampsia (PE) is a pregnancy-specific syndrome characterised by the appearance of hypertension (systolic blood pressure ≥ 140 mmHg or diastolic blood pressure ≥ 90 mmHg) and proteinuria (≥ 300mg per 24 hours) during the second half of pregnancy (after 20 weeks of gestational age). It may be variously associated with a myriad of other signs and symptoms, such as oedema, visual disturbances, headache, seizures (eclampsia), epigastric pain, HELLP syndrome (haemolysis, liver dysfunction and low platelet count), and it typically resolves after delivery.

PE is to be differentiated from other hypertensive disorders in pregnancy, both from a prognostic and a pathophysiological point of view. Under this respect, the NHLBI Working Group on Research on Hypertension During Pregnancy [[1]] distinguishes PE from:

- *gestational hypertension*: de novo hypertension arising after midpregnancy, in the absence of proteinuria. This category includes women who later satisfy diagnostic criteria for preeclampsia. However, in most cases, proteinuria never occurs, the course is relatively benign, and blood pressure normalizes postpartum;
- *chronic hypertension*: maternal hypertension recognised before pregnancy; it can also be assumed when hypertension is detected before mid-pregnancy and when it fails to normalize 12 weeks after delivery. Women with chronic hypertension are at increased risk to develop *superimposed preeclampsia* (25% risk) and the outcomes for the mother and infant with preeclampsia superimposed on existing hypertension are worse than with de novo preeclampsia.;

- *eclampsia* is a life-threatening complication of PE characterised by new-onset of seizures in a woman with PE. Such convulsions usually occur after mid-pregnancy, or during delivery, but about one third of eclamptic convulsions occur during the first 48 hours of the postpartum period.

The exact incidence of PE is uncertain, but it has been reported to be approximately 5-8% [[2]] and to be substantially higher in nulliparous women, and in women with multifetal pregnancies, history of PE in previous pregnancies, family history of PE, chronic hypertension, pregestational diabetes, antiphospholipid antibodies, obesity, age > 40 years. Paradoxically, cigarette smoking reduces the risk [[3]].

PE is one of the leading causes of maternal mortality in the developing countries and a cause of neonatal morbidity and mortality worldwide. Mortality from PE is largely preventable by delivery that stops the progression of the disease, so that the high rate of maternal mortality in developing countries is a marker of low quality of care, rather than disease frequency. Anyway, even in developed countries, PE puts the mother at risk for abruptio placentae, renal failure, pulmonary oedema, stroke and seizures (eclampsia).The reason for neonatal risks depends on the fact that, given the absence of an effective treatment, the only possibility to prevent further deterioration of maternal conditions is delivery, and preterm birth is associated with increased mortality and neurological disabilities. It is estimated that 15% of all preterm births are iatrogenic deliveries for preeclampsia[[4]]. Moreover, preeclampsia also increases the risk of fetal growth restriction (FGR) that, in turn, is an important cause of neonatal mortality and morbidity [[5]] and a recognised risk factor for long-term pathologies in adulthood, such as cardiovascular disease and insulin-resistance syndrome [[6]].

Preeclampsia: Pathogenesis

Despite considerable advances in research the ethiology of PE remains uncertain.

It has been known for a hundred years that PE depends on the presence of a *placenta*, and that particularly the trophoblast, is essential to the development of the pathology. This is demonstrated for instance by the fact that a condition such as hydatidiform mole, where the products of conception are almost exclusively trophoblastic, is at risk to develop PE.

Placentas from preeclamptic women are characterised by histological signs of hypoperfusion that are attributed to a defect in the vascular remodelling of the uterine compartment. In normal pregnancy, the spiral arteries, the branches of the uterine arteries that perfuse the placenta, are progressively transformed from small muscular vessels to large flaccid conduits without muscularis and elastic lamina, which results in a preferential increase in placental perfusion [7]. These physiological changes, that start with implantation and are completed by 20-22 weeks of gestational age, are due to a complex process of invasion of the decidua and the myometrium by the trophoblast [8]. The vascular remodelling is typically absent or faint in PE, as it is shown by histological studies on samples of placental beds [9], and by the finding of increased uterine vascular resistance at Doppler assessment. Moreover, spiral arteries of preeclamptic women are often characterized by the presence of a typical lesion known as *acute atherosis*; this lesion is very similar to those observed in atherosclerosis and is defined by fibrinoid necrosis of the vessel wall, accumulation of lipid-laden macrophages in the vessel wall, and infiltration of the perivascular space by mononuclear cells [7]. Acute atherosis is believed to occur only in vessels that have failed to undergo physiologic transformation.. The failure in the process of placentation, which depends on an anomalous interaction between the trophoblastic cells and the maternal environment, occurs in the first half of pregnancy, that is well before the clinical appearance of preeclamptic symptoms, usually in the third trimester.

Anyway failure in placentation is not sufficient to cause PE, as it can be associated with fetal growth restriction without hypertension and, occasionally, with uncomplicated pregnancies, so it is nowadays considered a predisposing factor, rather than the cause of PE [10], [11].

Whatever the nature of the placental anomalies, the maternal multi-systemic manifestations of the preeclamptic syndrome are currently ascribed to a generalized *endothelial dysfunction*, that is an impairment in the endothelial ability to orchestrate the dynamic balance between vasodilatation and vasoconstriction, inhibition and stimulation of smooth muscle cells proliferation and migration, thrombosis and fibrinolysis. The recurring histological findings in brain, liver and adrenal glands of women who experienced PE are necrosis and hemorrhage that are secondary to hypoperfusion. Endothelial dysfunction actually causes reduction in organ perfusion by vasoconstriction, micro-thrombosis due to activation of the coagulation cascade, and hypovolemia, secondary to the loss of proteins from the vascular compartment [11], [12].

There is growing evidence that the cause of endothelial dysfunction is a systemic inflammatory response: peripheral blood leukocytes from preeclamptic women show signs of activation comparable to those from non pregnant individual with proven sepsis [13], and the level of several pro-inflammatory cytokines, such as tumour necrosis factor-alpha (TNF-α) [14], interleukin-6 (IL-6) [[15], [16]], interleukin-8 (IL-8) [17], macrophage migration inhibitory factor (MIF) [18] result to be significantly increased. The inflammatory response also involves the coagulation and platelet activation, through the expression of intravascular tissue factors and leukocyte adhesion molecules, and through the down regulation of the fibrinolytic and protein C anticoagulant responses. Thus the inflammatory hypothesis can explain the presence of intravascular coagulation and micro-thrombosis in PE [19].

Surprisingly, the activation of the inflammatory system has been shown to be an attribute of normal pregnancy too, although with a milder intensity than in PE. It has been speculated that PE is the result of a decompensation of the normal inflammatory state of pregnancy due either to an excessive inflammatory stimulus or to an altered maternal reaction [20]. The most likely cause of such exaggerated maternal response is suspected to depend on an infectious status (even sublinical).

A simple attempt to resume the currently available data is the *two steps hypothesis*. According to this theory PE is the result of an initial placental trigger, due to a failure of the normal invasion of trophoblast cells leading to placental hypoxia, and a subsequent maternal systemic reaction, characterized by endothelial dysfunction, possibly on an inflammatory base, that produces the clinical signs and symptoms [21]. The link between reduced placental perfusion and the maternal syndrome remains basically unknown.

Preeclampsia and Cardiovascular Disease

A possible relationship between PE and essential hypertension in later life was reported for the first time by Adams and MacGillivray in 1961 [22]. In the following decades evidence about the association between PE and the risk for remote cardiovascular disease has been accumulating. Results from many of these studies, however, were criticisable because of inaccurate definition of PE, small sample size, shortness of follow-up, or lack of a suitable control group. A recently published meta-analysis of cohort studies [23], including a total of 3488160 women, intended to measure the association between PE and subsequent CVD, cancer, and mortality from any cause. Case-control studies were excluded because of their greater susceptibility to selection and recall bias. The results of the meta-analysis showed that women who experienced PE during one or more pregnancies have an increased risk of future hypertension, fatal and non fatal ischemic heart disease, haemorrhagic or ischemic stroke, venous thromboembolism, and mortality from any cause (table 1). As there was no difference in the relative risk of death from breast cancer or any other cancer, the major contribution to increased mortality was supposed to derive from CVD.

Although a part of the excess risk of CVD could be explained by the link between PE, hypertension and CVD, it is worth-noting that one of the studies [24], including over a million women, adjusted for prepregnancy hypertension, diabetes mellitus, obesity, dyslipidaemia, metabolic syndrome and smoking, obtaining a two-fold increase in the risk of CVD, very similar to the whole meta-analysis.

The observed association between PE and CVD might be explained by a common cause for the two syndromes, or by a deleterious effect of PE on maternal cardiovascular system, or both (figures 1 and 2).

Table 1. Association between PE and risk of cardiovascular disease, cancer, and mortality from any cause in later life. * = statistically significant (adapted from Bellamy et al. [[23]])

Outcome	Sample size (n)	Mean weighted follow-up (years)	Relative Risk	95% Confidence Interval
Hypertension	21030	14.1	3.70	2.70-5.05 *
Ischemic heart disease	2346997	11.7	2.16	1.86-2.52 *
Stroke	1671578	10.4	1.81	1.45-2.27*
Thromboembolism	427693	4.7	1.79	1.37-2.33 *
Breast cancer	776445	17	1.04	0.78-1.39
Any cancer	729025	13.9	0.96	0.73-1.27
Mortality	49049	14.5	1.49	1.05-2.14 *

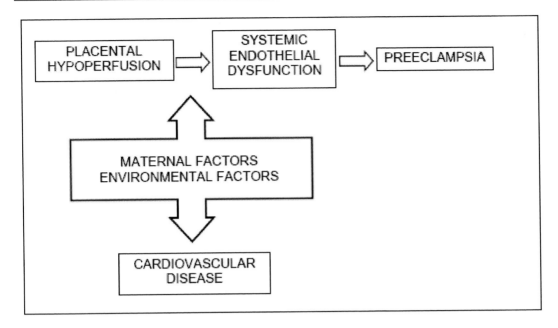

Figure 1. schematic representation of the hypothesis of a common cause for PE and CVD.

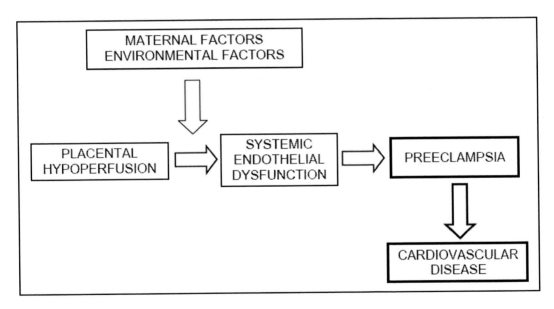

Figure 2. schematic representation of the hypothesis of the causal role of PE in the pathogenesis of CVD.

The hypothesis of the common causal link is supported by the fact that many disorders associated with endothelial dysfunction, such as hypertension, diabetes mellitus, antiphospholipid syndrome, inherited thrombophilias, are shared risk factors both for developing PE and CVD (a noteworthy exception is the protective effect of smoking on the risk of PE, in contrast with its negative effect on the risk of CVD). A recent prospective cohort study demonstrated that the presence of several cardiovascular risk factors before pregnancy, namely high body mass index and elevated levels of triglycerides, cholesterol, low density protein cholesterol and blood pressure, is associated with an increased risk to develop PE during pregnancy [25]. Under this respect, it is possible to think of PE as a first expression of the same unfavourable phenotype associated with the early development of CVD.

On the other side it is possible that the transient but severe endothelial dysfunction that characterizes PE could activate the cascade of events culminating, years later, in the manifestations of CVD. As a matter of fact, an impairment of endothelial function, defined by a reduction in endothelial-dependent vasodilatation, is are still detectable three years after PE has resolved [26], [27].

Inflammation as the Possible Link between CVD and PE

Whatever the chronological sequence between the events, the common factor between PE and CVD is, clearly, endothelial dysfunction [28].

Interestingly, a vast amount of evidence suggests a crucial role for inflammation in the pathogenesis of atherosclerosis, as we have just showed to be for PE. To simplify the cascade of events, an initial endothelial injury leads to a decreased production of nitric oxide (NO) – the most important mediator of endothelial-induced vasodilatation- and to the expression of endothelial cell surface receptors, which bind monocytes and T lymphocytes initiating an inflammatory reaction. Once migrated into the subendothelial space, the monocytes mature into macrophages, internalize lipoproteins (transforming themselves into *foam cells*), and produce proinflammatory cytokines, that maintain the chemotactic stimulus for circulating leucocytes. T lymphocytes, after penetrating into the intima, become activated in response to various antigens and begin secreting a range of cytokines. The inflammatory environment maintained within the intima acts as a stimulus for the smooth muscle cells to migrate from the media to the intima; here they undergo a change in their phenotype, reducing the content of contractile proteins and activating the production of proteinases, growth factors and matrix proteins (collagen, elastin) that result in the formation of the fibrous cap of the atheromatous lesion [29].

Several markers of inflammation are intensively studied both as risk factors and as prognostic factors for CVD. For an instance, moderately elevated levels of the acute-phase reactant C-reactive protein (CRP), are associated with increased risk of ischemic heart disease in a healthy population [30, 31, 32]. CRP is also a prognostic factor for coronary artery disease, as high levels of this marker are associated with higher rates of deaths [33, 34, 35]. High levels of CRP and others inflammatory markers (fibrinogen, IL-6, serum amyloid A, IL-7, IL-8, soluble CD40 ligand) are also found in patients with instable angina and myocardial infarction [36, 37, 38, 39, 40]. Moreover, it is now established that a part of the mechanism of action of statins, a class of drugs of proved efficacy for primary and secondary prevention of CVD, is to be ascribed to their anti-inflammatory effects, besides their lipid-lowering properties [29].

The Infectious Hypothesis

The increasing agreement about the role of inflammation in the pathogenesis of PE and CVD has independently stimulated research about a possible infective trigger in both pathologies.

Infectious agents could play their role either with a direct mechanism, by damaging the vascular endothelium, or with an indirect mechanism, by producing a systemic inflammatory environment.

As far as PE is concerned, evidences are interesting but not conclusive. A case-control study found, after multiple logistic regression, an increased risk of urinary tract infections in women with PE (Odds Ratio (OR) 1.6, 95% CI 1.1-2.5); the association was much stronger among primigravidae (OR 5.5, 95% CI 2.9-9.7) [41]. Two case-control studies have found an association between urinary and low genital tract infection with Ureaplasma urealyticum and Gardnerella vaginalis with the development of PE [42, 43].

A more recent cohort study demonstrated that the presence of a periodontal disease before 26 weeks of gestational age, doubled the risk for subsequent PE (OR 2.4; 95% CI 1.1-5.3) [44].

Several studies have arisen from sero-epidemological observations demonstrating a relation between the presence of antibodies against some infections and the incidence of PE. Women who were seronegative for *Herpes simplex virus type 2*, *Cytomegalovirus* and *Epstein-Barr virus* during the first trimester, resulted to be at higher risk to develop PE than controls, which suggest that acquiring a primary infection for these viral agents during pregnancy, is a risk factor for PE [45]. Other studies showed an association between PE and seropositivity for *Chlamydia pneumoniae* [46, 47, 48, 49], *Cytomegalovirus* [49], *Helicobacter pylori* [50], while a case-control study hypothesized that the association between certain alleles of the human leukocyte antigen system (HLA DRB1*06 or *08) and the infection from *Cytomegalovirus* (demonstrated by the presence of viral DNA in maternal blood) is a strong risk factor [51].

Another indirect finding supporting the role of infection comes from a cohort study that showed a lower incidence of PE in women treated with antibiotic for toxoplasmosis during pregnncy than controls.

Anyway, a meta-analysis of all observational studies investigating the relationship between infection or antimicrobial treatment and PE, concluded that a significant association with PE could be confirmed only for urinary tract infections and periodontal disease [53].

Interestingly the same infective agents that have been involved in the pathogenesis of PE are recurring subject of study for atherosclerosis and CVD. Particularly, both serological and histological studies have suggested some relationships between atherogenesis and infections from *Human Herpes virus*, *Cytomegalovirus*, *Chlamydia pneumoniae* and *Helicobacte pylori* [54]

Helicobacter pylori is an ubiquitous Gram-negative bacterium with a particular tropism for the gastric epithelium. It usually causes a life-long infection of the gastric mucosa, and it is the major cause of peptic ulcer disease. Several studies have investigated the correlation between *Helicobacter pylori* infection and CVD. The most positive results were obtained investigating the role of the most virulent strains, those bearing the cytotoxin-associated gene

A (*CagA positive*), and both ischemic heart disease and cerebrovascular disease [55]. Anti-CagA antibodies recognise antigens in the nuclei and cytoplasm of smooth-muscle cells and in the cell membranes of endothelial cells, which suggest a possible immuno-mediated mechanism of *Helicobacter pylori* infection in the progression of the atheromatous lesion [56]. Noteworthy the same preferential relationship was noticed between anti-*CagA positive* antibodies and PE [50]. Other potential pathogenic links between *Helicobacter pylori* and endothelial dysfunction rely on its ability to increase plasma level of cytokines and acute-phase reactants and to modify the serum lipid profile. Anyway the above-mentioned associations could not be reproduced by all studies[57].

Clinical and Research Implications

Further research is needed to clarify the nature of the association between PE and CVD, that could be a causal role of PE in the later development of CVD, or the presence of a common substrate for both diseases. The coexistence of both mechanism is also possible.

Whatever is the case, a history of PE during pregnancy should be considered as a risk factor in any screening program for CVD, and affected women could benefit from earlier implementation of preventive interventions for CVD.

On the other hand, if PE was recognized as an independent risk factor for subsequent CVD, the identification of preventive strategies or causal therapies for PE (such as, ideally, antibiotic treatment for an infective agent) could have important effects on the reduction CVD in the female population.

References

[1]   Roberts JM, Pearson GD, Cutler JA, Lindheimer MD. Summary of the NHLBI Working Group on Research on Hypertension During Pregnancy. *Hypertension.* 2003 ; 41(3):437-45

[2]   ACOG Practice Bulletin. Diagnosis and management of preeclampsia and eclampsia. *Int. J. Gynaecol. Obstet.* 2002; 77 (1): 67-75

[3]   Duckitt K, Harrington D. Risk factors for pre-eclampsia at antenatal booking: systematic review of controlled studies. *BMJ* 2005; 330 (7491): 565-72

[4]   Meis PJ, Goldenberg RL, Mercer BM, Iams JD, Moawad AH, Miodovnik M, Menard MK, Caritis SN, Thurnau GR, Bottoms SF, Das A, Roberts JM, McNellis D. The preterm prediction study. Risk factors for indicated preterm birth. *Am. J. Obstet. Gynecol.* 1998; 178: 562-67

[5]   Bernstein IM, Horbar JD, Badger GJ, Ohlsson A, Golan A, Stillman AL. Morbidity and mortality among very-low-birth-weight neonates with intrauterine growth restriction. *Am. J. Obstet. Gynecol.* 2000, 182(1 I): 198-206

[6]   Gluckman PD, Hanson MA, Pinal C. The developmental origins of adult disease. Matern Child Nutr. 2005;1 (3):130-41

[7] Espinoza J, Romero R, Kim YM, Kusanovic JP, Hassan S, Erez O, Gotsch F, Than NG, Papp Z, Kim CJ. Normal and abnormal transformation of the spiral arteries during pregnancy. *J. Perinat. Med.* 2006, 34: 447-58

[8] Pijnenborg R, Vercruysse L, Hanssens M. The uterine spiral arteries in human pregnancy: facts and controversies. *Placenta* 2006; 27: 939-58

[9] Robertson W, Brosens I, Landells WN. Abnormal placentation. *Obstet. Gynecol. Annual* 1985; 14: 411-26

[10] Papageorghiou AT, Yu CK, Cicero S, Bower S, Nicolaides KH. Second-trimester uterine artery Doppler screening in unselected populations: a review. *J. Matern Fetal Neonatal. Med.* 2002: 12(2):78-88.

[11] Redman CWG, Sargent IL. Pre-eclampsia, the placenta and the maternal systemic inflammatory response – a review. *Placenta* 2003; 24 Suppl A: S21-7

[12] Roberts JM, Lain KY. Recent insights into the pathogenesis of pre-eclampsia. *Placenta* 2002; 23:359-72

[13] Sacks GP, Studena K, Sargent K, Redman CWG. Normal pregnancy and preeclampsia both produce inflammatory changes in peripheral blood leukocytes akin of those of sepsis. *Am. J. Obstet. Gynecol.* 1998; 179: 80-86

[14] Serin IS, Ozcelik B, Basbug M, Kilic H, Okur D, Erez R. Predictive value of tumor necrosis factor-alpha (TNF-α) in preeclampsia. *Eur. J. Obstet. Gynecol. Reprod. Biol.* 2002; 100 (2): 143-5

[15] Vince GS, Starkey PM, Austgulen R, Kwiatkowski D, Redman CWG. Interleukin-6, tumour necrosis factor and soluble tumour necrosis factor receptors in women with preeclampsia. *Br. J. Obstet. Gynaecol.* 1995; 102: 20-25

[16] Teran E, Escudero C, Moya W, Flores M, Vallance P, Lopez-Jaramillo P. Elevated C-reactive protein and pro-inflammatory cyrokines in Andean women with preeclampsia. *In .J. Gynaecol. Obstet.* 2001; 75 (3): 243-49

[17] Ellis J, Wennerholm UB, Bengstsson A, Lilja H, Pettersson A, Sultan B, Wennergren M, Hagberg H. Levels of dimethylarginines and cytokines in mild and severe preeclampsia. *Acta Obstet. Gynecol .Scand.* 2001; 80: 602-8

[18] Todros T, Bontempo S, Piccoli E, Ietta F, Romagnoli R, Biolcati M, Castellucci M, Paulesu L. Increased levels of macrophage migration inhibitory factor (MIF) in preeclampsia. *Eur. J. Obstet. Gynecol. REprod. Biol.* 2005; 123 (2): 162-66

[19] Konijnenberg A, Stokkers EW, van der Post JA, Schaap MC, Boer K, Bleker OP, Sturk A. Extensive platelet activation in preeclampsia compared with normal pregnancy: enhanced expression of cell adhesion molecules- *Am. J. Obstet. Gynecol.* 1997; 176: 461-69

[20] Redman CW, Sacks GP, Sargent IL. Preeclampsia: an excessive maternal inflammatory response to pregnancy? *Am. J .Obstet. Gynecol.* 1999; 180: 499-506

[21] Walker JJ. Pre-eclampsia. Lancet 2000; 356:1260-6

[22] Adams EM, MacGillivray I. Long-term effect of preeclampsia on blood pressure. *Lancet* 1961; 2: 1373 5

[23] Bellamy L, Casas JP, Hingorani AD, Williams DJ. Pre-eclampsia and risk of cardiovascular disease and cancer in later life: systematic review and meta-analysis. *BMJ* 2007; 335 (7627): 974-86

[24] Ray JG, Vermeulen MJ, Schull MJ, Redelmeier DA. Cardiovascular health after maternal placental syndromes (CHAMPS): population-based retrospective cohort study. *Lancet* 2005; 366: 1797-803

[25] Magnussen EB, Vatten LJ, Lund-Nilsen TI, Salvesen KA, Davey Smith G, Romundstad PR. Prepregnancy cardiovascular risk factors as predictors of pre-eclampsia: population based cohort study. *BMJ* 2007; 335 (7627): 978-87

[26] Chambers JC, Fusi L, Malik IS, Haskard DO, De Sweit M, Kooner IS. Association of maternal endothelial dysfunction with preeclampsia. *JAMA* 2001; 285: 1607-12

[27] Agatisa PK, Ness RB, Roberts JM, Costantino JP, Kuller LH, McLaughlin MK. Impairment of endothelial function in women with a history of preeclampsia: an indicator of cardiovascular risk. *AJP-Heart Circ. Physiol.* 2004; 286 (4): HI389-HI393

[28] Forgione MA, Leopold JA, Loscalzo J. Roles of endothelial dysfunction in coronary artery disease. *Curr. Opin. Cardiol.* 2000; 15 (6) :409-15

[29] Mahmoudi M, Curzen N, Gallagher PJ. Atherogenesis: the role of inflammation and infection. *Histopathology* 2007; 50: 535-46

[30] Danesh J, Wheeler JG, Hirschfield GM, Eda S, Eiriksdottir G, Rumley A, Lowe GD, Pepys MB, Gudnason V. C-reactive protein and other circulating markers of inflammation in the prediction of coronary heart disease. *N. Engl. J. Med.* 2004; 350 (14): 1387-97

[31] Ridker PM, Cook N. Clinical usefulness of very high and very low levels of C-reactive protein across the full range of Framingham risk scores. *Circulation* 2004; 109: 1955-9

[32] Ballantyne CM, Hoogeveen RC, Bang H, Coresh J, Folsom AR, Heiss G, Sharrett AR. Lipoprotein-associated phospholipase A2, high-sensitivity C-reactive protein, and risk for incident coronary heart disease in middle-aged men and women in the Atherosclerosis Risk in Communities (ARIC) study. *Circulation.* 2004; 109: 837-42

[33] Toss H, Lindahl B, Siegbahn A, Wallentin L. Prognostic influence of increased fibrinogen and C-reactive protein levels in unstable coronary artery disease. 1997; 96(12): 4204-10

[34] Lindahl B, Toss H, Siegbahn A, Venge P, Wallentin L. Markers of myocardial damage and inflammation in relation to long-term mortality in unstable coronary artery disease. *N. Engl. J .Med.* 2000; 343 (16): 1139-47

[35] James SK, Armstrong P, Barnathan E, Califf R, Lindahl B, Siegbahn A, Simoons ML, Topol EJ, Venge P, Wallentin L; GUSTO-IV-ACS Investigators. Troponin and C-reactive protein have different relations to subsequent mortality and myocardial infarction after acute coronary syndrome: a GUSTO-IV substudy. *J. Am. Coll. Cardiol.* 2003; 41 (6): 916-24

[36] Liuzzo G, Biasucci LM, Gallimore JR, Grillo RL, Rebuzzi AG, Pepys MB, Maseri A. The prognostic value of C-reactive protein and serum amyloid a protein in severe unstable angina. *New Engl. J. Med.* 1994; 331 (7): 417-24.

[37] Biasucci LM, Vitelli A, Liuzzo G, Altamura S, Caligiuri G, Monaco C, Rebuzzi AG, Ciliberto G, Maseri A. Elevated levels of interleukin-6 in unstable angina. *Circulation.* 1996 ; 94 (5): 874-7

[38] Wilhelmsen L, Svärdsudd K, Korsan-Bengtsen K, Larsson B, Welin L, Tibblin G. Fibrinogen as a risk factor for stroke and myocardial infarction. *N. Engl. J. Med.* 1984; 311 (8): 501-5.

[39] Aukrust P, Müller F, Ueland T, Berget T, Aaser E, Brunsvig A, Solum NO, Forfang K, Frøland SS, Gullestad L. Enhanced levels of soluble and membrane-bound CD40 ligand in patients with unstable angina. Possible reflection of T lymphocyte and platelet involvement in the pathogenesis of acute coronary syndromes. *Circulation.* 1999; 100(6): 614-20.

[40] Damås JK, Waehre T, Yndestad A, Otterdal K, Hognestad A, Solum NO, Gullestad L, Frøland SS, Aukrust P. Interleukin-7-mediated inflammation in unstable angina: possible role of chemokines and platelets. *Circulation.* 2003; 107(21): 2670-6

[41] Mittendorf R, Lain KY, Williams MA, Walker CK. Preeclampsia. A nested, case-control study of risk factors and their interactions. *J. Reprod. Med.* 1996 ; 41 (7): 491-6

[42] Savidge JA, Gilbert GL, Fairley KF, McDowall DR. Bacteriuria due to Ureaplasma urealyticum and Gardnerella vaginalis in women with preeclampsia. *J. Infect. Dise.* 1983; 148: 605

[43] Gilbert GL, Garland SM, Fairley KF, McDowall DM. Bacteriuria due to ureaplasmas and other fastidious organisms during pregnancy: prevalence and significance. *Pediatr. Infect. Dis.* 1986; 5 (6 Suppl): S239- S43

[44] Boggess KA, Lieff S, Murtha AP, Moss K, Beck J, Offenbacher S. Maternal periodontal disease is associated with an increased risk for preeclampsia. *Obstet. Gynecol.* 2003; 101: 227-31

[45] Trogstad LIS, Eskild A, Bruu AL, Jeansson S, Jenum PA. Is preeclampsia an infectious disease? *Acta Obstet. Gynecol. Scand* 2001; 80: 1036-8

[46] Heine RP, Ness RB, Roberts JM. Seroprevalence of antibodies to *Chlamydia pneumoniae* in women with preeclampsia. *Obstet. Gynecol.* 2003; 101: 221-6

[47] Teran E, Escudero C, Calle A. Seroprevalence of antibodies to *Chlamydia pneumonite* in women with preeclampsia. *Obstet. Gynecol.* 2003; 102: 198-9

[48] von Dadelszen P, Magee LA, Krajden M, Alasaly K, Popovska V, Devarakonda RM, Money DM, Patrick DM, Brunham RC. Levels of antibodies against cytomegalovirus and Chlamydophila pneumoniae are increased in early onset pre-eclampsia. *BJOG.* 2003; 110 (8): 725-30.

[49] Goulis DG, Chappell L, Gibbs RG, Williams D, Dave JR, Taylor P, de Swiet M, Poston L, Williamson C. Association of raised titres of antibodies to Chlamydia pneumoniae with a history of pre-eclampsia. *BJOG.* 2005; 112 (3): 299-305

[50] Ponzetto A, Cardaropoli S, Piccoli E, Rolfo A, Gennero L, Kanduc D, Todros T. Pre-eclampsia is associated with Helicobacter pylori seropositivity in Italy. *J. Hypertens.* 2006 ;24 (12): 2445-9.

[51] Carreiras M, Montagnani S, Lyrisse Z. Preeclampsia : a multifactorial disease resulting from the interaction of the feto-maternal HLA genotype and HCMV infection. *AJRI* 2002: 48: 176-83

[52] Todros T., Verdiglione P, Oggè. G., Paladini D., Vergani P., Cardaropoli S. Low incidence of hypertensive disorders of pregnancy in women treated with spiramycin for toxoplasma infection. *British Journal of Clinical Pharmacology;* 2006, 61: 336-340

[53] Conde-Agudelo A, Villar J, Lindheimer M. Maternal infection and risk of preeclampsia: systematic review and metaanalysis. *Am. J. Obstet. Gynecol.* 2008; 198 (1): 7-22.

[54] Frishman WH, Issali A. Role of infection in atherosclerosis and coronary artery disease: a new therapeutic target? *Cardiol. Rev.*2002; 10 (4):199-210

[55] Franceschi F, Gasbarrini A. *Helicobacter pylori* and extragastric diseases. *Best Pract. Res. Clin. Gastroenterol.* 2007; 21(2):325-34.

[56] Franceschi F, Sepulveda AR, Gasbarrini A, Pola P, Silveri NG, Gasbarrini G, Graham DY, Genta RM. Cross-reactivity of anti-CagA antibodies with vascular wall antigens: possible pathogenic link between Helicobacter pylori infection and atherosclerosis. *Circulation.* 2002; 106 (4): 30-4

[57] Franceschi F, Leo D, Fini L, Santoliquido A, Flore R, Tondi P, Roccarina D,Nista EC, Cazzato AI, Lupascu A, Pola P, Silveri NG, Gasbarrini G, Gasbarrini A. *Helicobacter pylori* infection and ischemic heart disease: an overview of the general literature. Dig Liver Dis. 2005; 37 (5): 301-8.

In: Heart Disease in Women   ISBN 978-1-60692-066-4
Editor: B. V. Larner and H. R. Pennelton   © 2009 Nova Science Publishers, Inc.

Chapter IV

Diabetes and the Risk of Coronary Heart Disease among Women

*Gang Hu**

Department of Health Promotion and Chronic Diseases Prevention,
National Public Health Institute, Helsinki, and Department of Public Health,
University of Helsinki, Finland

Abstract

The number of diabetic patients in the world has been estimated to at least double during the next 30 years. Coronary heart disease is the leading cause of death among patients with type 2 diabetes. The associations of type 2 diabetes and hyperglycemia with the risk of coronary heart disease have been assessed by a number of prospective studies and the results are consistent. Patients with type 2 diabetes have a 2-4 times higher risk of coronary mortality than those without diabetes. Among the middle-aged general population, men have a 2 to 5 times higher risk of coronary heart disease than women. However, women with diabetes will lose their relative protection against coronary heart disease compared with men. In recent years, several studies compared the gender specific impact of diabetes and myocardial infarction at baseline on coronary mortality. These studies found that both diabetes and myocardial infarction at baseline increased coronary mortality. In women, prior myocardial infarction at baseline confers a lower risk on coronary mortality than prior diabetes does. The results of these studies have important implications for clinical practice. For future coronary heart disease risk we need to consider carefully the treatment strategies on individual disease status, particularly type 2 diabetes, in women.

---

* Correspondence to: Gang. Hu, MD, PhD, Department of Health Promotion and Chronic Diseases Prevention, National Public Health Institute, Mannerheimintie 166, FIN-00300 Helsinki, Finland, Tel: +358 9 19127366, Fax: +358 9 19127313, E-mail: hu.gang@ktl.fi.

Cardiovascular disease (CVD), especially coronary heart disease (CHD) and stroke, is the leading killer in western societies and its prevalence is also increasing dramatically in developing nations [1,2]. Preliminary mortality data show that CVD is an underlying cause of death accounted for 37.3% of all 2 440 000 deaths in 2003 or 1 of every 2.7 deaths in the United States [3]. CVD as an underlying or contributing cause of death (1 408 000 deaths in 2002) was about 58% of all deaths that year [3]. High blood pressure, smoking, dyslipidemia, overweight or obesity, physical inactivity, diabetes, chronic inflammation, hemostatic factors, psychosocial factors, perinatal conditions and several dietary factors are the main risk factors for CVD [3-5]. There is a significant difference in CVD risk between sexes [6,7]. Among middle-aged people, men have 2- to 5-times higher CVD mortality rates than women [7]. The sex difference in CVD mortality cannot be completely explained by abnormal levels of conventional CVD risk factors, such as high blood pressure, lipid abnormalities, smoking and obesity [7].

Diabetes is one of the fastest growing public health problems in both developing and developed countries [8]. It has been estimated that the number of individuals with diabetes among adults 20 or more years of age will double from the current 171 million in 2000 to 366 million in 2030 [8]. Much of the burden of diabetes is attributable to microvascular and macrovascular complications, such as retinopathy, nephropathy, CHD, and stroke. CVD accounts for more than 70% of total mortality among patients with type 2 diabetes [9]. Epidemiological studies have indicated that patients with type 2 diabetes have a 2-4 times higher risk of CVD mortality than those without diabetes [10-12]. The Framingham Study is the first one to point out that women with diabetes seem to lose their relative protection against CHD compared with men [13]. The reason for the higher relative risk of CHD in diabetic women than in diabetic men is still unclear. In this chapter, we summarize current results regarding the role of type 2 diabetes on the risk of CHD among women.

1. Diabetes and Women's CHD Risk

Type 2 diabetes is associated with an increased risk of CHD, cerebrovascular disease, and peripheral vascular disease [14,15]. Estimates of CHD mortality in diabetic men have varied from 1- to 3-fold of the rate in nondiabetic men [15-18], whereas estimates in diabetic women have ranged from 2- to 5-fold of the rate in nondiabetic women [15-18]. The variation in relative risk estimates of CVD makes it difficult to evaluate the strength of diabetes as a risk factor for either sex. Several studies compared the sex-specific risk of CHD and CVD mortality between diabetic men and women.

The 14-year follow-up of the Rancho Bernardo study showed that the multivariate-adjusted relative hazards of CHD mortality in diabetic compared with non-diabetic subjects was 3.3 in women and 1.9 in men [19]. An 11.6-year follow-up study in Scotland found asymptomatic hyperglycaemia (casual blood glucose > 7.0 mmol/l) to be a significant risk factor for CVD in both genders, but stronger in women than in men [20]. An early review about the impact of gender on the occurrence of atherosclerotic vascular disease in type 2 diabetes reported the overall relative risk for gender (men vs. women) in CHD mortality 1.46 (95%CI 1.21-1.95) in diabetic and 2.29 (2.05-2.55) in non-diabetic subjects [21]. A recent meta-analysis including prospective studies has indicated that the multivariate-adjusted summary odds ratio for CHD mortality due to diabetes was 2.3 (95% CI 1.9-2.8) for men and 2.9 (95% CI 2.2-3.8) for women [22]. There were no significant sex differences in the adjusted risk associated with diabetes for CHD and CVD mortality [22]. The result from DECODE study, including 8172 men and 9407 women without known diabetes, showed that newly diagnosed diabetic women had a higher relative risk for CVD death than newly diagnosed diabetic men [23]. This association is statistically independent of age, body mass index, systolic blood pressure, total cholesterol and smoking [23]. Moreover, in people who smoked, had hypertension, exhibited hypercholesterolaemia, or were overweight, the relative risk from CVD mortality was 1.3 to 2.1 times higher in diabetic women than in diabetic men compared with normoglycaemic women and men respectively. So we have suggested that hyperglycaemia could have a stronger additive or synergistic effect on smoking, hypertension, hypercholesterolaemia, and overweight in women than in men [23].

Moreover, most of these studies have presented the data on history of diabetes at baseline, and no study has the data on incident diabetes during follow-up. We evaluated prospectively the joint associations of history of hypertension at baseline and type 2 diabetes at baseline and during follow-up with the incidence of CHD and CHD mortality among 49,775 Finnish subjects aged 25-74 years without history of CHD and stroke [18]. During a median follow-up of 21.5 years, 5074 incident CHD events were recorded, of which 3134 were fatal. CHD incidence was increased by 23% (95% CI 1.10-1.37) in men with incident diabetes during follow-up and by 90% (95% CI 1.59-2.27) in men with history of diabetes at baseline compared with non-diabetic men. In women, CHD incidence was increased by 2.04 times (95% CI 1.80-2.30) and 3.7 times (95% CI 3.02-4.53), respectively. In the joint analyses, the multivariable-adjusted hazard ratios of CHD incidence were 1.25, 1.69, 1.25, 1.83, 1.85, 2.39, 2.15, and 3.31 (p for trend <0.001), respectively, among men with hypertension I (blood pressure 140-159/90-94 mmHg or using antihypertensive drugs at baseline but blood pressure <160/95 mmHg) only, with hypertension II (blood pressure ≥160/95 mmHg) only, with incident diabetes during follow-up only, with both hypertension I and incident diabetes, with both hypertension II and incident diabetes, with history of diabetes at baseline only, with both hypertension I and history of diabetes, and with both hypertension II and history of diabetes compared with men without either of these diseases (Table 1). The corresponding hazard ratios of CHD incidence among women were 1.52, 2.37, 2.45, 3.78, 4.56, 5.63, 6.10, and 7.41 (p for trend <0.001), respectively. The corresponding HRs of coronary mortality were 1.45, 2.06, 1.08, 1.43, 1.95, 3.09, 3.08, and 4.21 in men, 1.60, 2.70, 2.90, 3.34, 5.28, 7.85, 9.24, and 10.8 in women, respectively (Table 2). Compared with men and women without hypertension and diabetes, the relative risks of incident CHD and CHD mortality were higher in women than in men with any combination of hypertension and diabetes. This sex difference was however statistically significant for only CHD incidence among subjects with hypertension I only (χ^2=4.31, 1df, P<0.05), and for both CHD incidence and CHD mortality among subjects with hypertension II only (χ^2=20.46 and 9.0, 1df, P<0.001 and P <0.005), with incident diabetes during follow-up only (χ^2=8.47 and 10.36, 1df, both P<0.005), with both hypertension I and incident diabetes (χ^2=23.16 and 17.44, 1df, both P<0.001), with both hypertension II and incident diabetes (χ^2=50.46 and 34.64, 1df, both P <0.001), with history of diabetes at baseline only (χ^2=6.02 and 4.15, 1df,

P<0.025 and P <0.05), with both hypertension I and history of diabetes (χ^2=17.91 and 14.51, 1df, both P<0.001), and with both hypertension II and history of diabetes (χ^2=16.85 and 17.07, 1df, both P<0.001).

2. The Magnitude of the Effect of Diabetes and Myocardial Infarction on Women's CHD Risk

Another important question, whether a history of myocardial infarction (MI) carries a similar risk of CHD death as a history of type 2 diabetes does between men and women, is not fully understood. In recent years, several studies have compared the magnitude of the risk of a history of type 2 diabetes and MI on subsequent coronary mortality [16,17,24-29], but the results are inconsistent. The analyses from one Finnish cohort study [24] and from the Nurses' Health Study [25] found that the risk of CHD mortality among subjects with a history of diabetes without prior MI was similar to that in non-diabetic subjects with prior MI. The Health Professionals Follow-up Study [26], a Scottish population-based study [30], the Atherosclerosis Risk in Communities Study [28] and the Multiple Risk Factor Intervention Trial [29], consistently reported that the magnitudes of CHD and CVD mortality were weaker for prior diabetes at baseline than that associated with prior MI.

Five prospective studies compared CHD mortality associated with prior diabetes and established MI in men and women separately [16,17,27,31,32]. In the Hoorn Study, women with prior diabetes at baseline had a risk of CVD events that was similar to that of non-diabetic women with prior CVD, whereas, non-diabetic men with prior CVD conferred a higher risk of CVD events compared with men with prior diabetes and without prior CVD [31]. The analysis from the Framingham Study indicated that in men prior CHD at baseline signified a higher risk for CHD mortality than prior diabetes does; however, this was reversed in women, with prior diabetes being associated with a greater risk for CHD mortality [27]. In one Finnish cohort study [32], diabetes without prior MI and prior MI without diabetes indicated a similar risk for CHD death in men and women.

Recently, we also compared the magnitude of diabetes and MI at baseline and during follow-up on cause-specific and all-cause mortality [16,17]. For the baseline cohort with a mean follow-up period of 12.0 years, we identified 1,119 deaths from all causes among 2,416 patients with prior diabetes and MI at baseline, of which 591 deaths were coded as CHD, 781 deaths as CVD, and 338 deaths as non-CVD. Compared with men with prior diabetes at baseline, men with prior MI had a higher risk of death from CHD (HR 1.78, 95% 1.39-2.27), from CVD (HR 1.43, 95% CI 1.16-1.77), and from all causes (HR 1.22, 95% CI 1.03-1.44) (Table 3). In women, however, those with prior MI had a lower risk of death from CHD (HR 0.57, 95% CI 0.39-0.82), from CVD (HR 0.63, 95% CI 0.47-0.84), and from all causes (HR 0.55, 95% CI 0.43-0.70) compared with women with prior diabetes at baseline. These sex differences in HRs were statistically significant for CHD mortality (χ^2=23.58, 1df, P<0.001), CVD mortality (χ^2=21.21, 1df, P<0.001), and total mortality (χ^2=29.5, 1df, P<0.001). Men and women with both prior diabetes and MI at baseline showed the highest risks of death from CHD, CVD, and all causes.

Table 1. Hazard ratios for coronary heart disease incidence according to status of hypertension and diabetes [18]

| | Hazard ratios (95% Confidence intervals) | | | | | |
| | Men | | | Women | | |
	No hypertension	Hypertension I	Hypertension II	No hypertension	Hypertension I	Hypertension II
No diabetes						
Numbers of participants	8297	7142	6531	12 587	6055	5328
Numbers of cases	612	878	1327	212	370	697
Person-years	151 508	137 660	117 205	245 868	126 333	111 157
Adjustment for age and study year	1.00	1.35 (1.21-1.49)	1.98 (1.80-2.19)	1.00	1.61 (1.35-1.91)	2.61 (2.22-3.06)
Multivariable adjustment†	1.00	1.25 (1.13-1.39)	1.69 (1.53-1.87)	1.00	1.52 (1.28-1.81)	2.37 (2.01-2.79)
Incident diabetes during follow-up						
Numbers of participants	274	444	702	291	434	778
Numbers of cases	46	117	207	31	96	249
Person-years	6297	9496	14 434	7299	9862	17 284
Adjustment for age and study year	1.45 (1.07-1.96)	2.25 (1.85-2.75)	2.43 (2.07-2.84)	2.86 (1.96-4.17)	4.20 (3.28-5.36)	5.32 (4.40-6.42)
Multivariable adjustment†	1.25 (0.93-1.69)	1.83 (1.50-2.25)	1.85 (1.56-2.18)	2.45 (1.67-3.57)	3.78 (2.94-4.85)	4.56 (3.73-5.58)
History of diabetes at baseline						
Numbers of participants	121	144	196	117	135	199
Numbers of cases	26	34	67	13	30	62
Person-years	1732	2088	2413	1863	1887	2932
Adjustment for age and study year	2.54 (1.71-3.76)	2.28 (1.61-3.22)	3.65 (2.83-4.71)	5.88 (3.35-10.3)	6.65 (4.51-9.80)	8.66 (6.49-11.6)
Multivariable adjustment†	2.39 (1.61-3.55)	2.15 (1.52-3.04)	3.31 (2.56-4.28)	5.63 (3.20-9.88)	6.10 (4.13-9.02)	7.41 (5.53-9.94)

* No hypertension was defined as blood pressure <140/90 mmHg and without any antihypertensive drugs treatment at baseline; Hypertension stage I was defined as blood pressure 140-159 and/or 90-94 mmHg, or with any antihypertensive drugs treatment at baseline but blood pressure <160/95 mmHg; Hypertension stage II was defined as blood pressure ≥160/95 mmHg at baseline.

†Multivariable models were adjusted for age, study year, BMI, total cholesterol, education, smoking, alcohol drinking, physical activity, and family history of myocardial infarction.

Table 2. Hazard ratios for coronary heart disease according to status of hypertension and diabetes [18]

Hazard ratios (95% Confidence intervals)

	Men			Women		
	Non hypertension	Hypertension I	Hypertension II	Non hypertension	Hypertension I	Hypertension II
No diabetes						
Numbers of participants	8297	7142	6531	12 587	6055	5328
Numbers of cases	303	530	901	95	210	459
Person-years	154 598	141 929	123 140	246 859	128 163	113 835
Adjustment for age and study year	1.00	1.54 (1.34-1.77)	2.44 (2.14-2.78)	1.00	1.70 (1.33-2.17)	3.02 (2.41-3.79)
Multivariable adjustment†	1.00	1.45 (1.26-1.67)	2.06 (1.81-2.36)	1.00	1.60 (1.25-2.05)	2.70 (2.14-3.41)
Incident diabetes during follow-up						
Numbers of participants	274	444	702	291	434	778
Numbers of cases	22	55	128	20	53	183
Person-years	6527	10 283	15 548	7431	10 351	18 292
Adjustment for age and study year	1.28 (0.83-1.97)	1.82 (1.37-2.43)	2.60 (2.11-3.19)	3.49 (2.16-5.66)	3.78 (2.69-5.32)	6.40 (4.97-8.25)
Multivariable adjustment†	1.08 (0.70-1.67)	1.43 (1.07-1.91)	1.95 (1.57-2.42)	2.90 (1.78-4.71)	3.34 (2.36-4.71)	5.28 (4.05-6.90)
History of diabetes at baseline						
Numbers of participants	121	144	196	117	135	199
Numbers of cases	18	26	49	8	23	51
Person-years	1818	2155	2609	1906	1954	3100
Adjustment for age and study year	3.27 (2.03-5.26)	3.23 (2.16-4.83)	4.81 (3.55-6.52)	7.92 (3.84-16.3)	10.3 (6.49-16.4)	13.3 (9.39-18.8)
Multivariable adjustment†	3.09 (1.92-4.97)	3.08 (2.06-4.61)	4.21 (3.09-5.73)	7.85 (3.80-16.2)	9.24 (5.80-14.7)	10.8 (7.61-15.4)

* No hypertension was defined as blood pressure <140/90 mmHg and without any antihypertensive drugs treatment at baseline; Hypertension stage I was defined as blood pressure 140-159 and/or 90-94 mmHg, or with any antihypertensive drugs treatment at baseline but blood pressure <160/95 mmHg; Hypertension stage II was defined as blood pressure ≥160/95 mmHg at baseline.

†Multivariable models were adjusted for age, study year, BMI, total cholesterol, education, smoking, alcohol drinking, physical activity, and family history of myocardial infarction.

Table 3. Hazard ratios of coronary heart disease, cardiovascular, and total mortality according to the history of diabetes and myocardial infarction at baseline [17]

	Men			Women		
	Prior diabetes	Prior MI*	Prior diabetes and MI*	Prior diabetes	Prior MI*	Prior diabetes and MI*
No. of subjects	496	982	99	466	326	47
Person-years	6070	10529	859	6376	4731	479
Coronary heart disease mortality						
No. of deaths	85	320	42	74	53	17
Mortality rate/10,000 person-years†	117.3	208.5	365.9	88.7	55.6	226.3
Age and study year adjustment HR (95% CI)	1.00	1.87 (1.47-2.38)	2.93 (2.01-4.26)	1.00	0.58 (0.40-0.83)	2.73 (1.58-4.71)
Multivariate adjustment HR (95% CI)‡	1.00	1.78 (1.39-2.27)	2.97 (2.03-4.34)	1.00	0.57 (0.39-0.82)	2.26 (1.29-3.97)
Cardiovascular mortality						
No. of deaths	127	371	56	120	86	21
Mortality rate/10,000 person-years†	173.6	244.4	503.0	148.8	110.4	272.8
Age and study year adjustment HR (95% CI)	1.00	1.46 (1.19-1.79)	2.65 (1.92-3.65)	1.00	0.61 (0.46-0.81)	2.09 (1.30-3.36)
Multivariate adjustment HR (95% CI)‡	1.00	1.43 (1.16-1.77)	2.76 (2.00-3.81)	1.00	0.63 (0.47-0.84)	1.84 (1.13-3.00)
Total mortality						
No. of deaths	207	510	67	192	117	26
Mortality rate/10,000 person-years†	301.0	332.4	598.9	241.8	153.6	330.9
Age and study year adjustment HR (95% CI)	1.00	1.24 (1.05-1.46)	1.97 (1.49-2.61)	1.00	0.54 (0.42-0.68)	1.58 (1.04-2.40)
Multivariate adjustment HR (95% CI)‡	1.00	1.22 (1.03-1.44)	2.08 (1.57-2.76)	1.00	0.55 (0.43-0.70)	1.41 (0.92-2.16)

*MI=myocardial infarction; HR = hazard ratio; CI = confidence interval.

†Age-standardized mortality rate was calculated using a European standard population by 10-year age intervals.

‡Adjusted for age at baseline, study year, body mass index, systolic blood pressure, total cholesterol and smoking.

Table 4. Hazard ratios of coronary heart disease, cardiovascular, and total mortality according to incident diabetes and myocardial infarction during follow-up [17]

	Men			Women		
	Incident diabetes	Incident MI	Incident diabetes and MI	Incident diabetes	Incident MI	Incident diabetes and MI
No. of subjects	981	1308	171	1155	566	134
Person-years	6607	11215	971	9304	4646	662
Coronary heart disease mortality						
No. of deaths	102	365	47	146	126	39
Mortality rate/10,000 person-years†	150.4	301.7	506.9	123.7	190.5	496.7
Age and study year adjustment HR (95% CI)	1.00	2.04 (1.64-2.55)	3.42 (2.42-4.84)	1.00	1.57 (1.23-1.99)	4.18 (2.92-5.98)
Multivariate adjustment HR (95% CI)‡	1.00	2.15 (1.70-2.73)	3.24 (2.28-4.60)	1.00	1.65 (1.27-2.14)	3.91 (2.73-5.60)
Cardiovascular mortality						
No. of deaths	178	418	57	241	147	53
Mortality rate/10,000 person-years†	273.0	346.7	606.0	206.6	222.3	660.4
Age and study year adjustment HR (95% CI)	1.00	1.33 (1.11-1.59)	2.42 (1.79-3.27)	1.00	1.10 (0.90-1.36)	3.43 (2.53-4.63)
Multivariate adjustment HR (95% CI)‡	1.00	1.41 (1.16-1.71)	2.32 (1.71-3.14)	1.00	1.22 (0.98-1.53)	3.22 (2.38-4.36)
Total mortality						
No. of deaths	321	544	79	372	196	66
Mortality rate/10,000 person-years†	499.2	458.2	811.2	325.9	327.4	845.7
Age and study year adjustment HR (95% CI)	1.00	0.95 (0.83-1.10)	1.89 (1.48-2.42)	1.00	0.94 (0.79-1.12)	2.78 (2.13-3.62)
Multivariate adjustment HR (95% CI)‡	1.00	0.95 (0.82-1.11)	1.87 (1.46-2.40)	1.00	1.02 (0.84-1.23)	2.67 (2.05-3.48)

*MI=myocardial infarction; HR=hazard ratio; CI = confidence interval.

†Age-standardized mortality rate was calculated using a European standard population by 10-year age intervals.

‡Adjusted for age at diagnosed date, study year, body mass index, systolic blood pressure, total cholesterol and smoking.

For the follow-up cohort with a mean follow-up period of 7.7 years, we identified 1,578 deaths from all causes among 4,315 patients with incident diabetes or MI, of which 825 deaths were coded as CHD, 1,094 deaths as CVD, and 484 deaths as non-CVD (Table 4). Compared with men and women with incident diabetes, men and women with incident MI had higher multivariate-adjusted HRs of CHD mortality (2.15, 95% CI 1.70-2.73 in men; 1.65, 95% CI 1.27-2.14 in women) and CVD mortality (1.41, 95% CI 1.16-1.71 in men; 1.22, 95% CI 0.98- 1.53 in women), and almost similar HRs of total mortality (0.95, 95% CI 0.82-1.11 in men; 1.02, 95% CI 0.84-1.23 in women). There was no sex difference in CHD, CVD, and all-cause mortality (χ^2=1.30, 0.59, and 0.23, respectively, 1df, all P>0.1). Men and women with both incident diabetes and MI showed the highest risks of CHD and total mortality.

Conclusion

Diabetes is a major public health, clinical, and economical problem in modern societies, and also increases the risk of CHD among men and women. The combination of hypertension and diabetes increases the risk of CHD drastically. Diabetes and MI, either present at baseline or during follow-up, markedly increase the risk of CHD death. In men, MI at baseline or during follow-up confers a greater risk on CHD mortality than diabetes does. In women, prior MI at baseline confers a lower risk on CHD mortality than prior diabetes does, but incident MI during follow-up confers a greater risk than incident diabetes does. There is a gender difference of diabetes on the risk of CHD. The results of our study have important implications for clinical practice: First, we need to consider carefully the treatment strategies on individual disease status, particularly type 2 diabetes in women, for the future CVD risk. Furthermore, in order to reduce CVD mortality, more active management and prevention of diabetes are needed.

References

[1]   Murray, C. J. and Lopez, A. D. (1997) Mortality by cause for eight regions of the world: Global Burden of Disease Study. *Lancet.* 349, 1269-1276

[2]   World Health Organisation. Diet, nutrition, and the prevention of chronic diseases. WHO Technical Report Series 916. Geneva, World Health Organisation, 2003.

[3]   Thom, T., Haase, N., Rosamond, W., Howard, V. J., Rumsfeld, J., Manolio, T., Zheng, Z. J., Flegal, K., O'Donnell, C., Kittner, S., Lloyd-Jones, D., Goff, D. C., Jr., Hong, Y., Adams, R., Friday, G., Furie, K., Gorelick, P., Kissela, B., Marler, J., Meigs, J., Roger, V., Sidney, S., Sorlie, P., Steinberger, J., Wasserthiel-Smoller, S., Wilson, M. and Wolf, P. (2006) Heart disease and stroke statistics--2006 update: a report from the American Heart Association Statistics Committee and Stroke Statistics Subcommittee. *Circulation.* 113, e85-151

[4]   WHO Scientific Group: Cardiovascular disease risk factors: new areas for research. Geneva, World Health Organization, 1994.

[5]   Willett, W. C. (1994) Diet and health: what should we eat? *Science*. 264, 532-537

[6]   Tunstall-Pedoe, H., Kuulasmaa, K., Amouyel, P., Arveiler, D., Rajakangas, A. M. and Pajak, A. (1994) Myocardial infarction and coronary deaths in the World Health Organization MONICA Project. Registration procedures, event rates, and case-fatality rates in 38 populations from 21 countries in four continents. *Circulation*. 90, 583-612.

[7]   Jousilahti, P., Vartiainen, E., Tuomilehto, J. and Puska, P. (1999) Sex, age, cardiovascular risk factors, and coronary heart disease: a prospective follow-up study of 14 786 middle-aged men and women in Finland. *Circulation*. 99, 1165-1172.

[8]   Wild, S., Roglic, G., Green, A., Sicree, R. and King, H. (2004) Global prevalence of diabetes: estimates for the year 2000 and projections for 2030. *Diabetes Care*. 27, 1047-1053

[9]   Laakso, M. (1999) Hyperglycemia and cardiovascular disease in type 2 diabetes. *Diabetes*. 48, 937-942

[10]   Assmann, G. and Schulte, H. (1988) The Prospective Cardiovascular Munster (PROCAM) study: prevalence of hyperlipidemia in persons with hypertension and/or diabetes mellitus and the relationship to coronary heart disease. *Am Heart J*. 116, 1713-1724

[11]   Stamler, J., Vaccaro, O., Neaton, J. D. and Wentworth, D. (1993) Diabetes, other risk factors, and 12-yr cardiovascular mortality for men screened in the Multiple Risk Factor Intervention Trial. *Diabetes Care*. 16, 434-444

[12]   Hu, G., Jousilahti, P. and Tuomilehto, J. (2007) Joint effects of history of hypertension at baseline and type 2 diabetes at baseline and during follow-up on the risk of coronary heart disease. *Eur Heart J*.

[13]   Kannel, W. B. and McGee, D. L. (1979) Diabetes and cardiovascular disease. The Framingham study. *Jama*. 241, 2035-2038.

[14]   Muller, W. A. (1998) Diabetes mellitus--long time survival. *J Insur Med*. 30, 17-27

[15]   DECODE Study Group. (2001) Glucose tolerance and cardiovascular mortality: comparison of fasting and 2-hour diagnostic criteria. *Arch Intern Med*. 161, 397-405

[16]   Hu, G., Jousilahti, P., Qiao, Q., Katoh, S. and Tuomilehto, J. (2005) Sex differences in cardiovascular and total mortality among diabetic and non-diabetic individuals with or without history of myocardial infarction. *Diabetologia*. 48, 856-861

[17]   Hu, G., Jousilahti, P., Qiao, Q., Peltonen, M., Katoh, S. and Tuomilehto, J. (2005) The gender-specific impact of diabetes and myocardial infarction at baseline and during follow-up on mortality from all causes and coronary heart disease. *J Am Coll Cardiol*. 45, 1413-1418

[18]   Hu, G., Jousilahti, P. and Tuomilehto, J. (2007) Joint effects of history of hypertension at baseline and type 2 diabetes at baseline and during follow-up on the risk of coronary heart disease. *Eur Heart J*. 28, 3059-3066

[19]   Barrett-Connor, E. L., Cohn, B. A., Wingard, D. L. and Edelstein, S. L. (1991) Why is diabetes mellitus a stronger risk factor for fatal ischemic heart disease in women than in men? The Rancho Bernardo Study. *Jama*. 265, 627-631.

[20]   Janghorbani, M., Jones, R. B., Gilmour, W. H., Hedley, A. J. and Zhianpour, M. (1994) A prospective population based study of gender differential in mortality from

cardiovascular disease and "all causes" in asymptomatic hyperglycaemics. *J Clin Epidemiol.* 47, 397-405.

[21] Orchard, T. J. (1996) The impact of gender and general risk factors on the occurrence of atherosclerotic vascular disease in non-insulin-dependent diabetes mellitus. *Ann Med.* 28, 323-333.

[22] Kanaya, A. M., Grady, D. and Barrett-Connor, E. (2002) Explaining the sex difference in coronary heart disease mortality among patients with type 2 diabetes mellitus: a meta-analysis. *Arch Intern Med.* 162, 1737-1745

[23] Hu, G. (2003) Gender difference in all-cause and cardiovascular mortality related to hyperglycaemia and newly-diagnosed diabetes. *Diabetologia.* 46, 608-617

[24] Haffner, S. M., Lehto, S., Ronnemaa, T., Pyorala, K. and Laakso, M. (1998) Mortality from coronary heart disease in subjects with type 2 diabetes and in nondiabetic subjects with and without prior myocardial infarction. *N Engl J Med.* 339, 229-234.

[25] Hu, F. B., Stampfer, M. J., Solomon, C. G., Liu, S., Willett, W. C., Speizer, F. E., Nathan, D. M. and Manson, J. E. (2001) The impact of diabetes mellitus on mortality from all causes and coronary heart disease in women: 20 years of follow-up. *Arch Intern Med.* 161, 1717-1723.

[26] Lotufo, P. A., Gaziano, J. M., Chae, C. U., Ajani, U. A., Moreno-John, G., Buring, J. E. and Manson, J. E. (2001) Diabetes and all-cause and coronary heart disease mortality among US male physicians. *Arch Intern Med.* 161, 242-247

[27] Natarajan, S., Liao, Y., Cao, G., Lipsitz, S. R. and McGee, D. L. (2003) Sex differences in risk for coronary heart disease mortality associated with diabetes and established coronary heart disease. *Arch Intern Med.* 163, 1735-1740

[28] Lee, C. D., Folsom, A. R., Pankow, J. S. and Brancati, F. L. (2004) Cardiovascular events in diabetic and nondiabetic adults with or without history of myocardial infarction. *Circulation.* 109, 855-860

[29] Vaccaro, O., Eberly, L. E., Neaton, J. D., Yang, L., Riccardi, G. and Stamler, J. (2004) Impact of diabetes and previous myocardial infarction on long-term survival: 25-year mortality follow-up of primary screenees of the Multiple Risk Factor Intervention Trial. *Arch Intern Med.* 164, 1438-1443

[30] Evans, J. M., Wang, J. and Morris, A. D. (2002) Comparison of cardiovascular risk between patients with type 2 diabetes and those who had had a myocardial infarction: cross sectional and cohort studies. *Bmj.* 324, 939-942

[31] Becker A, Bos G, de Vegt F, Kostense PJ, Dekker JM, Nijpels G, Heine RJ, Bouter LM and CD., S. (2003) Cardiovascular events in type 2 diabetes: comparison with nondiabetic individuals without and with prior cardiovascular disease. 10-year follow-up of the Hoorn Study. *Eur Heart J.* 24, 1406-1413

[32] Juutilainen, A., Lehto, S., Ronnemaa, T., Pyorala, K. and Laakso, M. (2005) Type 2 diabetes as a "coronary heart disease equivalent": an 18-year prospective population-based study in Finnish subjects. *Diabetes Care.* 28, 2901-2907

In: Heart Disease in Women
Editor: B. V. Larner and H. R. Pennelton

ISBN 978-1-60692-066-4
© 2009 Nova Science Publishers, Inc.

Chapter V

The Impact of Heart Rate as a Cardiovascular Risk

*Taku Inoue and Kunitoshi Iseki**

Department of Clinical Pharmacology and Therapeutics, University of the Ryukyus,
Nishihara, Okinawa, Japan
*Dialysis Unit, University Hospital of the Ryukyus, Nishihara, Okinawa, Japan

Abstract

An elevated heart rate can indicate a patient's risk for cardiovascular disease. A large number of population-based studies have demonstrated an association between elevated heart rate and cardiovascular disease as well as all-cause mortality with and without diagnosed cardiovascular disease. Despite accumulating evidence of its significance, elevated heart rate remains neglected as a cardiovascular risk factor. From the preventive point of view, heart rate may be a useful biomeasurement for identifying subjects at risk for hypertension, metabolic syndrome, and cardiovascular events. By identifying subjects with these conditions, targeted and cost-effective cardiovascular disease prevention programs can be planned. Previous findings also suggest that heart rate modulation should be considered in the treatment of cardiovascular disease. There is a linear relationship between heart rate reduction and a reduction in mortality rate. Tachycardia is a strong marker of widespread abnormality of the autonomic control of the circulation. This autonomic nervous system imbalance could explain the association between elevated heart rate and hypertension, metabolic syndrome, and cardiovascular events. Unfortunately, lowering the heart rate is not currently a clinically recognized therapeutic goal. Prospective trials are needed to investigate the heart rate levels that should be considered hazardous and whether treatment of high heart rate can prevent cardiovascular events.

Introduction

Heart rate is an easily obtained source of biologic information that does not require special instruments or advanced techniques. As a sensitive indicator of autonomous nervous system activity, heart rate varies in response to positional, psychic, and environmental circumstances; thus, most physicians believe that heart rate is not a reliable prognostic marker and is therefore unsuitable for use in clinical research. Despite these issues, numerous studies have identified elevated heart rate as an independent risk factor for cardiovascular disease comparable with classical risk factors such as smoking, dyslipidemia, and hypertension. Pathophysiologic studies indicate that a relatively high heart rate has direct detrimental effects on the progression of coronary atherosclerosis, the occurrence of myocardial ischemia and ventricular arrhythmias, and on left ventricular function.

Among mammals, life expectancy can be represented by algometric scales that are based on heart rate. Heart rate in mammals represents an inverse semi-logarithmic relation to life expectancy: that is, smaller mammals have a higher heart rate and a shorter life span than do larger mammals [1] (Figure 1). In contrast to life expectancy, the number of heart beats per lifetime is incredibly constant. This suggests that life span is controlled by energetics. Table 1 indicates the cardiac parameters of one of the smallest mammals, a shrew weighing 2 g, and one of the largest mammals, a blue whale weighing 100,000 kg; despite their huge differences in size, stroke volume, and cardiac output, the total oxygen consumption and ATP usage per unit mass and lifetime and the total number of heart beats per lifetime are almost identical.

Table 1. Cardiac parameters of one of the smallest and one of the largest living mammalians

Parameter	Shrew	Blue whale	Fold difference
Body weight (kg)	0.002	100000	50000000
Heart weight (kg)	0.000012	600	50000000
Heart rate (bpm)	1000	6	170
Stroke volume (liters)	1.22×10^{-6}	350	300000000
Cardiac output (L / min)	0.0001	2098	2200000
Circulation time (s)	6	2236	370
Cardiac cycle (s)	0.06	10	170
Blood volume (L)	0.000116	8260	70000000
Maximum lifespan (years)	1	118	120
Maximum heart beats (beats / lifetime)	6.57×10^8	1.1×10^9	1.7
Mass-specific O_2 consumption (L O_2 / kg per h)	3.20	0.038	0.012
Total O_2 consumed (L O_2 / kg per lifetime)	35000	39300	1.1
Mol ATP / kg per lifetime	7813	8771	1.1
Total blood (L) pumped per lifetime (liter)	800	1.3×10^{11}	163000000
Blood (L) pumped / lifetime per kg heart	6.67×10^7	2.17×10^7	3.3

The aim of this paper is to review the data of the association of heart rate with cardiovascular risk, mortality, the possible pathophysiology of these associations, and the therapeutic utility of heart rate - lowering drugs for improving cardiovascular outcomes in a wide range of patients.

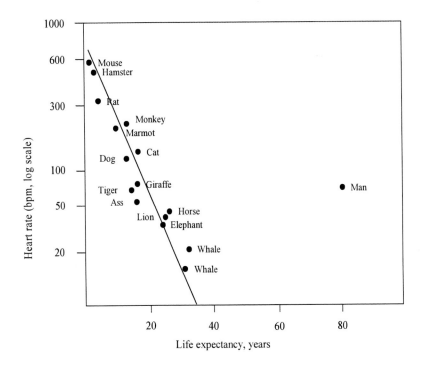

Figure 1. Relationship between resting heart rate in logarithmic scale and life expectancy in mammals.

1. Heart Rate as a Predictor of Risk for Cardiovascular Disorders: Epidemiologic Observations

The first evidence of an association between heart rate and cardiovascular mortality was demonstrated more than 60 years ago by Levy et al. [3], who reported that the incidence of cardiovascular death among subjects with sustained tachycardia was much higher than that in subjects with a normal heart rate. Since then, numerous studies have demonstrated that elevated heart rate is associated with cardiovascular and all-cause mortality. The predictive power of heart rate for cardiovascular disease is observed in general populations [4-10], elderly subjects [11-14], hypertensive cohorts 11 12 15 16, patients with stable coronary artery disease [17-19 20] (Table 2).

Table 2. Main studies on high resisting heart rate as cardiovascular risk factor

Authors	Study name	Reference
Coronary artery disease		
Wong et al.	Framingham	Am J Epidemiol 1989. 130. 469-480
Disegni et al.	SPRINT	J Clin Epidemiol 1995; 48: 1197-1205
Hjalmarson et al.		Am J Cardiol 1990.65.547
Diaz et al.	CASS	Eur Heart J 2005; 26:967-974
		Am J Epidemiol 1980;112:736-749
		Am Heart J 1985;109:876-885
		Am Heart J 1987;113:1489-1494
		Am Heart J 1988;116:163-174
		Am Heart J 1991; 121: 172-177
		Arch Intern Med. 1996;156:505-509
		Hypertension 1999;33:44-52
		Circulation 1996;99:1978-1983
		Am Heart J 1993; 125: 1148-1154
		Am J Cardiol 1996;78:1175-1176
		Hypertension 2001;37:1256-1261
		Arch Intern Med. 2002;162:2313-2321
Aronow et al.		Am J Cardiol 1996;78:1175-1176
Palatini et al.	CASTEL	Arch Intern Med.1999.159.181-
Moneotti et al.	FINE	J Clin Epidemiol 2001;54:680-686
Palatini et al.	Syst-Eur	Arch Intern Med. 2002;162:2313-2321
Benetos et al.	French ICP	J Hypertens. 2005;23:1803-1808

Table1 Cardiac parameters of one of the smallest and one of the largest living mammalians

Parameter	Shrew	Blue whale	Fold difference
Body weight (kg)	0.002	100000	50000000
Heart weight (kg)	0.000012	600	50000000
Heart rate (bpm)	1000	6	170
Stroke volume (liters)	1.22×10^{-4}	350	300000000
Cardiac output (L / min)	0.0001	2098	2200000
Circulation time (s)	6	2236	370
Cardiac cycle (s)	0.06	10	170
Blood volume (L)	0.000116	8260	70000000
Maximum lifespan (years)	1	118	120
Maximum heart beats (beats / lifetime)	6.57×10^8	1.1×10^9	1.7
Mass-specific O_2 consumption (L O_2 / kg per h)	3.20	0.038	0.012
Total O_2 consumed (L O_2 / kg per lifetime)	35000	39300	1.1
Mol ATP / kg per lifetime	7813	8771	1.1
Total blood (L) pumped per lifetime (liter)	800	1.3×10^{11}	163000000
Blood (L) pumped / lifetime per kg heart	6.67×10^7	2.17×10^7	3.3

2. Risk of Elevated Heart Rate on Cardiovascular Mortality in General Population

To examine the potential of heart rate as a prognostic factor for cardiovascular and coronary heart disease mortality, three epidemiologic studies were conducted 20 years ago 5. The associations between heart rate and death from cardiovascular diseases, coronary artery disease, and sudden cardiac death from coronary heart disease, as well as death from all causes, were studied prospectively in middle-aged white male employees: 1233 men aged 40 to 59 years followed for 15 years in the Chicago Peoples Gas Company study; 1899 men aged 40 to 55 years followed for 17 years in the Chicago Western Electric Company study; and 5784 men aged 45 to 64 years followed for 5 years in the Chicago Heart Association Detection Project in Industry study. Univariate analysis revealed that mortality from cardiovascular or noncardiovascular causes increased with an increase in heart rate. Cox regression analysis controlling for age and risk factors demonstrated that elevated heart rate was a significant risk factor for sudden death due to coronary heart disease and non-cardiovascular disease in two of the three studies.

The Framingham Heart Study [7], in which 5070 individuals free of cardiac disease were enrolled, demonstrated a relationship between heart rate and cardiovascular mortality. During the 30-year study period, a total of 1876 subjects died, of which 894 were cardiovascular death. In both sexes, all-cause, cardiovascular, and coronary artery disease mortality increased progressively in relation to the baseline heart rates, independent of preexisting cardiac damage. A substantial excess of noncardiovascular deaths at high heart rates was also observed.

In the NHANES I Epidemiologic Follow-up Study[9], 7594 black and white subjects aged 25 to 74 years old at the time of the initial survey were screened and followed up for an average of 9.9 years for white subjects and 10.3 years for black subjects. The adjusted relative risk for coronary heart disease incidence was significantly higher in white men and women, with a pulse rate over 84 beats/min, than in those with a pulse rate under 74 beats/min. The adjusted risks for death from all causes, cardiovascular diseases, and non-cardiovascular diseases were also elevated for white men, but not women, with raised pulse rate. The adjusted risks for death from all causes and cardiovascular diseases were also increased in black men and women with an elevated pulse rate.

Benetos et al. studied a large French population (19 386; 12 123 men, 7263 women), aged 40 to 69 years to assess the effects of heart rate on mortality in different subgroups [10]. Their result indicated that heart rate was a significant predictor of noncardiovascular mortality in both sexes. In men, djusted relative risk for cardiovascular death in the highest quartile was approximately 2.2 times higher than those in the lowest quartiles. In women, however, there was no heart rate-mortality relation observed. The association of heart rate with cardiovascular mortality in men was independent of age and hypertension, and strongly associated with coronary, but not cerebrovascular mortality.

Risk of Elevated Heart Rate for Hypertension and in the Elderly

Hypertensive patients generally have a higher heart rate than do comparable normotensive persons [8]. Gillman et al. followed 4530 hypertensive patients aged 35 to 74 years old from the Framingham Heart Study for 36 years [15]. They demonstrated that the adjusted odds ratios (95% confidence intervals) for each 40 beats/min increment in heart rate were: for all-cause mortality, 2.18 (1.68-2.83) for men and 2.14 (1.59-2.88) for women; and for cardiovascular mortality, 1.68 (1.19-2.37) for men and 1.70 (1.08-2.67) for women. Excluding the subjects that died within the first 2 or 4 years did not change the results. This means that elevated heart is not merely an indicator of preexisting illness, but that it is an independent risk factor for cardiovascular death in those with hypertension. The impact of heart rate on mortality is consistent in patients with known coronary heart disease [7 9] and those who survived myocardial infarction [17]. These data suggest that treatment regimens for hypertension may need to include heart rate-lowering drugs.

Aronow et al. [11] prospectively examined 1311 elderly patients (60-100 years, mean age 81 years) who had hypertensive or other forms of heart disease for 48 months. They evaluated the risk for high heart rate and the incidence of new coronary events. Their data indicated that a 5 beats/min heart-rate increase leads to a 1.14 times higher probability of developing a new coronary event.

In the Syst-Eru Trial [12], a total of 4682 elderly subjects with systolic hypertension were studied to examine the association of heart rate with total, cardiovascular, and noncardiovascular death. An elevated baseline heart rate was positively associated with a worse prognosis for total, cardiovascular, and noncardiovascular mortality among the 2293 men and women taking a placebo. Subjects with heart rates higher than 79 bpm had a 1.89 times greater risk of mortality than subjects with heart rate of 79 bpm or less. Cox regression analysis also indicated that heart rate is a significant predictor of time to death.

The risk of elevated heart rate for cardiovascular death in the elderly was evaluated in the CASTEL study 14. Palatini et al. examined 763 white men and 1175 women aged 65 years or older and evaluated the association between heart rate and mortality. They showed that the relative risk (95% confidence intervals) for cardiovascular death in men was 1.38 (0.94 - 2.03) in the top quintile of heart rate and 0.82 (0.52 - 1.28) for those in the bottom quintile. In the Cox analysis, heart rate was a predictor of time to cardiovascular death ($p < 0.001$). The heart rate-mortality association, however, was not evident in women. Benetos et al. evaluated the predictive value of clinical and biologic parameters assessed in subjects aged 60 to 70 years of age, in the survival to 80 years for men and 85 years for women 21. The multivariate analysis revealed that the odds ratio (95% confidence intervals) of late survival with a heart rate > 80bpm was 0.77 (0.66 - 0.91) after adjustment for age, sex, personal history of cardiovascular disease, and forced expiratory volume.

Recent Epidemiologic Data Relating Heart Rate and Outcome

Three large recent studies expanded our understanding of the importance of heart rate. In the Paris Prospective Study I [22], a total of 5713 middle aged working men, none of whom had known cardiovascular disease, were followed up for 23 years. The risk of sudden death from myocardial infarction was increased in subjects with a resting heart rate greater than 75 bpm (RR 3.92; 95% CI, 1.91 - 8.00). After adjustment for potential confounding variables, a resting elevated heart rate remained strongly associated with an increased risk of sudden death, as well as a moderate but significantly increased risk of death from any cause, but no increased risk of nonsudden death from myocardial infarction. Diaz et al. explored the prognostic value of heart rate in 24913 patients with coronary artery disease from the Coronary Artery Surgery Study registry with a median follow-up of 14.7 years [19]. All-cause and cardiovascular mortality and cardiovascular re-hospitalizations were significantly increased with an increase in heart rate. Patients with a resting heart rate ≥ 83 bpm at baseline had a significantly higher risk for total mortality (Hazard ratio 1.32, 95% CI 1.19-1.47) and cardiovascular mortality (Hazard ratio 1.31, 95% CI 1.15-1.48) after adjustment for multiple clinical variables when compared with the reference group. Iddo Z et al. noted the importance of heart rate reduction during sleep evaluation of 3957 patients aged 55±16 years, 58% of which were treated for hypertension [23]. They demonstrated that heart rate measures during sleep, and in particular the absence of heart rate slowing, were independently associated with all-cause mortality.

Gender Difference

The resting heart rate in women is 6 to 14 bpm faster than that of men throughout all age ranges, even after adjustment for multiple variables[8]. A number of previous studies in younger subjects have shown that the association between heart rate and all-cause and cardiovascular mortality was weaker or even absent in women [7 14 24]. Recent data from the France IPC study also demonstrated that men, but not women, with heart rate > 80 bpm had a 20% lower probability of surviving after the age of 80 years (odds ratio 0.80, 95% confidence interval 0.69-0.90) as compared to subjects with a heart rate ≤ 80 bpm[21]. Several hypotheses may explain this sex difference in heart rate. The mechanisms for an elevated heart rate can differ among men and women [25]. The sex difference may, in part, be explained by heart rate-blood pressure interaction. The muscle sympathetic nerve activity of female subjects was significantly lower than that of male subjects instead of having same heart rate. In male but not female subjects with faster heart rates, higher levels of muscle sympathetic nerve activity are associated with higher blood pressure[26]. Further, due to their hormonal state, premenopausal women are thought to be protected from the 'deleterious' effects of an elevated heart rate.

Heart Rate and Cardiovascular Risk Factors, Risk Stratification

Numerous studies report that elevated heart rate correlates with increased blood pressure [3 27] and is also a predictor of the future development of hypertension [3 27-29]. Individuals with tachycardia have characteristic features of insulin resistance syndrome, including high blood pressure, obesity, increased blood glucose and insulin levels, and an abnormal lipid profile [30], as well as clustering of these features [31]. This suggests that an increased heart rate can be indicative of a patient's risk for cardiovascular disease, and thus, metabolic syndrome. Tomiyama et al. reported that elevated heart rate predicts the development of metabolic syndrome in middle-aged Japanese men (age: 41±8 years). According to their 3-year follow-up study, the adjusted odds ratio for developing metabolic syndrome in subjects with an elevated heart rate (≥69 bpm) was approximately 3.6 times higher than those with lower heart rate (<69 bpm) [32].

There have been various attempts to integrate the clinical variables into a risk model for identifying the subjects at moderate to high cardiovascular risk [33-36]. Risk stratification is important for determining the prognosis of subjects at moderate to high cardiovascular risk and planning targeted and cost-effective cardiovascular disease prevention programs. These risk scores require blood samples to determine serum lipid levels to include in the calculation, in addition to anthropometric measurements. Moreover, calculation of the risk score is somewhat complicated for routine clinical use. Measuring heart rate is a simple process that does not require special instruments or advanced techniques, and is thus an easy way to identify individuals with high cardiovascular risk and those who may therefore benefit to a greater extent by preventive treatments. Higher heart rate should be considered an indicator of the potential to develop metabolic syndrome, as well as cardiovascular events and death.

Pathophysiologic Mechanisms

The pathogenetic mechanisms connecting elevated heart rate with hypertension, atherosclerosis, and cardiovascular events are well-studied. An elevated heart rate is caused by an imbalance in central nervous system activity, leading to increased sympathetic and decreased parasympathetic tone. This autonomic nervous system abnormality might explain the connection between heart rate and cardiovascular events. Elevated heart rate, which is representative of sympathetic over-activity, is closely associated with blood pressure; levels of fasting glucose, insulin and serum lipids [37]; and clustering of several risk factors [31]. This autonomic imbalance also plays a critical role in potentially lethal cardiac arrhythmias [38] and may cause ventricular arrhythmia and sudden death.

Elevated heart rate not only serves as a marker of cardiovascular risk factors or clustering of risk factors, but also causes mechanical damage to the cardiovascular system. Experimental data indicate that blood flow changes associated with elevated heart rate are favorable for the formation of atherosclerotic lesions. An elevated heart rate itself intensifies pulsatile stress, which may cause endothelial injury [39]. A heart rate reduction can delay the progression of coronary atherosclerosis in monkeys [40 41]. Beere et al. also demonstrated that male cynomolgus monkeys subjected to sinus node ablation or those with naturally low heart rates had significantly less coronary atherosclerosis than animals with higher heart rates [40].

The hemodynamic stress produced by an increase in heart rate intensifies cardiac work and oxygen consumption, shortens the diastolic period, which regulates the coronary flow, a situation that is especially crucial for individuals with coronary artery disease. Clinical data reveal that an elevated heart rate may facilitate coronary plaque disruption, whereas beta blocker therapy has a protective effect [42]. Heart rate elevation also deteriorates arterial stiffness. Lantelme et al. demonstrated the effect of heart rate changes on arterial stiffness accessed by measuring pulse wave velocity at five different pacing frequencies in elderly men [43]. Their results indicated that pulse wave velocity increased gradually with an increase in heart rate and the average difference between pulse wave velocity at 100 and 60 bpm was 1.36 ± 2.9 m/s.

A high heart rate increases myocardial oxygen consumption and shortens the diastolic period, which leads to decreases in coronary perfusion time, both of which can induce or exacerbate myocardial ischemia. Since the fast heart rate per se causes cardiovascular damage, all drugs that lower the heart rate have the potential to further reduce cardiovascular events in patients with an elevated heart rate.

Heart Rate-Lowering Therapy

Reduction of heart rate appears to be a reasonable additional goal of antihypertensive therapy, especially in subjects with augmented sympathetic tone. To date, there are only retrospective analyses of clinical trials performed to demonstrate the effect of lowering heart rate using beta blockers in patients with acute myocardial infarction or congestive heart failure [44 45] (Figure 2); heart rate-lowering therapy using beta blockers was effective only in subjects with a high baseline heart rate and was completely ineffective in those with a low baseline heart rate in both clinical settings. This finding is because of the lack of relationship between sympathetic activity and blood pressure in subjects with a lower heart rate [26]. The heart rate-lowering effect remains the main determinant of the anti-ischemic action by beta blockers. Lowering the heart rate leads to reduced myocardial oxygen consumption. Moreover, lowering the heart rate prolongs the diastolic period, which leads to increased coronary perfusion time, both of which reduce myocardial ischemia.

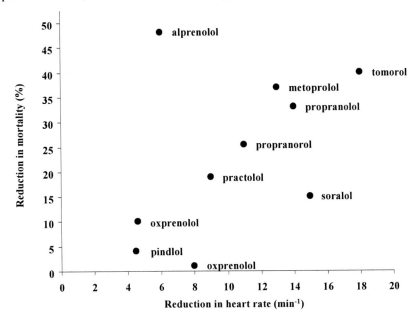

Figure 2. Relationship between reduction in heart rate and reduction in mortality from several large prospective double-blind trials with beta blockers.

Besides heart rate-lowering drugs, it is important to note that heart rate is also affected by lifestyle related factors. Lifestyle modification such as fish consumption is associated with a lower heart rate. Dallongeville et al. examined 9758 men, age 50 to 59 years, without coronary heart disease to examine the association between fish consumption and heart rate [46]. According to their results, heart rate decreased across the categories of fish intake (P<0.0001). After adjustment for age, center, education level, physical activity, smoking habit, alcohol consumption, body mass index, and antiarrhythmic medications, heart rate among fish consumers remained significantly lower than that among non-consumers (P for trend <0.0001). The docosahexaenoic acid content of erythrocyte phospholipids was inversely correlated with heart rate (P<0.03). Endurance training increases parasympathetic activity and decreases sympathetic activity in the human heart at rest [47].

Recent studies in patients with coronary artery disease indicate that exercise therapy led to superior event-free survival, lower costs, reduced rehospitalizations and repeat revascularizations compared with percutaneous coronary intervention [48]. We therefore should consider the non-pharmacological approach for reducing heart rate in patients with coronary artery disease.

Unlike the mounting evidence for elevated heart rate as a potent predictor of cardiovascular morbidity and mortality, there are no objective evidence for establishing the optimal heart rate for a growing individual. Previous results of studies performed in general populations or hypertensive subjects indicated that a value between 80 and 85 bpm is a reasonable cut-off level [49] (Table 3). Recent data from 106 patients that underwent coronary angiography demonstrated that a heart rate greater than 80bpm facilitates coronary plaque disruption, whereas beta blocker therapy had a protective effect[42]. More recently, the 83-bpm cut-off point identified by Diaz et al. [19] is consistent with previous results. This means that heart rate-lowering therapy for those with a heart rate over 80 to 85 bpm might be beneficial. However, we have no prospective results indicating that heart rate-lowering therapy may be beneficial for the subjects in this condition.

Conclusion

The clinical and experimental data reviewed here provide the association between elevated heart rate and cardiovascular risk factors, metabolic syndrome, developing atherosclerosis, increased incidence of mortality in persons with coronary artery disease, hypertension, elderly, and general population. Heart rate is considered as a useful and cost-effective bio-measurement for identifying the subjects at risk of cardiovascular disease. Physicians should pay attention to elevated heart rate as a harmful sign of health, especially subjects with coronary artery disease, hypertension, and elderly. Heart rate lowering therapy should be taken into account in the medical treatment strategy. As the heart rate lowering is not recognized as a clinical target, the effect of heart rate lowering has never been examined in randomized clinical trials in such patients with stable coronary artery disease or hypertension. Prospective trials examining whether heart rate lowering therapy can prevent cardiovascular events, especially in hypertensive patients, are warranted.

References

[1]   Levine HJ. Rest heart rate and life expectancy. *J. Am. Coll. Cardiol.* 1997;30(4):1104-6.

[2]   Dobson GP. On being the right size: heart design, mitochondrial efficiency and lifespan potential. *Clin. Exp. Pharmacol. Physiol* .2003;30(8):590-7.

[3]   Levy RL, White PD, Stround WD, Hillman CC. Transient tachycardia: prognostic significance alone and in association with transient hypertension. *JAMA* 1945;129:585-588.

[4]   Jouven X, Desnos M, Guerot C, Ducimetiere P. Predicting sudden death in the population: the Paris Prospective Study I. *Circulation* 1999;99(15):1978-83.

[5]   Dyer AR, Persky V, Stamler J, Paul O, Shekelle RB, Berkson DM, et al. Heart rate as a prognostic factor for coronary heart disease and mortality: findings in three Chicago epidemiologic studies. *Am. J. Epidemiol.* 1980;112(6):736-49.

[6]   Kannel WB, Wilson P, Blair SN. Epidemiological assessment of the role of physical activity and fitness in development of cardiovascular disease. *Am. Heart J.* 1985;109(4):876-85.

[7]   Kannel WB, Kannel C, Paffenbarger RS, Jr., Cupples LA. Heart rate and cardiovascular mortality: the Framingham Study. *Am. Heart J.*1987;113(6):1489-94.

[8]   Gillum RF. The epidemiology of resting heart rate in a national sample of men and women: associations with hypertension, coronary heart disease, blood pressure, and other cardiovascular risk factors. *Am. Heart J.* 1988;116(1 Pt 1):163-74.

[9]   Gillum RF, Makuc DM, Feldman JJ. Pulse rate, coronary heart disease, and death: the NHANES I Epidemiologic Follow-up Study. *Am. Heart J.* 1991;121(1 Pt 1):172-7.

[10]   Benetos A, Rudnichi A, Thomas F, Safar M, Guize L. Influence of heart rate on mortality in a French population: role of age, gender, and blood pressure. *Hypertension* 1999;33(1):44-52.

[11]   Aronow WS, Ahn C, Mercando AD, Epstein S. Association of average heart rate on 24-hour ambulatory electrocardiograms with incidence of new coronary events at 48-month follow-up in 1,311 patients (mean age 81 years) with heart disease and sinus rhythm. *Am. J. Cardiol.*1996;78(10):1175-6.

[12]   Palatini P, Thijs L, Staessen JA, Fagard RH, Bulpitt CJ, Clement DL, et al. Predictive value of clinic and ambulatory heart rate for mortality in elderly subjects with systolic hypertension. *Arch. Intern. Med.* 2002;162(20):2313-21.

[13]   Menotti A, Mulder I, Nissinen A, Giampaoli S, Feskens EJ, Kromhout D. Prevalence of morbidity and multimorbidity in elderly male populations and their impact on 10-year all-cause mortality: The FINE study (Finland, Italy, Netherlands, Elderly). *J Clin Epidemiol* 2001;54(7):680-6.

[14]   Palatini P, Casiglia E, Julius S, Pessina AC. High heart rate: a risk factor for cardiovascular death in elderly men. *Arch. Intern. Med.* 1999;159(6):585-92.

[15]   Gillman MW, Kannel WB, Belanger A, D'Agostino RB. Influence of heart rate on mortality among persons with hypertension: the Framingham Study. *Am. Heart J.* 1993;125(4):1148-54.

[16]   Thomas F, Rudnichi A, Bacri AM, Bean K, Guize L, Benetos A. Cardiovascular mortality in hypertensive men according to presence of associated risk factors. *Hypertension* 2001;37(5):1256-61.

[17]   Hjalmarson A, Gilpin EA, Kjekshus J, Schieman G, Nicod P, Henning H, et al. Influence of heart rate on mortality after acute myocardial infarction. *Am. J. Cardiol.* 1990;65(9):547-53.

[18]   Wong ND, Cupples LA, Ostfeld AM, Levy D, Kannel WB. Risk factors for long-term coronary prognosis after initial myocardial infarction: the Framingham Study. *Am. J. Epidemiol* .1989;130(3):469-80.

[19]   Diaz A, Bourassa MG, Guertin MC, Tardif JC. Long-term prognostic value of resting heart rate in patients with suspected or proven coronary artery disease. *Eur. Heart J.* 2005;26(10):967-74.

[20]   Disegni E, Goldbourt U, Reicher-Reiss H, Kaplinsky E, Zion M, Boyko V, et al. The predictive value of admission heart rate on mortality in patients with acute myocardial

infarction. SPRINT Study Group. Secondary Prevention Reinfarction Israeli Nifedipine Trial. *J. Clin. Epidemiol.* 1995;48(10):1197-205.

[21] Benetos A, Thomas F, Bean KE, Pannier B, Guize L. Role of modifiable risk factors in life expectancy in the elderly. *J. Hypertens* .2005;23(10):1803-8.

[22] Jouven X, Empana JP, Schwartz PJ, Desnos M, Courbon D, Ducimetiere P. Heart-rate profile during exercise as a predictor of sudden death. *N. Engl. J. Med.* 2005;352(19):1951-8.

[23] Ben-Dov IZ, Kark JD, Ben-Ishay D, Mekler J, Ben-Arie L, Bursztyn M. Blunted heart rate dip during sleep and all-cause mortality. *Arch Intern Med* 2007;167(19):2116-21.

[24] Thomas F, Bean K, Provost JC, Guize L, Benetos A. Combined effects of heart rate and pulse pressure on cardiovascular mortality according to age. *J. Hypertens.* 2001;19(5):863-9.

[25] Ryan SM, Goldberger AL, Pincus SM, Mietus J, Lipsitz LA. Gender- and age-related differences in heart rate dynamics: are women more complex than men? *J. Am. Coll. Cardiol* 1994;24(7):1700-7.

[26] Narkiewicz K, Somers VK. Interactive effect of heart rate and muscle sympathetic nerve activity on blood pressure. *Circulation* 1999;100(25):2514-8.

[27] Julius S. Transition from high cardiac output to elevated vascular resistance in hypertension. *Am. Hear. J.* 1988;116(2 Pt 2):600-6.

[28] Selby JV, Friedman GD, Quesenberry CP, Jr. Precursors of essential hypertension: pulmonary function, heart rate, uric acid, serum cholesterol, and other serum chemistries. *Am. J. Epidemiol.* 1990;131(6):1017-27.

[29] Inoue T, Iseki K, Iseki C, Kinjo K, Ohya Y, Takishita S. Higher heart rate predicts the risk of developing hypertension in a normotensive screened cohort. *Circ. J.* 2007;71(11):1755-60.

[30] Palatini P, Casiglia E, Pauletto P, Staessen J, Kaciroti N, Julius S. Relationship of tachycardia with high blood pressure and metabolic abnormalities: a study with mixture analysis in three populations. *Hypertension* 1997;30(5):1267-73.

[31] Inoue T, Oshiro S, Iseki K, Tozawa M, Touma T, Ikemiya Y, et al. High heart rate relates to clustering of cardiovascular risk factors in a screened cohort. *Jpn. Circ. J.* 2001;65(11):969-73.

[32] Tomiyama H, Yamada J, Koji Y, Yambe M, Motobe K, Shiina K, et al. Heart rate elevation precedes the development of metabolic syndrome in Japanese men: a prospective study. *Hypertens Res.* 2007;30(5):417-26.

[33] Wilson PW, D'Agostino RB, Levy D, Belanger AM, Silbershatz H, Kannel WB. Prediction of coronary heart disease using risk factor categories. *Circulation* 1998;97(18):1837-47.

[34] Executive Summary of The Third Report of The National Cholesterol Education Program (NCEP) Expert Panel on Detection, Evaluation, And Treatment of High Blood Cholesterol In Adults (Adult Treatment Panel III). *Jama* 2001;285(19):2486-97.

[35] Wood D, De Backer G, Faergeman O, Graham I, Mancia G, Pyorala K. Prevention of coronary heart disease in clinical practice: recommendations of the Second Joint Task Force of European and other Societies on Coronary Prevention. *Atherosclerosis* 1998;140(2):199-270.

[36] Conroy RM, Pyorala K, Fitzgerald AP, Sans S, Menotti A, De Backer G, et al. Estimation of ten-year risk of fatal cardiovascular disease in Europe: the SCORE project. *Eur Heart J* 2003;24(11):987-1003.

[37] Palatini P, Julius S. Heart rate and the cardiovascular risk. *J. Hypertens.* 1997;15(1):3-17.

[38] Schwartz PJ, La Rovere MT, Vanoli E. Autonomic nervous system and sudden cardiac death. Experimental basis and clinical observations for post-myocardial infarction risk stratification. *Circulation* 1992;85(1 Suppl):I77-91.

[39] Gordon D, Guyton JR, Karnovsky MJ. Intimal alterations in rat aorta induced by stressful stimuli. *Lab. Invest.* 1981;45(1):14-27.

[40] Beere PA, Glagov S, Zarins CK. Retarding effect of lowered heart rate on coronary atherosclerosis. *Science* 1984;226(4671):180-2.

[41] Kaplan JR, Manuck SB, Adams MR, Weingand KW, Clarkson TB. Inhibition of coronary atherosclerosis by propranolol in behaviorally predisposed monkeys fed an atherogenic diet. *Circulation* 1987;76(6):1364-72.

[42] Heidland UE, Strauer BE. Left ventricular muscle mass and elevated heart rate are associated with coronary plaque disruption. *Circulation* 2001;104(13):1477-82.

[43] Lantelme P, Mestre C, Lievre M, Gressard A, Milon H. Heart rate: an important confounder of pulse wave velocity assessment. *Hypertension* 2002;39(6):1083-7.

[44] Kjekshus J. Comments-Beta-blockers: Heart rate reduction a mechanism of benefit. *Eur Heart J.* 1985;6(suppl A):S29-S30.

[45] Palatini P. Heart rate as a risk factor for atherosclerosis and cardiovascular mortality: the effect of antihypertensive drugs. *Drugs* 1999;57(5):713-24.

[46] Dallongeville J, Yarnell J, Ducimetiere P, Arveiler D, Ferrieres J, Montaye M, et al. Fish consumption is associated with lower heart rates. *Circulation* 2003;108(7):820-5.

[47] Carter JB, Banister EW, Blaber AP. Effect of endurance exercise on autonomic control of heart rate. *Sports Med* .2003;33(1):33-46.

[48] Hambrecht R, Walther C, Mobius-Winkler S, Gielen S, Linke A, Conradi K, et al. Percutaneous coronary angioplasty compared with exercise training in patients with stable coronary artery disease: a randomized trial. *Circulation* 2004;109(11):1371-8.

[49] Palatini P. Need for a revision of the normal limits of resting heart rate. *Hypertension* 1999;33(2):622-5.

In: Heart Disease in Women
Editor: B. V. Larner and H. R. Pennelton

ISBN 978-1-60692-066-4
© 2009 Nova Science Publishers, Inc.

Chapter VI

Women in a World of Men's Disease: The Case of Female Cardiac Patients

Michal Rassin[*]

Assaf Harofeh Medical Center, Zrifine, Beer- Yakov, 70300, Israel

Abstract

The central purpose of the study was to examine differences between women and men, ages 30-50 years, in their responses to heart disease, and to identify the factors influencing them in the fields of health and illness. The study was conducted using a qualitative method. The participants in the study included 30 men and 30 women who suffered from coronary heart disease. The study findings suggest that women delayed seeking treatment and that when they did seek treatment they were not initially diagnosed as suffering from heart disease due to physicians' perceptions that heart disease is a men's disease. The recovery period for women was characterized by their quick return to daily home making before their physical condition permitted it. Conversely, the men extended their recovery period and received support from their families. As part of the return to normal life, the men were strict in following the instructions of the health regimen, whereas most of the women ignored it. The women, compared to the men, received less support from their spouses and families, and they noted that social expectations concerning their role were high. Our study concludes that heart disease varies between men and women in the characteristics of its symptoms and in the attitude of medical staff and the public, as well as of patients themselves, towards the disease. The role of the cardiac patient is based on male characteristics and, as a result, men are legitimized and receive social support in all that relates to the disease; consequently, men adhere to the health regimen, whereas women are less inclined to. This study can advance insights on the influence of the gender variable on responses to heart disease, as well as supply information on therapeutic intervention for male and female cardiac patients and the nature of the different measures used for each.

[*] Correspondence concerning this article should be addressed to: Dr. Michal Rassin, R.N, PhD, Research Unit, Nursing Care Management, Asaf Harofe Medical Center, Zrifinn, Bear Yaakov, 70300, ISRAEL. Tel- 972-8-9779114; fax- 972-8-9779551; Email address: rasinm@asaf.health.gov.il.

Key words: gender, coronary heart disease, diagnosis, recovery, health regimen

Introduction

Coronary heart disease (CHD) is the leading cause of mortality and morbidity in developing countries (Grace et al, 2002; Weidner, 2000). For many years, coronary heart disease was considered mostly a male illness. However, current data show that it is also the main cause of mortality among women (Efre, 2004; Gottlieb, 2005). Once heart disease reaches clinical expression, the quality of life and prognosis for women are worse than for men (Helitz et al, 2002; Hochner et al, 2002; Lukkarine & Hentinen, 1998). Research indicates that this is due not only to biological and genetic factors but also to gender differences in personal and social responses to the illness (McKinlay, 1996; Weidner, 2000).

Efforts in coping with the illness are especially remarkable among young cardiac patients between the ages of 30 and 50, despite the fact that in these ages there is an increasing difficulty in combining the major tasks of life, such as work and raising children, with the demands of the illness. However, these age groups have been neglected in the sphere of research, in particular women, who have been neglected due to the misguided assumption that heart disease is a disease of elderly men (McKinlay, 1996; Uuskuela, 1996). A comparison of male and female responses to the illness, and identification of the factors affecting them, can contribute to a deep appreciation of the aspects related to quality of life among male and female cardiac patients, as well as provide nurses with information on the necessity of therapeutic intervention and the nature of its specific measures for women and men.

Gender Differences in the Response to Heart Disease

Studies on the differences between the sexes in the field of health habits suggest that women, more than men, participate in health-promoting activities. Women often seek help from the health system, receive more medical services, and maintain a healthier lifestyle (Courtenay, 2000; Verbrugge, 1985, 1986). However, where heart diseases are concerned, women delay seeking medical services despite the appearance of symptoms, resulting in a worsening of their condition (Ashton, 1999; Evanoski, 1997; Foster & Millik, 1998). In addition, physicians diagnose and treat women less than men for heart disease (Brink, Karlson & Hallberg, 2002; Efre, 2004; Ferrara, Williamson, Karter, Thompson & Kim, 2004). Furthermore, female cardiac patients are less responsive to a health regimen than men, especially among those 55 years of age and younger, and thus have a much worse prognosis (Drori, 1999, Foster & Mallik, 1998; Keller & Lemberg, 2000; King & Koop, 1999; Lieberman et al, 1998; Mark, 2000; Noris, 1998; Remennick & Raanan, 2000)., Among young female cardiac patients ages 50 years and younger, the mortality rates are twice as high in comparison to those of male patients of the same ages (Efre, 2004).

According to the System Contribution Model, which is a model specific to heart disease, women are discriminated against, especially by the medical system. The American sociologist John McKinlay (1996), who developed this model, explains that cardiologic services exemplify markedly the way gender stereotypes turn women into second-rate patients, causing them to further neglect their cardiac disease. McKinlay demonstrates that physicians ignore coronary events among young women due to the common belief that the estrogen hormone has cardiac protective influences. As such, they often do not diagnose cardiac conditions among women, even in the presence of symptoms. When women are eventually diagnosed, they are admitted less to intensive care, are referred less to a cardiologist, and receive less medication and treatment in comparison to men. This leads to the conclusion that physicians make their clinical decisions based on gender biases. This phenomenon is most obvious among patients 30 to 50 years of age, a time of life known to be a person's most productive. The appearance of illness at this time of life makes it difficult to deal with the numerous and demanding tasks of these years such as family, parenting, and employment (Bury, 1982; Verbrugge, 1985). Nonetheless, these ages have been neglected in the research, apparently due to the common belief that heart diseases appear only at older ages. This belief is misguided, as evidenced by statistical data (McKinlay, 1996; Uuskuela, 1996).

Most studies dealing with heart disease have examined its influences mainly on older male patients, and the studies that have dealt with younger patients have examined far fewer women than men (Ashton, 1999; Rosenfeld, 2000). The current study wishes to change this. Up until now, the factors and responses examined have over-emphasized physiological and psychological aspects and have neglected the influences of social factors such as the medical establishment, employers, friends, and family (Brezinka & Kittel, 1996; Ladwing et al, 2000).

All of the above suggests that critical questions concerning gender differences in the diagnosis and treatment of heart disease are still unresolved. The current study wishes to broaden this body of knowledge.

Purpose of Study

The central purpose of the current study was to examine the differences between women and men, ages 30 to 50, in their responses to heart disease, and to identify the factors influencing them in the areas of health and illness.

Design

The study used a qualitative design and was conducted using narrative investigation. The illness narratives, gathered using in-depth interviews, were analyzed by thematic analysis. Narrative is especially suitable for studying cardiac patients, while providing a sense of order in terms of causality and direction of progress. The interviewee was asked to reconstruct his/her past by presenting a chronological sequence of events linking the dimensions of past, present, and future as well as body, self, and society.

Sample

The study included 60 Israeli patients with coronary heart disease, 30 females and 30 males, selected using a convenience-sampling method. Most participants were native Israelis, married and with children (*see Table 1*). The participants were chosen according to the following criteria: 1) patients classified in one of the following states: patients who had undergone myocardial infarction, patients who had undergone coronary artery bypass grafts, or patients suffering from ischemic heart disease; 2) patients within the age range of 30 to 50; and 3) patients with a period of three or more years from the time of diagnosis of the illness, (as it is reasonable to assume that experienced patients can provide much more information than inexperienced patients). For the purposes of comparing the groups of men and women, they were matched according to the variables of clinical status, age, and illness experience (*see Table 2*).

Table 1. Sociodemographic Variables, Comparison of Women and Men

Variable	Category	Women – N (%)	Men – N (%)
Marital Status	Married	21 (70%)	25 (83%)
	Divorced	6 (20%)	5 (15%)
	Single	3 (10%)	-------
Number of Children	Average	2.8	3.3
	Range	1-6	1-8
Country of Origin	Israel	22 (73.4%)	17 (56.6%)
	Russia	3 (10%)	5 (16.6%)
	Morocco	3 (10%)	3 (10%)
	South America	2 (6.6%)	5 (16.6%)
Education	Average Years of Study	12.9	14.8
	Range of Years of Study	10-18	8-19
Employment	Employed	24 (80%)	27 (90%)
	Unemployed	3 (10%)	1 (3.3%)
	Retired (due to illness)	3 (10%)	2 (6.6%)
Self-Defined Economic State	Very Good	-------	6 (20%)
	Fair (give or take)	24 (80%)	18 (60%)
	Not Good	6 (20%)	6 (20%)
Religious Background	Secular	17 (56.6%)	20 (66.6%)
	Traditional	10 (33.3%)	6 (20%)
	Orthodox	3 (10%)	4 (13.3%)

Methods

Data collection was carried out for 10 months. The participants were located with the help of two senior physicians working in large cardiology clinics in Israel. The physicians contacted candidates who met the criteria for participating in the study. The telephone numbers of suitable candidates who agreed to participate were delivered to the researcher. The researcher met with and explained to the candidates the purpose of the study. Participants were promised complete confidentiality. The meetings lasted for two hours, and when this was not sufficient an additional meeting was held. Meetings were held in the participants' homes when requested. The interviews contents were recorded with the consent of the participants.

Table 2. The Variables Correlated Between Women and Men

| Gender | Diagnosis Age Average | Time from Diagnosis Average (years) | Clinical Status in Diagnosis | | |
			Myocardial Infarct	Coronary Artery Bypass Graft	Ischemic heart disease
Women	42.8	4.7	20	8	2
Men	40.8	5.7	20	8	2

Data gathering was conducted using in-depth interviews. The interview started with a general question: "Could you tell me how it all started and what happened later?" The interview included coverage points, topics that reminded the researcher what the question should encompass; for example, "What were your sensations and how did you respond?", "What made you respond?", and "How did the illness affect your function at work and home?" The interview also included probing questions, such as "What do you mean?" and "Can you give an example?" (Berg, 1998). These questions were asked only when the interviewees' answers were superficial and demanded more details, or when he or she digressed.

The interview with the participants was carried out by the researcher using a qualitative method. "The man as a research tool", a term coined by Lincoln & Guba (1985) illustrates the special role of researchers in the qualitative study, seeing human beings as the only "tools" flexible enough to comprehend the complexity of the human experience. Human beings vary from other tools in that humans respond to context, changing their methods according to the circumstances and dealing with and adjusting to various responses.

Analysis of Data

Findings from the interviews were analyzed using thematic analyses. In the first stage, the recorded interviews were transcribed and the analytic work was begun with a preliminary reading of each interview in order to gain some general impressions.

The second stage consisted of an additional reading of each interview in order to identify themes, or units, which appeared to be the central building blocks of the narrative. Identification of themes in the narrative investigation is particularly characterized by a process termed "over-reading," implying a meticulous, educated, and sensitive reading during which the narrative is examined several times by the researcher in order to identify repetitions; inconsistencies; metaphors; side comments; defensive statements; latent relations; nuances; endings; and silences all of which can constitute an index for interpreting the narrative (Good & Good, 1994; Poirier & Lioness, 1997; Sandelowski, 1991). As is customary in qualitative studies, theme conceptualization is bound to the process of data organization (Berg, 1998); it requires the organization of data in a systematic filing system in which prominent topics arising from the participants' narratives are classified. Each topic in the study was coded on a separate list. Each list, in turn, was related to the original interview material, referencing the number of the interviewee, the page number in the interview, and an abstract of the segment. Similarly, relevant sub-topics were classified according to various themes.

Each theme title chosen was based on what seemed the most logically related to the information it represented; initially, a temporary name was chosen, and only later was a permanent name decided on. Straus and Corbin (1992) claim that theme titles should be related as closely as possible to the expressions the participants used in vivo. These are usually catchy phrases that attract one's attention and embody and summarize the phenomenon. In this tenor, most titles given in the current study were taken from the natural language of the participants.

In the third stage, the themes were reorganized according to the chronological order of events on a continuum, as narratives presented by interviewees are often inconsistent and lack causality. In such cases, some claim it is allowed, and even required, to cut and reorganize the narrative segments, provided the content and meaning of the narrative are not changed (Franzosi, 1998; Kleinman, 1988; Poirier & Lioness, 1997).

In the fourth stage, the themes collected from the male and female groups were compared, and gender patterns were marked in a manner that would demonstrate similarities and differences between the two groups. Similarities and differences between the groups were then identified and explained.

In the fifth stage, occurrences (quotes from the participants) were copied below their respective themes and sub-themes. The themes were characterized by a narrative segment, accounting for a discursive organization of time and causality (Bury, 2001; Riessman, 1990). As the central purpose of the narrative approach is to provide explanations of given descriptions (Franzosi, 1998; Sandelowski, 1991), special attention was given to the detailed explanation of the events, contexts, and comparisons suggested from the study data. Combining these conditions, the thematic framework included a reference to the chronological order of the factors, as well as responses, analysis of the connections between them, and comparison of the files from the women's group to those from the men's group.

In the final stage, as in the discussion section, there was an attempt to link the personal narratives to a broader discourse dealing with themes resulting from the concepts and theories developed (Franzosi, 1998; Silverman, 1993).

Standards of trustworthiness were obtained using peer debriefing, incorporating into the findings an additional study colleague familiar with the qualitative method, as well as peer review. Two interviewees, chosen according to their interest and desire to see the findings, were re-interviewed for their feedback on the study conclusions (Lincoln & Guba, 1985). In addition to standards of trustworthiness, relationships of confidence and rapport formed with the participants during the meetings helped in obtaining authentic reports (Berg, 1998).

Findings

In analyzing the narratives provided by the female and male participants in the study, eight different themes were identified. The themes characteristic of the women were then compared to those characteristic of the men. Events were classified in terms of causality into three main time periods: diagnosis and hospitalization, recovery, and return to normal life. The study findings point to gender differences in both the nature of some of the responses and the factors that shaped them.

a) Diagnosis and Hospitalization

--"Young Women Don't Expect to Get a Heart Attack, It Has Always Been a Men's Disease"

The women who participated in the current study sought help from the health system only after many hours, sometimes days, had passed since the appearance of symptoms. All female participants interpreted the symptoms as originating from logical causes linked to everyday activities, such as muscle aches due to hard work, digestive problems due to spoiled food, etc. Despite the numerous causes the female participants attributed to their symptoms, it never crossed their minds that these symptoms might be related to heart disease. Several factors led to this, including an unrealistic perception of related symptoms and the women's perception that their young age and feminine sexuality protected them from illness

*(Female, age 38) – It started with aches in my hands and shoulders. I thought it was because of the work, since I had just finished with the Passover Spring cleanings. At first I didn't take it seriously, because I occasionally get an ache here and there. I said to myself, "forget about it, you're young, it'll pass". I took an Acamol here, an Optalgin there. Who would have thought of the heart, because young women don't expect to get a heart attack, it has always been a men's disease... A few days later, when it hadn't passed, I saw my GP. He laughed and said "Passover's a dangerous holiday for women." He gave me Moscul and a Voltaren gel to apply. Meanwhile, several more days passed and the aches didn't go away. One day, I came to work feeling aches in my back and shoulders, dizziness and nausea, and the world around me turned black and white, colorless... A co-worker who passed by was alarmed by how I looked. She asked me "do you feel alright?"... I answered: "I'll rest a bit and it'll pass," but she decided to call an ambulance and they took me to the hospital... My condition was so bad they had to admit me. Then they started talking about it maybe being something with the heart. The EKG showed disturbances, yet they told me, "look, at such a young age we don't suspect women as having heart problems." The next morning they sent me for mapping. The physician insisted that the mapping showed a shadow on the breast: "We'll have another mapping in three months and see", he said... In the evening my condition deteriorated. They took me right away for catheterization. There they found blocks of 95%. I was operated on within a week...

--"Men at the Age of 40 Get Glasses, and at 50 They Get a Heart Attack"

While it was a noticeable fact among the female participants that none of them related their symptoms to the heart, most of the male participants reported immediately relating their symptoms to the heart. As a result, the time that passed from the appearance of symptoms to their receiving medical help was shorter for the men, and within the time range defined as critical for minimizing damage to the heart. The interviewees' descriptions suggest that the quick diagnosis, which prevented unnecessary suffering, resulted from the legitimacy given to men by health system workers, according to which a man can have a heart attack even if he is young:

> *(Male, age 45) – One day I was climbing up the stairs and started feeling all kinds of recurrent pressures in my chest. I sat on the couch. The A.C. was working full force, and I was sweating buckets and nothing helped… When I saw after half an hour that the pain was severe and would not pass, I realized it was the heart. I called an ambulance, alerted my wife, and arrived at the E.R. There they shocked me, attached me to all sorts of equipment, and sent me right away to the I.C.U… After that, as a present for my 45th birthday, I subscribed to a cardiac patients' service. Well, I'm a man, and a smoker, and you know what they say - men at the age of 40 get glasses, and at 50 they get a heart attack.

--"How Come I Got a Heart Attack?"

Upon receiving their diagnosis, all participants expressed crisis responses, exhibited by shock, mistrust, and denial. However, the women's crisis responses were more noticeable inasmuch as the women, in contrast to the men, had not thought that they might develop heart disease. The shock response was accompanied by feelings of anger, self pity, and an explicit accusation of malpractice on the part of the medical system.

> *(Female, age 34) – The director of the catheterization unit looked at me and said "I want her in my unit." He admitted me to the I.C.U. I was hospitalized at 8:30 in the morning. In the evening, after the blood tests, he talked with me and said I had had a heart attack. I was in shock. I said: "how come I got a heart attack? How come? I'm young and healthy, I never had any problems. All my brothers and sisters are well. And I don't even smoke"… I was shocked; I took it very badly, thinking of my very young kids. I started thinking about what would happen to them, who would take care of them. I felt I was loosing my ability to control my life. I went out and had a good cry. I felt my world come crashing down… I blamed the GP in the clinic for not taking me seriously; maybe if he had done something straight away all of this would've been avoided. When I got to the ward all the doctors and nurses started coming in. They came to see the 'case' and were buzzing around me all day because I was the youngest there and it was very strange to see a woman in my condition. It was very stressful…

The men participating in the study also responded intensely to the diagnosis, even though most saw heart attacks as a part of life for men. The men's shock resulted from the fact that they had not expected heart disease at such a young age, and mainly from a feeling that the illness had cut short their plans and threatened their lives. Unlike the women's narratives, the men chose to concentrate more on facts than feelings in describing the diagnostic process. Another aspect of the men's narratices, noticeable in its absence, was that, despite the fact that the men had children, they did not mention them, whereas in the women's accounts children were a central issue.

*(Male, age 42) – After this, they took me for catheterization. The doctor told me that there were two blocks and they would have to operate. Until I was 44, I hadn't thought about my health. I hadn't thought something would happen to me. My father died of a heart attack when he was 60, but I didn't know what cholesterol and blood-pressure were... So maybe the risk was there under the surface. The crisis was serious because I was in the middle of my plans at work and it cut it all short. I understood I had no choice and needed to be operated on. I tried to focus on the facts...

b) Recovery

--"Women Are Someplace Else in Terms of Home and the Family"

Although the female participants noted that they had received medical instructions concerning the recommended recovery period, the response pattern characteristic of most of the women was nonetheless a quick return to all of their familial roles and homemaking tasks. A minority of them checked into a rehabilitation center upon discharge, but these were mostly from the group of women who had had surgery. Even these women, however, who suffered from pains due to difficult surgery, waited anxiously for the end of their time in the rehabilitation center in order to return home and continue to function as mothers and wives:

*(Female, age 42) – Before the heart attack I was a healthy, strong woman who worked long hours and worried about everyone. After the heart attack, I felt that everything was difficult for me. I was discharged on Friday and on Sunday I was back working at home. It was hard but I didn't make allowances for myself. I forced myself to do things. I started washing the dishes, dusting, all by myself...

*(Female, age 46) – I quickly returned to functioning because I worried so much about the house. Generally, women are someplace else in terms of the home, the family, the kids, and doing their responsibilities... Ten days after the surgery I was still recovering, and when I returned home after a fortnight I did everything by myself until I felt physical pain... I told them, "Now you have a refurbished maid." At first my daughters told me, "Mom, don't work, mom sit, don't do this," but they sort of enjoyed me doing the work, so that's not much help. Even my husband stopped helping me pretty quickly. So I found myself standing in the kitchen frying his steaks, and preparing sandwiches for the kids in the morning. But then again, that's me. I need to do everything by myself like I like to do. A month after the surgery I even hosted all of our friends and thanked them... When they saw my husband put the dishes in the dishwasher they were very impressed. I thought to myself, "Do I need to have something like a heart attack to get some help around here?"

The men, in comparison, were using the rehabilitation centers as much as possible, and some even extended their stay beyond the period subsidized by the HMO. Other male interviewees chose complete physical rest at home, during which they received substantial support from wife and family. Support was expressed, among other things, in preparing special foods, administering medication, keeping them rested, and freeing them from all household chores:

*(Male, age 42) – I stayed a little bit longer at Kfar Hamacabia (a rehabilitation center), and when I returned home I was taken care of. They kept me lying down all the time so that I wouldn't strain myself or lift heavy things. My wife made me special low-fat foods and called me from work to remind me to take my pills…

c) Normal Life

--"Returning to Living Normally"

After the recovery period, both female and male participants started dealing with their condition by returning to normal lives. However, the return to normalcy among the women was quick, concise, and more extreme than for the men, in some cases so extreme that they denied ever being ill:

*(Female, age 43) – In the first few months life revolves around the disease. You invest yourself in how to rebuild your life, doing sports, meticulous tests each month, all those diets, and having intense thoughts. And they help too, with more mapping and more ergometry. So you can't repress the illness. You have to run to your checkup and talk about it with everyone. Then it ended all at once. I stopped going to the institute; it didn't suit me anymore. I returned to the couple of years before the illness, to the routine, the work. I had no time to be ill and forgot about my heart. I asked myself, "Why shouldn't I live normally, why should I eat hard cheese only once a month? Everything is either not allowed or not recommended…" So I decided to return to normal life.

Among the men, the return to normal life was not expressed as succinctly but with gradual and cautious progress. In their narratives, the male participants reported how elements from the sphere of illness penetrated their everyday life, integrating with other aspects to produce a normal life but with a different perspective compared to before the diagnosis:

*(Male, age 42) – It's safe to say that six months later I returned to normal life, but more cautiously and more aware of my health. Once I used to do what I felt like doing, smoking and eating what I wanted, but all of this changed. I continue as before but with the addition of taking pills, and keeping fit. In short, today I'm more alert and conscious of my condition.

--"With Time They Forgot I was Ill and They Don't Give Me Any More Allowances"

Complete return to normal life and maintaining stability for an extended period of time was made possible due to several factors. The first and central factor was a noticeable improvement in the physical feeling of the participants. The second factor was the message of the physicians that their condition was now good. The third included the expectations of family and other relatives that it was time to return to normal life. The women, in particular, expressed that family expectations of them to return to full function, both at home and work, were tremendous. Moreover, they noted that their family members virtually forgot the fact that only a few months before they had been ill and in grave danger:

*(Female, age 47) – After a year people forgot I had had a heart attack. All settled back into routine. They were less interested, less caring and less supportive. You no longer carry the "title" of a cardiac patient. Eventually, you are left to face it all alone, by yourself, with no support, as if you are no longer ill. At home I get no allowances. I remain both homemaker and working wife. I live at home with four uninterested people (a husband, two daughters, and one son) and no one so much as lifts a finger around the house. It doesn't seem awkward to them that I pick up after them; if they drop something they won't even bother to pick it up. As far as they're concerned, if the physician said from now on everything's fine and I'm healthy then it's all back to where they left it…

d) Health Regimen

--"You Can't Live Under Constant Warning"

Most of the study participants reported that they were given medical recommendations regarding a health regimen that included quitting smoking; a low-cholesterol diet; rehabilitative physical activity; medication according to instructions; and being under medical supervision. However, the women dismissed the health regimen almost entirely. While some clearly specified that they were aware of not following physicians' orders, others reported that they were following them. In actual fact, it turned out that these women were only partially following physicians' orders, which usually amounted to taking pills and following up medically. Aside from not maintaining adequate finances, quitting smoking, or exercising, most serious was the issue of discontinuing medication. The women reported various causes for such behaviors, including difficulty following the strict recommendations, a desire to enjoy life without constraints, and a lack of social support. They also mentioned aesthetic and health reasons. Above all, however, the participants demonstrated a strong will to be distracted from the illness and not to dwell on it. Thus, by partially or completely avoiding any illness-related activities, they managed to remain distracted, preserving their inner feeling that they were maintaining ordinary and normal lives like anyone else:

*(Female, age 45) – I hadn't quite changed my health habits. The sports thing – sweating isn't for me. Besides, you are always warned don't eat, don't smoke, don't, don't, don't! … You can't live under constant warning. So I eat salt, buy cakes and ice-creams, smoke cigarettes, and do as I please…

*(Female, age 47) – After a year or so, you are left to deal with it alone. There's less support from your surroundings. They're not interested anymore if you've been to your checkups. So I ignore this too, I don't go to checkups or anything. I've become indifferent…

*(Female, age 38) – After three months they referred me for rehabilitation; I was there one time, and one time only. As I entered I saw they were all old and men. They gave me a look like "what are *you* doing here." So there was nothing for me… Six months after surgery I decided to stop with the medication. The pills stressed me out from the get-go. I used to sit each morning by the pile of pills and cry because of having to take them, because a healthy person doesn't take pills. Taking pills is being sick, and I had never taken a pill in my life. Even when I had headaches I wouldn't…

--"Perseverance for me is Like Life Insurance"

In contrast to the women, most of the male participants in the study adhered to a health regimen and were cooperative with the medical staff:

> *(Male, age 45) – I quit smoking right away, and I used to smoke two to three packs a day. I've been at it for seven years. Every three months I see the GP for a checkup and take the medication that he tells me to. Even my physical fitness has improved because I exercise. All in all, today I live better then I ever did.

> *(Male, age 38) – From that day I quit smoking and stopped eating butter. I went to see a dietitian and I was in a follow-up group. Since the heart attack I practice in the Institute (for Heart Rehabilitation) twice a week. I realize that if I don't have a framework I won't do a thing, so I prefer to pay. I get up everyday at 6 o'clock to practice, rain or shine, and it's not easy. But perseverance for me is like life insurance.

Following a health regimen strengthened the feeling among the participants that they had recovered and were doing their best to stay alive. The men's reaction seems in opposition to that of the women's described above; however, it, too, was aimed at distracting their minds from the possibility that the illness would recur or that their condition would deteriorate. Ultimately, both women's and men's reactions and ways of coping are meant to preserve the "healthy self" with the passage of time.

Discussion

The study findings suggest that the participants' reactions to the diagnosis of heart disease were particularly influenced by the social legitimacy they are given in assuming the "sick role." Parsons (1951), in coining this term, explained that humans are not to be blamed for their illness and so are exempt from normal social duties. However, they should understand that illness is not a desirable thing and that they are to seek help in improving their condition so that they can return to their normal social role. Thus, the first duty defined by the sick role is to seek appropriate help by turning to the medical system.

Social legitimacy for the sick role requires the seal of approval of a medical diagnosis; however, before this, the individual is required to acknowledge that the symptoms demand help. The findings of the current study showed that women, as opposed to men, sought help much later because they had not thought of the symptoms as originating from the heart, and in most cases they attempted to deal with them on their own. As mentioned, the men did not delay seeking medical treatment, and some immediately attributed their symptoms to the heart.

Seeking immediate medical help during a heart attack has well-known importance, for it improves survival and prevents complications (Clark, 2001). However, some linger and therefore do not receive treatment in time. Numerous studies that examine this phenomenon among young cardiac patients identify that the main causes for this delay result first and foremost from a misinterpretation of the symptoms, attributing them to more familiar conditions such as stomach aches, muscle aches, etc. Secondly, the social image of the heart disease as a disease of the elderly, and myths that relate heart disease to loss of consciousness and sudden death, create disparities between people's expectations and the symptoms they actually experience. However, others who reach the hospital quickly perceive themselves as being at high risk for developing heart disease and so are aware of a wide range of illness-related symptoms (Alonzo & Reynolds, 1998; Clark, 2001; Johnson & Morse, 1990; Maclean & Cockshutt, 1979; Ruston, Clayton & Calnan, 1998).

The symptoms reported by the women in the current study, together with findings from other studies, indicate that in most cases women tend to report pains in areas other than the chest, such as hands; shoulders; neck; jaw; stomach; and back. Men, however, mainly report pain in the chest area (Efre, 2004; McSweeney, Cody & Crane, 2001; Meischke, Larsen & Eisenberg, 1998; Miller, 2002; Philipott et al, 2001). Although evidence clearly points to different pain locations in women and men, the medical textbooks continue to treat these pain locations as atypical. Philpott et al (2001), read "atypical" as relating to "not like men." The failure of the health system in the timely diagnosis of heart disease among women is documented in the current study, as it has been in previously published studies. This failure is illustrated in the careless disregard of women's complaints, even relating these complaints to psychiatric problems. In addition, the medical system still maintains that heart disease among young women is a rare phenomenon, based on the common misperception that female hormones protect against this illness (Efre, 2004; Ferrara et al, 2004; Foster et al, 1998; McKinlay, 1996; Philpott et al, 2001; Rosenfeld, 2000; Van-Tiel et al, 1998).

The conclusion of the current study, which is consistent with that of many previously published studies, is that social legitimizing of the sick role of the cardiac patient is gender related. This is due to the perception of heart disease as a men's disease. This provides the main explanation for the difficulty female participants experienced in achieving personal, medical, and social legitimacy regarding their diagnosis as cardiac patients. It also explains their delay in turning to health services upon the appearance of symptoms.

Another factor to be considered in the sick role is that entering into this role is especially difficult for women, as traditionally a woman's role is perceived as being engaged in helping others; women are not expected to be sick themselves (Johansson et al, 1999; Maclean & Cockshutt, 1979; Miles, 1991). In a survey conducted in Israel among a random sample of 839 women, average age 38, the women were asked to describe how they respond to not feeling well. More than 70% answered that they "ignore" it, that they decide it is "nothing" and wait for it to pass. Avgar and Gordon (1997) explain the findings of this survey in the context of considering the tremendous commitments these women carry; they might not have the time to be sick. However, there still persists the common misperception of women as hypochondriacs, constantly complaining and using health services excessively (Courtenay, 2000; Lorber, 1997).

During the recovery period, the participants in the study reassumed their social functions. Particularly noticeable among the women was the tension between their sick role and their role as woman. The women's families had only partly legitimized their sick role, while their maternal and domestic functions were viewed as superior. A similar picture is reported in numerous other studies, in which women note an early return to domestic tasks during the recovery period. Furthermore, they feel a withdrawal of social support, and in some cases unrealistic expectations are reported by recovering women regarding the extent of their involvement in domestic tasks. In comparison, men assume the sick role perfectly and it is fully legitimized by their family members (Fleury, 2001; Hawthorne, 1992; Johnson & Morse, 1990; King & Koop, 1999; King, 2001; Rose et al, 1996; Uuskuela, 1996).

Factors concerning self were also identified during the current study, prompted by the women's feelings of guilt that, due to their illness and dysfunction, their families were suffering. These feelings served as the main factor in driving these women quickly back to their domestic tasks. Research indicates that women's severe perceptions of their failure to function as mothers and wives drives them back to their domestic tasks, even before fully recovering physically (Brink, Karlson & Hallberg, 2002; Miles, 1991). This, however, is a simplistic perspective, since it ignores the origin of the women's private feelings of guilt – they were brought up with these social expectations. Izraeli (1990) explains that a woman's decision to give priority to the family seems to be her personal preference and will. In effect, this interpretation ignores the power of the subconscious ideology, that which demands that women give precedence to the requirements of family life over anything else. For instance, in all that pertains to Israeli society, Berkowitz (1999) claims that women's position and status were designed during the first decades of the fledgling state, their full citizenship being granted in exchange for their contribution to the collective as mothers and wives. This role has been fixated since then in the national consciousness as the central one for the woman in Israeli society. Izraeli (1990) adds that the family institution is particularly demanding for the women, and that questions about having children or a career are alien to the Israeli cultural milieu, which is dominated by the assumption that career and family will be combined. This perspective can explain why the women in the current study found themselves "trapped" between the sick role and the roles of mother and wife. This can explain also why they did not receive full social legitimacy for their sick role, as was granted the men.

Return to normal life following the recovery period was marked by all the research participants leaving the crisis-response pattern that had characterized their diagnosis and hospitalization. The female participants' narratives generally described a sharper return than the males to life as it had been before the diagnosis.

Miles (1991) states that there are negotiations between the patient, the physician, and the patient's social group about the period of retirement from social roles. The timing of return to normal life depends, of course, on the absence of symptoms; however, this too, is a consequence both of one's social group's expectations as well as of the patient's commitments to his/her normal roles.

The structure of normal life, and normalcy in general, are the most favorable and dominant social principles in Western society. Being normal means being productive within society (Anderton, Elfert & Lai, 1989). It follows that the role of the norm is to contribute to society, in complete opposition to the sick role, which does not contribute. Therefore, stories of "normalization" are most favorable among the sick and disabled, even when this illusion of normalcy turns out to be counterproductive, preventing them from obtaining support, talking about their problems, or asking for allowances when tired or under the weather (Anderton et al, 1989; Robinson, 1993).

Two variations on the return to normal life were demonstrated by the participants in the current study. Most of the men carried on with the lifestyles that had preceded their illness, incorporating into them their medical regimens, which they perceived would protect and maintain their health. Based on this, they could present themselves as healthy. In contrast, the women employed a different strategy. An examination of their behaviors shows that most of the women ignored the medical regimen and instead reverted to the lifestyles that had preceded their illness. Thus, the women preserved a sense of health and normal life by avoiding any illness-related activities such as taking pills. In relation to this strategy, Bury (1982, 2001) differentiates between normalization and normal life. Normalization, he asserts, is the preservation of the lifestyle preceding the illness by way of maintaining a large proportion of previous activities and minimizing the influences of the illness on life, often by actively denying the illness and by adopting an opposing lifestyle. Conversely, normal life is expressed by redesigning one's lifestyle to accommodate the illness; in other words, it is a combination of the previous lifestyle and the demands of the illness.

In a study conducted among 3523 cardiac patients, it was found that 50% of their mortality resulted from unwillingness to follow their health regimen. The same study also suggested that this unwillingness was particularly marked among the young group, ages 55 and under (Noris, 1998). In another study comparing women and men, it was found that the willingness of female cardiac patients to maintain their health regimen was lower than that of the male patients, thus worsening their prognosis (Keller & Lemberg, 2000; Lieberman et al, 1998). In interviews held with 30 HIV carriers, it was found that women in particular employed the approach of continuing normal life, which revolved around the concept of not needing to change anything because of the illness (Pierret, 2001). Another study, conducted among cystic fibrosis patients, examined why the women's prognoses were much worse than the men's (the men had a life expectancy of 14 years, on average, more than the women). The researchers state clearly that even though it is customary to explain this disparity between the sexes in physiological terms such as women's lower weight, different microbiology of the airways, etc., in actuality, willingness versus unwillingness to follow the recommended health regimens underlies this disparity. In principle, the men in the study incorporated their health regimens into their lives by following recommendations regarding physiotherapy, exercise, diet, and antibiotic courses, whereas the women ignored their regimens completely and were less active physically, less strict with their diet, and in some cases did not take their medications or simply ignored the illness altogether (Willis, Miller & Wyn, 2001).

These findings closely resemble the findings of the current study, even though the patient populations vary. Again, it seems that, in all that relates to the gender variable, there are identical response patterns among same-sex patients, even when they suffer from different illnesses.

The literature, in numerous instances, notes that the willingness to observe, and maintenance of, a health regimen are directly linked to the level of social support a patient receives (Barefoot, Gronbæk, Jensen, Schnohr & Prescott, 2005; Chafetz, 1996; Charmaz, 1991; Twaddle & Hessler, 1987). Sick women receive less social support from their spouses and families compared to sick men. And when a woman does receive support, it is curtailed shortly thereafter, at which point she is expected to resume her previous roles, primarily the role of providing support for her family members (Miles, 1991). Managing a health regimen requires that the family encourage the patient so that he/she can persist in it despite hardships. It is therefore not surprising that women turn less than men to heart rehabilitation programs, and when they do it is only short lived (Drori, 1999). This phenomenon has been found to be significantly linked to a lack of support and encouragement from family members (Lieberman et al, 1998).

In conclusion, heart disease varies between men and women in the nature of its symptoms and the attitudes of medical staff, the public, and even the sick person towards the illness. The role of the cardiac patient is traditionally based on male characteristics, thus offering men social legitimacy and support in all that relates to the illness. Consequently, men are much more willing to maintain a health regimen than women. This finding contradicts the prevalent theories that present women as obedient and adapting to a healthier lifestyle than men.

This study concludes that social factors, mainly the legitimacy of sick roles, is different for men than for women, and specifically that men are afforded much more legitimacy than women regarding sick roles. The findings of this study are very consistent with explanations of the system-contribution approach regarding gender differences in heart disease. This approach states that the reason for under-diagnosis of heart disease among young women results from physicians' perception of heart disease as a male illness. This perception, in turn, creates a societal gender delineation of the illness as a men's disease, leading to social legitimacy of the sick role only for men.

This study, following the qualitative approach, can provide insights into the phenomenon of heart disease among women and men. The qualitative approach hypothesizes that a social phenomenon draws its meaning from the way people who are related to it interpret it. This study provides information on the extent to which therapeutic intervention is necessary for cardiac patients, including specific measures, which differ between women and men. In addition, social factors influencing patients' responses are identified in the study, which could help in locating target populations requiring intervention. While the responses and factors are expressed from the perspectives of both women and men, these personal points of view can bridge the gap between caregivers' and patients' perceptions regarding heart disease. As the current study was based on a convenience sample, which included only 60 participants from one country, it is highly recommended that additional studies be conducted, aimed at exploring further the claim on gender-based differences in diagnosis and treatment among young cardiac patients.

References

Alonzo, A., & Renolds, N. (1998). The structure of emotions during acute myocardial infarction: A model of caring. *Social Sciences and Medicine, 46*, 1099-1110.

Anderton, J. M., Elfert, H., & Lai, M. (1989). Ideology in the clinical context: Chronic illness, ethnicity and the discourse on normalisation. *Sociology of Health & Illness, 11*, 253-278.

Ashoton, K. C. (1999). How men and women with heart disease seek care: The delay experience. *Progress in Cardiovascular Nursing, 14*(2), 53-60

Avgar, A., Gordon, K. (1997). Your health: The results and conclusions. *At, 97*, 62-65 [Hebrew].

Barefoot, J. C., Gronbæk, M., Jensen, G., Schnohr, P., & Prescott., E. (2005). Social network diversity and risks of ischemic heart disease and total mortality: Findings from the Copenhagen city heart study. *American Journal of Epidemiology. 161, 960-971.*

Berg, B. L. (1998). *Qualitative research: Methods for the social science.* London: Viacom.

Berkowitz, N. (1999). A woman of valor who can find? Women and citizens in Israel. *Israeli Sociology, B*(1), 277-318 [Hebrew].

Brezinka, V., & Kittel, F. (1996). Psychosocial factors of coronary heart disease in women: A review. *Social Science and Medicine, 42,* 1351-1365

Brink, E., Karlson, B. W., & Hallberg, L. R. M. (2002). Health experiences of first time myocardial infarction: Factors influencing women's and men's health related quality of life after five months. *Psychology Health and Medicine, 7* (1), 5-

Bury, M. (1982). Chronic illness as biographical disruption. *Sociology of Health and Illness, 4,* 165-182.

Bury, M. (2001). Illness narratives: Fact or fiction? *Sociology of Health and Illness, 23,* 263-285.

Chafetz, L. (1996). The experience of severe mental illness: A life history approach. *Archives of Psychiatric Nursing, 10*(1), 24-31.

Charmaz, K. (1991). *Good days, bad days: The self in chronic illness and time.* New Brunswick, NJ: Rutgers University Press.

Clark, A. M. (2001). Treatment decision- making during the early stages of heart attack: A case for the role of body and self in influencing delays. *Sociology of Health and Illness, 23*(4), 425-446.

Corbin, J. M., & Strauss, A. (1992). A nursing model fore chronic illness management based upon the trajectory framework. In P.Woog, (Ed), *The chronic illness trajectory framework,* (pp. 9-28). New- York, NY: Springer Publishing Company

Courtenay, W. H. (2000). Constructions of masculinity and their influence on men's well-being: A theory of gender and health. *Social Science and Medicine, 50,* 1385-1401.

Drori, I. (1999). Cardiac rehabilitation among women: The desirable and available. *Ha-Rephuah, 137*(e-f), 228-232 [Hebrew].

Efre, A. J. (2004). Gender bias in Acute Myocardial Infarction. *Nurse Practitioner, 29*(11) 42-51.

Evanoski, C. (1997). Myocardial infarction: The number one killer of women. *Critical Care Nursing of North America, 9,* 489-496.

Ferrara, A., Williamson, D. F., Karter, A. J., Thompson, T. J.,& Kim, K. (2004). Sex differences in quality of health care related to ischemic heart disease prevention in patients with diabetes: The translating research into action for diabetes (TRIAD) study, 2000-2001. *Diabetes Care, 27,* 2974-2977.

Fleury, J., Sedikidies, C., & Lunsford, V. (2001). Women's experience following a cardiac event: The role of the self in healing. *Journal of Cardiovascular Nursing, 15*(3), 71-82.

Foster, S., & Mallik, M. (1998). A comparative study of differences in the referral behaviour patterns of men and women who have experienced cardiac related chest pain. *Intensive and Critical Care Nursing, 14,* 192-202.

Franzosi, R. (1998). Narrative analysis — or why (and how) Sociologists should be interested in narrative. *Annual Review of Sociology, 24,* 517-554

Good, B., & Good, M. (1994). In the subjunctive mode: Epilepsy narrative in Turkey. *Social Science and Medicine, 38*, 835-842.

Gottlieb, S. H. (2005). Dose sex matter? Diabetes, heart disease and gender. *Diabetes Forecast, 58*(2), 33-36.

Grace, S. L., Abbey, S. E., Shnek, Z. M., Irvine, J., Franch, R. L., & Stewart, D. E. (2002). Cardiac rehabilitation I: Review of psychosocial factors. *General Hospital Psychiatry, 24*(3), 121-126.

Hawthorne, M. H. (1992). Using the trajectory framework: Reconceptualizing cardiac illness. In P.Woog, (Ed), *The chronic illness trajectory framework,* (pp. 29-39). New- York, NY: Springer Publishing Company.

Herlitz, J., Karlson, B. W., Lindqvist, J., & Sjolin, M. (2002). Prognosis and risk indicators of death during a period of 10 years for women admitted to the emergency department with a suspected acute coronary syndrome. *International Journal of Cardiology, 82*, 259-269.

Hochner-Celnikier, D., Manor, O., Gotzman, O., Lotan, H., & Chajek-shaul, T. (2002). Gender gap in coronary artery disease: Comparison of the extent, severity and risk factors in men and women aged 45-65. *Cardiology, 97*(1), 18-23.

Izraeli, D. (199). Women, work, family and public policy. In Globerzon et al., (Eds.), *Human Resources and Labor Relationships in Israel – New Routes* (pp. 228-232). Tel-Aviv: Ramot (Hebrew). .

Johnson, J. L., & Morse, J. M. (1990). Regaining control: The process of adjustment after myocardial infarction. *Heart & Lung, 19,* 126-135.

Johanson, E. E., Hamberg, K., West, G., & Linder, G. (1999). The meaning of pain: An exploration of women's description of symptoms. *Social Science and Medicine, 48*, 1791-1802.

Keller, K. B.,& Lemberg, L. (2000). Gender differences in acute coronary events. *American Journal of Critical Care, 9*, 207-209.

Kim-Kyungeh, A. (2000). *Gender differences in the associations between anxiety early after acute myocardial infarction and subsequent in hospital complications.* Dissertation Abstracts.

King, K., & Koop, P. M. (1999). The influence of the cardiac surgery patient's sex and age on care giving received. *Social Science and Medicine, 48*, 1735-1742.

Kleinman, A. (1988). *The illness narratives.* New York, NY: Basic Books.

Ladwing, K. H., Muhlberger, N., Walter, H., Schumacher, K., Popp, K., Holl, R., et al. (2000). Gender differences in emotional disability and negative health perception in cardiac patients six months after stent implantation. *Journal of Psychosomatic Research, 48*, 501-508.

Levine, T. B., Levine, A. B., Raminski, P., & Stom, R. J. (2000). Reversal of heart failure remodeling in women. *Journal of Women's Health and Gender Based Medicine, 9*, 513-519

Lieberman, L., Mena, M., & Stewart, D. (1998). Cardiac rehabilitation: Gender differences in factors influencing participation. *Journal of Women's Health, 7,* 717-723.

Lincoln, Y., & Guba, E. (1985). *Naturalistic inquiry.* Beverly Hills, CA: Sage Publications.

Lorber, J. (1997). *Gender and the social construction of illness.* Thousand Oaks, CA: Sage Publications.

Lukkarinen, H., Hentinen, M. (1998). Asessment of quality of life with the Nottingham health profile among women with coronary artery disease. *Heart and Lung: Journal of Acute & Critical Care, 27*, 189-199.

Maclean, U., & Cockshutt, A. (1979). How women cope with their men-folk's heart attacks. *New Society, 26*, 183-185.

Mark, D. B. (2000). Sex bias in cardiovascular care: Should women be treated more like men? *Journal of the American Medical Association, 283*, 659-661.

McKinlay, J. B. (1996). Some contributions from the social system to gender inequalities in heart disease. *Journal of Health and Social Behavior, 37*(1), 1-26.

McSweeney, J. C., Cody, M., & Caren, P. B. (2001). Do you know them when you see them? Women`s prodromal and acute symptoms of myocardial infraction. *Journal of Cardiovascular Nursing, 15*(3), 26-38.

Meischke, H., Larsen, M. P., & Eisenberg, M. S. (1998). Gender differences in reported symptoms for acute myocardial infarction: Impact on pre-hospital delay time interval. *American Journal of Emergency Medicine, 16*, 363-366.

Miles, A. (1991). *Women, health and medicine.* Great Britain: Open University Press.

Miller, C. L. (2002). A review of symptoms of coronary artery disease in women. *Journal of advanced Nursing, 39*(1), 17-23.

Norris, R. M. (1998). Fatality outside hospital from acute coronary events in three British heart districts, 1994-5. *British Medical Journal, 316*, 1065-1070.

Parson, T. (1951). *The social system.* London: Routledge & Kegan Paul.

Phillpott, S., Boynton, M. P., Feder, G., & Hemingway, H. (2001). Gender differences in descriptions of angina symptoms and health problems immediately prior to angiography: The ACRE study. *Social Science and Medicine, 52*, 1565-1575.

Pierret, J. (2001). Interviews and biographical time: The case of long- term HIV nonprogressor. *Sociology of Health & Illness, 23*, 159-179.

Poirier, S., & Lioness, A. (1997). Ending, secrets and silences: Overreading in narrative inqury. *Research in Nursing and Health, 20*, 551-557.

Remennick, L. I., & Raanan, O. (2000). Institutional and attitudinal factors involved in higher mortality of Israeli women after coronary bypass surgery: Another case of gender bias. *Health , 4*, 455-478.

Riessman, C. K. (1990). Strategic uses of narrative in the presentation of self and illness: A research note. *Social Science and Medicine, 30*, 1195-1200.

Robinson, C. A. (1993). Managing life with a chronic condition: The story of normalization. *Qualitative Health Research, 3*(1), 6-28.

Rose-Gail, L., Suls, J., Green, P., & Lounsbury, P. (1996). Comparison of adjustment, activity and tangible social support in men and women patients and their spouses during the six months post myocardial infarction. *Annals of Behavioral Medicine, 18*, 264-272.

Rosenfeld, J. A. (2000). Heart disease in women: Gender specific statistics and prevention strategies for a population at risk. *Postgraduate Medicine, 107*, 111-116.

Ruston, A., Clayton, J., & Calnan, M. (1998). Patient's action during their cardiac event: Qualitative study exploring differences and modifiable factors. *British Medical Journal, 316*, 1060-1064.

Sandelowski, M. (1991). Telling stories: Narrative approaches in qualitative research. *Image, 23,* 161-167.

Silverman, D. (1993). Theory and method in qualitative research (chapter 1). *Interpreting Qualitative Data: Methods for Analyzing Tallk, Text and Interaction.* Thousand Oaks, CA: Sage Publication.

Twaddle, A. C., & Hesslers, R. M. (1987). The sickness career. *A Sociology of Health.* (2nd Edition), (pp 143-161). New York, NY: Macmillan.

Uuskuela, M. (1996). Psychological differences between young male and female survivors of myocardial infarction. *Psychotherapy and Psychosomatics, 65,* 327-330.

Vakili, B.A ., Kaplan, R. C., & Brown, D. L. (2001). Sex-based differences in early mortality of patients undergoing primary angioplasty for first acute myocardial infarction. *Circulation, 104*(25), 3034-3038

Van Tiel, D., Van Vliet, K. P., & Moerman, C. J. (1998). Sex differences in illness beliefs and illness behaviour in patients with suspected coronary artery disease. *Patient Education & Counseling, 33,* 143-147.

Verbrugge, L. M. (1985). Gender and health: An update on hypotheses and evidence. *Journal of Health and Social Behavior, 26,* 156-182.

Verbrugge, L .M. (1986). From sneezes to adieux: Stages of health for American men and women. *Social Science and Medicine, 22,* 1195-1212.

Wenger, N. K. (1996). The high risk of CHD for women: Understanding why prevention is crucial. *Madscape Womens Health, 1*(11), 6.

Weidner, G. (2000). Why do men get more heart disease than women? An international perspective. *Journal of American College Health, 48,* 291-294.

Willis, E., Miller, R., & Wyn, J. (2001). Gendered embodiment and survival for young people with cystic fibrosis. *Social Science and Medicine, 53,* 1163-1174

In: Heart Disease in Women
Editor: B. V. Larner and H. R. Pennelton

ISBN 978-1-60692-066-4
© 2009 Nova Science Publishers, Inc.

Chapter VII

Thromboembolism and Coronary Heart Disease: In Which Aspects are Women Different?

Sigrid Nikol[1,] and Katharina Middendorf[2]*
[1]Department for Cardiology and Angiology, Klinikum
Westfälische Wilhelm University, Münster, Germany
[2]Clinic for Gynecology and Obstetrics, Klinikum Großhadern,
Ludwig Maximilian University, Munich, Germany

Abstract

Young women are at a 3-fold higher risk of experiencing venous thromboembolism compared to young men. This risk is further increased by oral contraceptives, smoking, hereditary thrombophilia and/or low socioeconomic status. There are also hints for gender specific differences in the arterial system. Coronary heart disease which is particularly important develops in women 10-15 years later than in men. However, the clinical course in women is often more complicated. In women, thrombophilic predispositions play a more important role before menopause and metabolic risk factors after menopause, compared to men.

Thrombus formation needs to be initiated by disturbances of at least one element of the Virchow trias. There is principally no difference between men and women. However, all three elements are influenced by estrogen, resulting in gender specific differences. There is a favourable influence on blood flow by the inhibition of atherogenesis and on the endothelial function by increased NO release, and an unfavourable influence on hemostasis resulting in hypercoagibility. Thus, particularly non-selective hormone replacement therapy for the inhibition of atherogenesis may be questionable due to increased thrombogenicity. The solution may be more selective estrogen receptor

* Correspondence to: Univ.-Prof. Dr. med. Sigrid Nikol, Medizinische Klinik und Poliklinik C, Universitätsklinikum, Albert-Schweitzer-Str. 33, D-48129 Münster, Germany, Telefon: +49 251 834 8501, Fax: +49 251 834 5101, E-mail: nikol@uni-muenster.de

modulators. Clinical trials are still needed for both, hormone replacement therapy and the therapy of venous and arterial thromboembolism which has been thus far studied in predominantly male patient cohorts.

Key words: Estrogen, hormone replacement therapy, venous thromboembolism, arterial thromboembolism, myocardial infarction, arteriosclerosis

Introduction

Over many years, sex-specific investigations in physical medicine were restricted to the fields of gynecology and andrology. Although 44% of cardiological in-hospital patients suffering from coronary heart disease (CHD) are women it was not before the sixties that the different pathogenesis and clinical course of CHD in women were investigated. Furthermore, until the end of the nineties only 25% of patients included in large interventional trials for myocardial infarction and unstable angina were women (Lee et al., 2001). Large interventional studies for the prevention and treatment of CHD, and its complications, contained only 1.7% women. Clinical trials with statines, ß-blockers to lower cholesterol and ACE inhibitors to lower arterial blood pressure were also performed predominantly with male probants (Harris and Douglas, 2000). However, being female represents an additional risk factor for those patients suffering from CHD, and that also requires therapies adapted for women. This is particularly true for arterial and venous thromboembolism because women are more prone to thrombophilia than men due to certain selectional advantages meant particularly to protect younger women with childbearing potential.

Here we will review the particularities of arterial and venous thromboembolism and arteriosclerosis in women and point out potential diagnostic and therapeutic consequences. We will emphasize differences in the course of the disease and behavioural differences as well as the problems related to the way clinical trials have been conducted.

Background

Particularities of Anatomy, Physiology and Biomechanics in Women

The muscle mass in women is only 25% (men 35-40%) and there is also a histological difference in fat content and structure of muscle fibres. Physical stress delays the growth of girls to the age of 12 years. The coordination of different muscle groups and the flexibility of the body are better developed in women. Girls reach maximal static power earlier than boys (16-17 years). However, the higher the velocity of movement the smaller is the difference between men and women.

Anaerobic and aerobic efficiencies are also consistently different. Women dominate sports with anaerobic stress (e.g. short marathons, 100 km runs, long-distance swimming and recently also the 10-fold triathlon). In performances that require aerobic endurance, women burn fat faster and in more volume than men, preserving their glycogen stocks. Therefore, muscle acidosis appears later.

Pharmacogenetics, Pharmacokinetics and Pharmacodynamics of Cardiovascular Drugs in Women

Psychosocial and hormonal differences influence the metabolism of medications. The hormonal cycles are particularly important for their resorption and distribution. Gender-based therapeutics is the recognition that the dose of a medication should be different for a female, not only because of differences in body size, but also because of the gender of the patient. Gender-based therapeutics is also the selection of one drug over another, or perhaps no drug at all, because of gender. In addition, it encompasses the monitoring of a patient's reaction to a medication in a certain way because of that patient's gender. This is essential when there are side-effects of drugs that are more likely to occur in one gender (Woosley, 1998).

There are numerous gender differences in the handling of drugs in the body (pharmacokinetics) and in drug response (pharmacodynamics) that have been reported. Reviews by Harris et al. (Harris et al., 1995) and by Berg (Berg, 1995) cite ample evidence that one or more of the relevant pharmacokinetic parameters (absorption, distribution, clearance, half-life, metabolic or renal clearance, and protein binding) for a specific drug may be different between man and women, which may be clinically relevant. Clinical relevance depends very much on the narrowness of therapeutic indices, with little differences in detectable responses being more important in those drugs where the range of dosage required for efficacy is near the dosage that causes side effects.

Although there are many gender differences demonstrated in the pharmacokinetics of drugs (Harris et al, 1995), one cannot always assume that these differences will predict the existence or magnitude of pharmacodynamic differences accurately. Experience with the drug propranolol is most instructional. In the National Institutes of Health-sponsored *Beta-blocker Heart Attack Trial* (*Beta-blocker Heart Attack Trial* Research Group, 1982), there were clear indications that women had higher plasma concentrations of propranolol that men given equivalent dosages (the same effect has been much also shown later for metoprolol which demonstrated a 2-fold increased plasma concentration with the same dose in women (Luzier et al., 1999)). Subsequent studies found women to have a lower clearance for propranolol than men (Walle et al, 1989). The natural response to these data would be to recommend that women be given lower dosages of propranolol to correct for their lower clearance of the drug. However, when the actual degree of the ß-adrenoceptor blockade produced by propranolol was compared in men and women using an isoproterenol exchange infusion, it was found that women had lower sensitivity to propranolol that compensated for the higher concentrations in women. This difference negates the need for lower doses, which might have reduced the overall efficacy of this life-saving drug (Woosley, 1998).

For several other cardiovascular medications, a gender-specific difference in metabolism influenced by endogeneous hormones and further enhanced by the application of exogeneous hormones (oral contraceptives, hormone replacement therapy) has been demonstrated. Such differences may result in higher risk for some undesired side-effects or lack of efficiency of some of these drugs. It has become apparent in recent years that sex hormones have effects on many more tissues than just those involved in reproduction. Even heart muscle has receptors for sex hormones, and exposure to these hormones can alter the expression of ion channels responsible for cardiac repolarization and the QT interval on the electrocardiogram (Drici et al., 1996; Stumpf, 1990) which may explain differences in cardiac response to drugs. Such gender-specific differences in conduction lead to more drug-induced torsades-depointes in women, who physiologically have longer QT-intervals than men (Makkar et al., 1993). Sex hormones prolong the QT interval and, thus, down regulate potassium channel expression (Drici et al., 1996). Thus, potassium channel expression and sensitivity to drugs is regulated by sex hormones (Drici et al, 1996). A large number of drugs from diverse classes, such as antiarrhythmic drugs, antihistamines (terfenadine, astemizole), antibiotics (erythromycin, halofantrine), and gastrointestinal prokinetics (cisapride) have the potential to induce such potentially lethal cardiac arrhythmia, torsades des pointes (Lazzara, 1996). These drugs further block potassium channels already down regulated by female hormones (Makkar et al, 1993) a regulation also dependent on the menstrual cycle (Rosano et al, 1996). A gender-specific reaction to digoxin in heart failure patients has only recently become known, leading to an increased rate of death in women (Rathore et al., 2002).

Also important for the prevention of thromboembolism is the 61% higher clearance of acetylsalicylic acid in men compared to women, which explains a 50% extended half-life for acetylsalicylic acid in women. However, when using oral contraceptives, the clearance of acetylsalicylic acid becomes more similar to that of men (Miners et al., 1986). In contrast, the aggregation of thrombocytes is clearly less inhibited in women compared to men and is similar to men following orchiectomy (Spranger et al., 1989). Testosterone, not estrogen, causes the difference in aggregation of thrombocytes. The clinical relevance of this finding is not very well known, especially since important studies, e.g. for the use for coumarines versus acetylsalicylic acid following myocardial infarction, were performed only in men or postmenopausal women (*Coumadin Aspirin Reinfarction Study CARS* Investigators, 1997).

Influence of Estrogen on the Coagulation System

The dual system of blood coagulation consists of a procoagulatoric and an anticoagulatoric part. The antithrombotic system prevents the transition of a physiological thrombus formation to a pathological thrombosis (thrombophilia). Thrombophilia can be based on hereditary or acquired pathologies. Acquired reasons may be diseases (e.g. malignoma, myeloproliferative disease and abnormalities with lupus anticoagulans), recent surgery or trauma, immobilization, oral contraceptives, pregnancy or smoking.

If venous thrombosis occurs at a young age, in the case of recurrent thromboembolic events, or if there is a trait for hereditary venous thrombosis, chances for a biological defect causing thrombophilia are high. Hereditary reasons comprise mutations leading to a preponderance of the procoagulatoric system: factor V mutation (50%), deficiency of antithrombin (5%), protein S (5%) and protein C (5%). However, about 35% of hereditary underlying causes are still unknown.

Factor V Leiden is the most important cause of hereditary thrombophilia and is associated with 50% of familial thrombophilias. Inactivation of activated factor V (Va) by activated protein C (APC) is inhibited due to this mutation. Factor V Leiden alone does not cause thromboembolic events. Additional risk factors for thrombosis are necessary and in women, particularly, oral contraceptives and hormone replacement therapy play an important role. In thrombophilic women, the first venous thrombotic events occur at the age of 25 (10-40) years, at which heterozygotes show a 5-7-fold and homozygotes a 50-100-fold increased risk. Age in women is significantly lower compared to men for the first thrombotic event.

Even without mutation, women show an increased estrogen-dependent physiological thrombophilia due to a selectional advantage leading to a shorter bleeding time. Thus, loss of iron during menstruation, birth and trauma is reduced (Rees et al., 1995). Additionally, physiological thrombophilia may be advantageous for fetal implantation (Majerus, 1994) and improving placental function (Hajjar, 1994). This tendency toward thrombophilia is based on the role of estrogen in hemostasis. Factor VII, antithrombin, PAI-1 activity and the inactivation rate of factor Va by APC (activated protein C) are lower and the activity of protein C and protein S, thrombin and potentially fibrinogen is increased by estrogen (Samsioe, 1998). Therefore, hypercoagulability is more common in pregnant women or women using oral contraceptives.

Estrogens also influence activated protein C (APC). The average APC activity in men is significantly higher than in women. Moreover, premenopausal women show a lower APC ratio than postmenopausal women, which is even lower during pregnancy or estrogen therapy (Kiechl et al., 1999). The lower APC ratio of women under the influence of oral contraceptives may be explained by a shorter activated partial thromboplastin time (aPTT) and an increase of factor VIIIc and IXc (Lowe et al., 1999). Thus, fertile women demonstrate a thrombophilic tendency. Increased APC ratios have been reported following consumption of alcohol (Kiechl et al., 1999) which may explain in part its vasculoprotective effect.

In the presence of additional cardiovascular risk factors typical for the Western world and improved medical care, the selectional advantage of more efficient coagulation becomes less relevant and the originally protective thrombophilia becomes disadvantageous for women.

Influence of Estrogen on the Endothelial Function

An intact and well-functioning endothelium is necessary for vascular resistance against thrombosis. Damage of the vascular endothelium leads to a reduction of agents which prevent coagulation and exposure of the microfibrillar, subendothelial tissue with its characteristic adhesiveness for thrombocytes and activation of coagulation. Toxins reaching the endothelium via blood flow (e.g. endotoxine, ischaemia, inflammation) and perivascular lesions to the vessel (e.g. trauma, necrosis, inflammation, atheroma) can cause such endothelial damages.

Male and female experimental animals show differential endothelial functions: the basal rate of nitric oxide (NO) release is higher in females than in males. After ovarectomy, this favourable vasodilatating effect is absent. The NO-mediated vasodilation depends on the control of the hormonal cycles (Hernandez et al., 2000). Increased NO release is observed following application of estrogens or selective modulators of estrogen receptors after ovarectomy, or in transgenic hypertensive rats (Hernandez et al., 2000; Ma et al., 2000).

While hypercholesterinemia has no influence on vascular function in premenopausal women, postmenopausal women reveal the same influence of lipid profiles on microcirculation as men. This may be caused by a decrease of the density of estrogen receptors after menopause. Good results were shown with substitution of estrogen alone. The combination with gestagen showed no further improvement regarding hypercholesterinemia and microcirculation, although there was a reduction of the risk for carcinoma of the endometrium.

Manifestatiosn of Thromboembolism and Arteriosclerosis

Venous Thromboembolism

Venous thromboembolism becomes clinically apparent as thrombophlebitis or phlebothrombosis, with its complication pulmonal embolism. Overall, one out of a thousand persons experiences a venous thrombosis per year (Majerus, 1994).Iin the USA alone, there are 300,000 patients suffering from deep vein thrombosis with or without pulmonal embolism per year. The latter results in its main complication of deep vein thrombosis and 5-10% of all cases of in-hospital deaths and women are more often affected than men (Stein et al., 1999).

The risk is increased 3-fold in young women compared to young men and remains increased until the age of 45 years (Winkler, 1997). In combination with oral contraceptives the risk increases 4-fold, in combination with smoking 7-fold. The relative risk for a lethal pulmonal embolism caused by oral contraceptives is as high as 9.6 per 1 million women years in New Zealand (Parkin et al., 2000). In the presence of an additional genetic defect causing thrombophilia, the risk increases 6-30-fold (Winkler, 1997). Hormone replacement therapy increases the risk for venous thrombembolism 2-3-fold (Oger and Scarabin, 1999), especially in women with a history of thrombosis (Hoibraaten et al., 2000).

Arterial Thromboembolism

Arterial thromboembolism comprises embolic disease with emboli from the left heart causing cerebral ischaemia and stroke, but also affecting all larger aortic branches and tissues perfused by these arteries. Some emboli, however, originate from the venous system and cross the atrial septum due to an open oval foramen.

In contrast, there are acute vascular occlusions which are caused by local thrombosis following plaque rupture. Typical events with this pathogenesis are myocardial infarction and acute leg ischemia and are usually due to an underlying arteriosclerosis.

Peripheral Embolism including Stroke

Patients with severe cardiac failure are at a 0.9-5.5% risk per year to suffer from thromboembolic events. Women are more often affected than men (2.4% vs. 1.8%), if the sinusrhythm is preserved (Dries et al., 1997). Atrial fibrillation is another frequent reason for peripheral embolism including stroke, especially in women older than 75 years. Moreovber, women show more proarrhythmic effects caused by antiarrhythmic drugs and have more benefit from anticoagulation for the prevention of stroke (Michelena and Ezekowitz, 2000).

Diabetes and arterial hypertension are more important risk factors for stroke in women than in men, similarly for CHD (Keller and Lemberg, 2000). In all age groups stroke is more frequent in men (Moulin et al., 1997; Wyller, 1999), but mortality is higher in women (Moulin et al., 1997) and they seem to be more functionally handicaped if they survive. This may be due to the higher age when women experience their first stroke compared to men and the age-dependent success of rehabilitation after stroke (Wyller, 1999). Over 80 years, prevalence becomes higher in women compared to men.

Coronary Heart Disease (CHD)

The *Framingham Heart Study*, which began in 1948, is a longitudinal prospective study of cardiovascular disease involving several thousand men and women. According to this study, CHD is one of the main causes of death in the industrial world (Sytkowski et al., 1990). The prevalence of CHD is 20% in middle-aged men, and in women CHD becomes more common after menopause because of estrogen deficiency. A 50-year-old woman has a 46% risk of having CHD and a 31% risk of dying from it (Schenk-Gustafsson 1996). Female CHD patients have a distinct clinical presentation, which includes more thromboembolic disease without coronatry arteriosclerosis. Lipid profiles differ between men and women. Women have higher levels of HDL (high density lipoprotein) and lower levels of LDL (low density lipoprotein) cholesterol compared with men. Due to the protection afforded by female hormones, particularly, estrogen, fertile women are at a lower risk for arteriosclerosis. Postmenopausal women loose this protection, and the course of CHD is then even more complicated than in men. Therefore, since 1984 more women then men in the USA died due to cardiovascular disease per year—more than 450,000 because of cardiac disease, 250,000 of the latter due to CHD (Giardina, 2000).

Male gender is an independent risk factor for arteriosclerosis and thus, for CHD. The ratio for men over women is 2 to 3 over 1. The vasoprotection of estrogen during the fertile period leads to its lower prevalence in women. The *PEPI-study* group investigated the influence of estrogens on lipids in 875 healthy postmenopausal women (45-64 years). Estrogen significantly lowered atherogenic LDL and increased protective HDL cholesterol levels in plasma by 10-20% each. Lipid-dependent mechanisms such as increased NO and prostacyclin as well as reduced endothelin and thromboxan A2 release are anti-atherogenic (Taubert, 1998). The combination with gestagen lowers the positive effect of estrogen on HDL cholesterol. The increase of triglycerides, the size of VLDL (very low density lipoprotein) cholesterol, decrease of apolipoprotein B and the size of LDL cholesterol induce potentially atherogenic changes.

While estrogen protects young women against atherogenesis, the gender-specific difference regarding morbidity for CHD decreases with age (Vogels et al., 1999). CHD becomes more important to female life over time due to the longer life expectancy of women in contrast to men (1999: women 81 and men 74 years; 22% women but only 10% of men reach the age of 90 years). Cardiovascular risk factors become more important, while the physiological thrombophilia of the fertile age disappears.

The distribution of risk factors show gender-specific differences: in the *Nurses Health Study* (80,000 women, follow-up 14 years) "low risk" was defined as: no history of diabetes, arterial hypertension or CHD in combination with a cholesterol level of below 200 mg/dl. All other women were at "normal risk". Only 30% of the nurses were in the low risk group, among those only 0.17% suffered from severe coronary events in contrast to 1% of women at high risk. Smoking and bad nutrition increased the coronary risk to 13 and 16%, respectively. In the presence of the same risk factors, there is a higher cardiovascular mortality in women compared to men (Stampfer et al., 1991a).

The major problem for women is the coincidence of different atherogenic parameters of the metabolic syndrome due to a more severe adipositas in ageing women compared with men. 35% of women with a body mass index (BMI) > 30 kg/m^2 have at least 2 or more risk factors. Decrease of estrogen additionally increases the risk profile. An increase of triglycerides is a more important risk factor in women than in men. Compared with male cardiovascular risk, women with diabetes show a 6-fold, with smoking a 4-fold, with arterial hypertension a 2-fold and with unemployment a 1.9-fold increased risk for CHD (Keller and Lemberg, 2000; Sullivan et al., 1994). Particularly, socioeconomic status seems to be more important in women than in men (Vogels et al., 1999). In addition, women are over-represented among patients with type II diabetes. CHD appears 10-15 years later in women, but women with CHD have more risk factors then men at the same age. When women become symptomatic, they hesitate to visit a physician, which in itself often results in a more complicated course of the disease. Referrals to a specialist are almost twice as common in men compared to women (Vogels et al., 1999).

In 1972 the natural history of angina was reported based on data from the *Framingham study* and several sex differences emerged (Kannel et al., 1972). Compared with men, angina was the most common presentation of CHD in women (65% vs 37% in men) although the clinical course was less complicated. The 26-year follow-up of the Framingham population, reported in 1986 (Lerner et al., 1986), demonstrated that the incidence of angina pectoris increased in men with age, peaking between 55 and 65 years and then declining in older men. In contrast, the rate in women increased in parallel with men until 55 to 65 years, when it continued to rise, making angina a predominately female disease over the age of 75 years. The mean age at onset of angina was consequently greater in women than in men (64 years vs. 61 years).

Diagnostics of CHD are more difficult to interpret in women than in men. The exercise test is considered less reliable in women than in men both for diagnostic and prognostic purposes. Exercise testing is a non-invasive, readily available and low-cost method for assessment of chest pain syndromes. However, evaluations of this test for several indications have mostly been performed in male patients (Severi et al., 1988; Nyman et al., 1993). Only 32% of women, but 70% of men show a typical stress-induced angina. In contrast, syndrome X with normal vessels in the coronary angiography and typical angina is found in 48% of women and only 32% of men. Stress tests for ischemia are false positive in 40% of women (but only 10% of men) (Foussas et al., 1998). Although the prevalence of CHD in women is lower than in men, particularly in the pre-menopausal years, the prevalence of ST depression is higher in women younger than 45 years. This high prevalence of false-positive findings has been attributed to the presence of a higher estrogen level. There is evidence that estrogen may be a vasoconstrictor to coronary arterioles. It has a chemical structure similar to that of digitalis, which has also been demonstraed to be a vasoconstrictor. Men receiving large doses of estrogen for carcinoma of the prostate have increased degrees of ST depression (Degre, 2000). Overall, misinterpretations of exercise tests in both directions are found in 30-70% of the cases (Sullivan et al., 1994). Stress echocardiography in women shows a sensitivity and specificity of 75 and 87%, respectively, but stress myocardial scintigraphy with Tc[99m] Sestamibi is more suitable due to the possibility of applying stress until physicial limits are reached (Takeuchi et al., 1996) and interpretations are thus even more valid in women than in men (Hachamovitch et al., 1996). Women represent only 23% of patients who undergo angiography due to chest pain but coronary angiography performed when CHD was suspected showed no coronary stenosis in only 8-13% of men, but in 31-41% of women (Sullivan et al., 1994; Kirchgatterer et al., 1999). Likewise, the diagnosis of myocardial infarction as a complication of CHD is more difficult in women (Arslanian-Engoren, 2000). Pre- or postmenopausal women, with or without estrogenic treatment, with atypical chest pain in the presence of risk factors for CHD, must be submitted, if a doubt persists about the diagnosis of CHD after the non-invasive investigations, to coronary angiography more quickly than men.

Myocardial Infarction

A myocardial infarction (MI) which appears in pathological findings as a coagulation necrosis, can occur, if perfusion via an arteriosclerotically narrowed vessel suddenly halts due to an occlusion by a thrombus. Thrombus formation takes place in vascular lesions caused by atheromas formed in patients with certain cardiovascular risk factors. The fissure, rupture or ulceration of an atherosclerotic plaque in combination with local or even systemic thrombophilia usually ends in a fixed thrombus, that occludes the coronary vessel and finally leads to a myocardial infarction. There is an increased risk for rupture in atherosclerotic plaques with a lipid rich core and a thin fibrous cap.

Men and women have a different risk of suffering a MI: The Framingham Study demonstrated that myocardial infarction was twice as likely in men with angina compared to women (Kannel et al., 1972). The risk for MI increases at the age of 50-55 years in women, but already at 40-45 years in men. The incidence of MI increases in women who smoke in the age range of 35-54 years. Throughout Europe, the lowest risk for MI was found in the South (Spain) and the highest in the North (Scotland).

According to the Framingham report published in 1993 (Murabito et al., 1993), women were more likely to present with angina (47%) then either recognized MI (18%) or unrecognized MI(14%), unstable angina (7%) or death due to CHD (14%). In contrast, MI (recognized or unrecognized) accounted for nearly half of the first presentations in men (46%), followed by angina (32%), death (16%) and unstable angina (6%).

There are some reasons for the postmenopausal increase of myocardial infarction. The increase in weight may be due to the decrease of the ovarial function: after 55 years the BMI rises in women more than in men. This may result in an increased insulin resistance with an increase of the incidence of diabetes at an age of 45-65 years in women. Therefore, women predominate in type II diabetes. Furthermore, postmenopausal women show an increase of blood pressure and a disadvantageous statin-reversible change in lipids. Maximum LDL cholesterol levels are found in women at an age of 65 years, in men already at 45 years. After menopause, the LDL profile shifts to more atherogenicity, with more abundant LDL cholesterol and Apolipoprotein B. Moreover, proaggregatory factors become more abundant (Peters et al., 1999).

Also in the event of a MI or acute coronary syndrome, men and women demonstrate different behaviours, similar to the gender-specific behaviour in the case of angina: women request emergency treatment later than men and, therefore, they also receive thrombolysis later. Consequently, the course of MI in women reveals more complications (e.g. ventricular fibrillation, AV block, heart failure following MI) (Barakat et al., 2000; Keller and Lemberg, 2000). There is an increased lethality due to MI in women under 75 years, even in-hospital. Lethality is particularly high in young women in the first days after MI. Women receive thrombolytic therapy not only later but also more rarely than men (Yarzebski et al., 1996). Thrombolysis in women is also associated with more complications than in men, due to an overdose caused by a lack of adaption to dosages taking into account their average lower weight (Keller and Lemberg, 2000). Standards are still based on investigations in men mainly because women were under-represented or not separately evaluated in the large clinical trials available. Furthermore, coronary interventions and bypass surgery are associated with more complications in women (Malenka et al., 1999; Keller and Lemberg, 2000). Most notable in the case of MI, intervention and bypass surgery, are that women are at a higher age and suffer more often from arterial hypertension or diabetes resulting consequently in more complex coronary heart disease, often combined with preexistant heart failure (Fiebach et al., 1990). Not surprisingly, prognosis after MI is worse for women than for men. There is speculation that women form less vascular collaterals than men.

The role of hereditary disorders of the coagulation system in relation to MI is still controversial, and, particularly, a gender-specific role can only be deducted from a few clinical investigations. Thus, we investigated a possible association between the most frequent congenital thrombophilia, factor V Leiden, and MI (Middendorf et al., in press): The patient population analyzed comprised 507 patients with documented MI, 77.5% (393/507) were men and 22.5% (114/507) were women. Among patients with MI, 44 showed a factor V Leiden (p< 0.001), 68.2% (30/44) were men and 31.8% (14/44) women representing a statistically non-significant trend towards a higher prevalence of MI in women with this mutation (Nikol et al., data not shown). As expected, independent of the mutation, women with MI showed a tendency towards lower APC ratios than men. Patients with MI had a mean age of 56.1 years at the first MI, similar to the 44 patients with additional factor V Leiden with 54.5 years. The subgroup of women with the mutation showed a much lower age at first MI than the group without factor V Leiden (Table 1).

Table 1. Age-wise Distributon of Patients Following Myocardial Infarction with and without Factor V LEIDEN (Nikol et al., data not published)

All patients with MI		+Factor V Leiden	-Factor v leiden
Women	60.1 (18-84) years	53.9 (37-74)	61.0 (18-84)
Men	55.0 (21-86) years	54.8 (35-84)	55.0 (21-86)

This is in contrast to some publications which stated no association between factor V Leiden and the incidence of MI. Again, most of these trials included almost exclusively men (Emmerich et al., 1995; Inbal et al., 1999; Ridker et al., 1995). Other authors, however, did find a positive association between this mutation and acute MI. According to Baranovskaya et al. (Baranovskaya et al., 1998), factor V Leiden is particularly an important risk factor for MI in elderly patients with atherosclerosis as the main underlying cause of cardiovascular disease. Doggen et al. (Doggen et al., 1998) even noted that the risk for MI was 40-fold increased by this mutation. The presence of additional cardiovascular risk factors further augmented the risk, e.g. smoking resulted in a 6-fold increased risk.

Holm et al. described two young women suffering from acute MI (Holm et al., 1994). Both showed normal plasmatic values of protein C, protein S, antithrombin, fibrinogen, von-Willebrand-factor, factor VII-activity, cholesterol and triglycerides, but were homozygous for factor V Leiden. In coronary angiography, one had normal coronary arteries with transitory vasospasms indicating a possible role of resistance against APC on endothelial dysfunction.

Rosendaal et al. investigated the prevalence of factor V Leiden in young females with MI (Rosendaal et al., 1997a): 84 women (18-44 years) with first MI, among those 15% postmenopausal women. The control group comprised 388 age-matched women without MI from the same region. Women with factor V Leiden had a 2.5-fold increased risk for MI. In the presence of additional metabolic risk factors such as adipositas, arterial hypertension, hypercholesterinemia or diabetes, the risk was 25-fold increased in comparison to women without this mutation and risk factors (Rosendaal et al., 1997b). Smoking women with factor V Leiden even had a 32-fold risk for MI compared with non-smoking women without this mutation. Therefore, according to the authors, smoking is a precondition for an increased risk due to factor V Leiden as both represent complete or at least partial prothrombotic factors.

In summary, biochemical gender-dependent differences for the etiology of MI are suspected. Factor V Leiden represents a risk factor for MI especially in women. Independent from the presence of factor V Leiden, endo- and exogeneous estrogen increases the APC resistance in women and additionally lowers the inactivation rate of factor V by APC. The increased risk for MI in women on oral contraceptives is clearly further augmented by smoking.

Therapeutic Consequences

Particularities of thromboembolism and coronary heart diseases in women demand specific therapeutic consequences. This chapter will give an overview based on evidence available at this point in time. Many clinical trials with fertile and postmenopausal women included are certainly still needed.

Anticoagulation

An increased thrombophilia in young women possibly requires a more aggressive anticoagulatory therapy, in particular in the presence of prothrombotic mutations and a history of venous or arterial thromboembolism which represents a clearly increased risk compared to men. However, the association between certain risk factors and the actual increased number of events has been proven only for repeated venous thromboembolism. For arterial thromboembolism, no consensus has been reached so far. There are indications, however, that women with atrial fibrillation have more benefit regarding the prevention of strokes following anticoagulation (Michelena and Ezekowitz, 2000).

For the dosing of acetylsalicylic acid, the 50% extended half-life in women has to be taken into account, which is, however, not true for women using oral contraceptives (Miners et al., 1986).

Thrombolysis

The higher complication rate of thrombolysis of venous and arterial thromboembolism in women clearly requires adapted dosages. Present standards are based on data almost exclusively obtained in men or without separate analysis of the female subgroup. Thus randomized clinical trials for the female population are still needed.

Screening before Oral Contraceptives

Because of the increased risk of venous thromboembolism in women with inherited thrombophilia, the initiation of appropriate screening for genetic defects before prescription of oral contraceptives has been extensively discussed. These mutations, especially factor V Leiden causing 50% of the defects, affect particularly Caucasions, but rarely Asians and Africans. Winkler et al. (Winkler, 1997) investigated almost 6 million women on oral contraceptives. In this group, 840 thromboembolic complications were found, among them only 235 (28%) in women with APC resistance and 60 (7.2%) with an inhibitor deficiency (antithrombin, protein S, protein C). Therefore, 545 women suffering from thromboembolism showed no known mutation for thrombophilia. On the contrary, there was a prevalence of APC resistance (5.7%) and inhibitor deficiency (0.5%) which relates to an absolute number of 371,966 women with one of these mutations, who did not suffer from any thromboembolic complications (Winkler, 1997). Because of the high costs of such genetic screening, and under the conditions that not every genotypically positive person actually suffers from a phenotypic thrombophilia, it was recommended to limit this screening to women with a history of venous thromboembolism or clear hereditary taint (Winkler, 1997).

Hormone Replacement Therapy (HRT)

Initial indications comprised prevention of climacteric symptoms and postmenopausal disturbances. Repeately, there were also reports about the reduction of osteoporosis and arteriosclerosis in some of the women treated. With increasing age, there is an almost exponential increase for risk of hip fracture, stroke and coronary heart disease in women. 12% of women from 45-64 years of age have clincial signs of CHD and 33% over 65 years (Collins, 2002). Ovarectomized premenopausal women have a 2-fold increased risk for CHD and women beyond menopause suffer from more complicated courses of disease, even if they reveal the same risk profile like men. This, according to the findings from the *Framingham Study*, CHD accounts for more deaths due to cardiovascular disease in women compared to men (Sytkowski et al 1990). The change of risk for CHD following menopause is apparently associated with the reduction of levels for estrogen and estrogen receptors as well as the reaction of microcirculation towards pathological lipid profiles which becomes more men-like. The *Postmenopausal Estrogen/Progestin Interventions (PEPI)* then demonstrated in a randomized trial that LDL cholesterol was in women on HRT over 3 years 0,37-0,46 mmol/L lower compared to placebo (The Writing Group for the PEPI Trial, 1995). And the *Women's Ischemia Syndrom Evaluation (WISE)* observational trial demonstrated in 453 pre-, peri- und postmenopausal women who underwent coronary angiography for myocardial ischemia, that low cholesterol levels with or without statin therapy are not associated with low reproduction hormone levels (Bairey Merz et al., 2002). Due to all these findings, 38% of postmenopausal women were in 1996 on HRT and in the year 2000 Premarin (estrogen) was prescribed 46 million times and became the second most prescribed drug in the USA (Keating et al., 1999; Kreling et al., 2001). Premarin, together with Prempro (estrogen in combination with medroxyprogesteronacetate), accounted in 2002 for more than 2 billion US$ sales for the Wyeth company.

Table 2. Recommendation of the American Heart Association (AHA) Regarding Hormone Replacement Therapy (HRT) Based on Standard Doses (Mosca et al., 2001)

Primary Prevention
- Firm clinical recommendations for primary prevention await the results of ongoing randomized clinical trials.
- There are insufficient data to suggest that HRT should be initiated for the sole purpose of primary prevention of cardiovascular disease.
- Initiation and continuation of HRT should be based on established noncoronary benefits and risks, possible coronary benefits and risks, and patient preference.

Secondary Prevention
- HRT should not be initiated for the secondary prevention of cardiovascular disease.
- The decision to continue or stop HRT in women with cardiovascular disease who have been undergoing long-term HRT should be based on established noncoronary benefits and risks and patient preference.
- If a woman develops an acute cardiovascular disease event or is immobilized while undergoing HRT, it is prudent to consider discontinuance of the HRT or to consider venous thromboembolism prophylaxis while she is hospitalized to minimize risk of venous thromboembolism associated with immobilization. Reinstitution of HRT should be based on established noncoronary benefits and risks, as well as patient preference.

For about a decade, data regarding HRT to inhibit postmenopausal atherogenesis and to avoid cardiovascular events were controversial while only observational studies were available (Table 3) (Stampfer and Colditz, 1991b; Grady et al., 1992; Grodstein et al., 1996b; Sullivan et al., 1990; O'Brien et al., 1996). For primary prevention of CHD, the most important trial among those observational studies was the prospective, non-randomized *Nurses' Health Study*. This trial was performed from 1976 until 1996 including 70,533 healthy postmenopausal women. Among those women, 1,258 non-fatal MIs were registered. The risk for a severe coronary event while taking HRT was 39% lower than in women who had never been on hormones. An atheroprotective effect was already observed after a short period of hormone therapy, but clearly diminished with time following disruption of such HRT (Grodstein et al., 2001). However, this study demonstrated some weaknesses. Nurses have high medical knowledge and, therefore, are not representative of the general population. The decision to be on hormones was voluntary and, therefore, not the result of randomization. Women who decided to be on HRT usually live a more healthy lifestyle and, therefore, have less risk factors. In addition, a combination with progestin is necessary to prevent carcinoma of the endometrium, which was not considered in this study with estrogen monotherapy.

Table 3. Important Observational Clinical Trials to Study Hormone Replacement Therapy for Cardiovascular Disease in Women

Primary prevention
- CHD: Stampfer et al., 1991b
- CHD + life expectancy: Grady et al., 1992
- Cardiovascular disease: Grodstein et al., 1996b

Secondary prevention
- CHD: Sullivan et al., 1990
- Restenosis: O'Brien et al., 1996

The need for randomized placebo-controlled trials became evident, particularly when trials demonstrated a life-threatening risk related to HRT. The prospective observational *Nurses' Health Study* had been extended to evaluate the risk for breast cancer with 121,700 nurses 30-55 years of age included, and resulted in 725,550 women years follow-up. During this period of time, 1,935 cases of breast cancer were found. The relative risk was 1.32 for estrogen alone and 1.41 for estrogen combined with progesteron (Colditz et al., 1995). The relative risk for breast cancer correlated with the age of patients as well as with the duration of HRT. There was also an increased risk of venous thromboembolism which was demonstrated by the double-blind randomized placebo-controlled *Estrogen in Venous Thromboembolism Trial (EVTET)*. In this trial, 140 women following venous thromboembolism were included. The trial was disrupted when 8 vs.1 case of venous thromboembolism (deep vein thrombosis or pulmonary embolism) became apparent in the verum group versus placebo. Thus, the incidence of venous thromboembolism was more than 4-fold (10.7% vs. 2.3%) in the HRT group versus the placebo group (Hoibraaten et al., 2000). Other authors have also noted in previous publications an estrogen-induced increase of venous thrombogenesis with a thrombogenic influence even at low doses of hormones, with an overall 2-4-fold increased risk of deep vein thrombosis and pulmonary embolism (Grodstein et al., 1996a; Oger and Scarabin, 1999).

Only recently have data from randomized, placebo-controlled trials for primary prevention of CHD become available (Table 4). The most important among these trials is the *Women's Health Initiative (WHI)*, a trial with 16,608 healthy postmenopausal women, 50-79 of age who received estrogen alone or in combination with progestin vs. placebo. The estrogen/progestin arm of this trial had to be disrupted after 5.2 years follow-up when risks for this therapy became apparent (planned follow-up was 8.5 years). Increased risk was most likely due to prothombotic and proinflammatory effects of progestin. The study arm with estrogen therapy alone versus placebo is still continuing. So far, the overall mortality has not increased due to HRT in this trial (Rossouw et al., 2002; Hays et al., 2003). Increased risk per 10,000 women years comprised coronary events (+7), stroke (+8), pulmonary embolism (+8), invasive breast cancer (+8) and decreased risk was recorded for colon carcinoma (-6) and hip fracture (-5). Thus, the net effect was +20 major adverse events per 10,000 women years, or in other words, 2 per mille. Older women and women on HRT over 5 years were particularly at risk. Subgroup analyses revealed that even women with a familial risk for colon carcinoma

(1.4 events/1,000 women years HRT) and osteoporosis T score < -2,5 (1.5 events/1,000 women years HRT) and women with reduced osteodensity following fracture of the spinal column (compensation of other serious adverse events, however, other effective therapies available) had no overall benefit from HRT (Rossouw et al., 2002; Grady 2003). In addition to the risks noted above, final results from the *Women's Health Initiative Memory Study (WHIMS)*, an ancillary study to the *WHI*, have shown that combination therapy with estrogen and progestin is associated with a 2-fold increase in dementia compared to placebo (Shumaker et al., 2003).

Table 4. Randomized Clinical Trials to Study Hormone Replacement Therapy for Cardiovascular Disease in Women

Primary prevention:
- WHI Women's Health Initiative Study: Rossouw et al., 2002; Hays et al., 2003; Grady, 2003
- WISDOM Women's International Study of Long-Duration Oestrogen After Menopause: Vickers et al., 1995

Secondary prevention:
- HERS Heart and Estrogen/Progestin Replacement Follow-Up Study: Hulley et al., 1998
- PHASE Papworth Hormone Replacement Therapy Atherosclerosis Survival Enquiry: Clarke et al., 2000
- WEST Women's Estrogen and Stroke Trial: Viscoli et al., 2001
- ESPRIT Estrogen in the Prevention of Reinfarction Trial: Cherry et al., 2002
- WHISP Women's Hormone Intervention Secondary Prevention: Khan et al., 2000

Angiographic endpoints:
- WAVE Women's Atherosclerosis Vitamin/Estragen Trial: Waters et al., 2002
- ERA Estrogen Replacement and Atherosclerosis Study: Herrington et al., 2000
- WELL-HART Women's Estrogen/Progestin and Lipid Lowering Atherosclerosis Regression Trial (unpublished)
- EAGAR Estrogen and Graft Atherosclerosis Regression Trial (unpublished)

Evaluation of quality of life was conducted in a subgroup of 1,511 women. Only 12% of those women had symptoms which were only slightly improved in some cases 1 year following HRT (sleeping disturbance, body function, body pain). Most of these complications disappeared 3 years after HRT, except for sleeping disturbances. Overall, HRT for the improvement of quality of life was noted as clinically relevant not justified (Hays et al., 2003).

Results from the *Women's International Study of Long-Duration Oestrogen after Menopause (WISDOM)* for the clinical evaluation of HRT in primary prevention are still awaited

For secondary prevention, there have been a number of observational trials (Table 3) (Sullivan et al., 1990; O'Brien et al., 1996,) among those the prospective observational extension of the *Nurses' Health Study* for secondary prevention. 2,489 women with documented atherosclerosis or MI were included. During follow-up, 213 new MIs occurred. The relative risk for short-term HRT was 1.25, however, for long-term HRT 0.38, overall

0.65. There was a trend towards reduced risk for recurrent cardiovascular events (p = 0.002). However, there was no difference for estrogen alone versus the combination with progestin (Grodstein et al., 2001). Finally, the randomized, double-blind, placebo-controlled *Heart and Estrogen/Progestin Replacement Study (HERS)* with 0.625mg estrogen in combination with 2.5mg medroxyprogesterone acetate (MPA) and 4.1 years follow-up was performed (Hulley et al., 1998). 2,763 postmenopausal women with CHD, 55-80 years of age (mean age 67.7 years) were included. There was no decrease in mortality or coronary events (relative risk 0.99). The risk of MI in the first year was even increased by 52%, which then decreased during years 3 to 5 of the trial. In the first phase of hormone effects, prothrombotic effects were assumed and in a later phase a lowered progression of atherosclerosis, analogously to some of the large lipid studies which did not show any protection in the first two years. In addition, an increase in venous thromboembolic events (relative risk 2.89) and gallbladder disease (relative risk 1.38) were observed. However, there was no difference in number of fractures and cancer and overall mortality and no improvement of cognitive functions (Hulley et al., 1998; Grady et al., 2002b). Weaknesses of this study included the higher age of women included compared to other studies, thus leading to more morbidity, a study population infrequently prescribed with HRT and the use of a quite unfavourable type of gestagen. In addition, the follow-up period was too short, which became obvious when the last year of observation showed a clear trend towards a decrease of events in the treated group, a difference which became even more significant for the subgroup of women with high Lp(a)levels which were reduced by HRT (Shlipak et al., 2000). Lp(a) influenced the course of the trial and turned out to be an independent risk factor in the placebo group (Furberg et al., 2002). It is noteworthy is that the use of statines in the study population led to a reduction of cardiovascular events, thromboembolism and overall mortality which was, however, independent from the use of HRT (Herrington et al., 2002).

Follow-up of the *HERS trial* was then extended to 6.8 years (*HERS II*) with open-label use of HRT left to the discretion of the 2,321 women participating. The aim was to demonstrate persistence of the beneficial effects of HRT during years 3 to 5 in the HERS trial. However, results clearly demonstrated no significant overall difference in coronary events (relative risk for MI and cardiac death was 1.00 for *HERS II* alone and 0.99 for *HERS* and *HERS II* together). The relative risk for venous thrombosis was 1.4 and for gallbladder surgery 1.48, which was even higher in older women. There was a trend towards more carcinomas (Grady et al., 2002a, Hulley et al., 2002).

Another negative randomized placebo-controlled trial for secondary prevention was the *Estrogen in the Prevention of Reinfarction Trial (ESPRIT)*. Following their first MI, 1,017 women, 50-69 years of age were included and received estrogen versus placebo. End points were re-infarction, cardiac death and overall mortality during a follow-up period of 24 months. There was no significant difference for all 3 end points (Cherry et al., 2002).

ESPRIT confirmed results which had been earlier obtained by a secondary analysis of the *Coumadin Aspirin Reinfarction Study (CARS)* database. 524 postmenopausal women who had started HRT during the study phase immediately following MI had been analyzed retrospectively and compared to women who had never used HRT. Endpoints were MI, cardiac death and unstable angina. There were 41% vs 28% events for HRT vs women who had never used HRT (p=0.001, relative risk=1.44), and a particularly increased incidence of unstable angina (39% vs 20% p=0.001), which represented an endpoint not evaluated in the previously described trials. Estrogen combined with progestin was better than estrogen alone (relative risk 0.56) (Alexander et al., 2001).

Noteworthy is also the *Women's Estrogen and Stroke Trial (WEST)*, a randomized double-blind placebo-controlled study for secondary prevention with endpoints of stroke and death. 644 women following stroke or transitory ischemic attack (TIA) were included and received oral 17-ß Östradiol vs. placebo over a follow-up period of 2.8 years. Again, there was no benefit from HRT (relative risk 1.1 for estradiol). The risk for fatal stroke was even increased (relative risk 2.9) (Viscoli et al., 2001)There are also a number of randomized placebo-controlled trials with angiographic instead of clinical endpoints (Table 4). The *Estrogen Replacement and Atherosclerosis* (ERA) *trial,* was a double-blind, study with conjugated estrogen in combination with medroxyprogesterone acetate (MPA) with a follow-up of 3.2 years (Herrington et al., 2000). 309 postmenopausal women with CHD and a mean age of 65 years were included. A reduction of atherosclerotic progression in coronary angiography was seen. However, a possible proinflammatory effect of hormone replacement therapy with increased CRP (C reactive protein) levels was observed. In contrast, other trials such as the *Women's Angiographic Vitamin and Estrogen (WAVE)* trial did not demonstrate any beneficial effect on angiographic endpoints. In this randomized, double-blind, placebo-controlled trial for secondary prevention, 423 postmenopausal women with at least one 15-75% coronary stenosis in coronary angiography were included. They received estrogen in combination with progestin vs. placebo, and vitamine E vs. placebo. Repeat coronary angiography was performed after an average 0.9 years. There was a trend towards a decrease of minimum lumen diameter (MLD) compared to a baseline of 0.047mm for HRT vs. 0.024 mm for placebo per year (p=0.17) und 0.044 for vitamin E vs. 0.028 for placebo (p=0.32). And there was a significant increased risk for MI and death for the HRT group and as a trend for the vitamin E group (Waters et al., 2002).

Taken together, in all randomized trials on HRT for cardiovascular indications, there was no benefit regarding primary and secondary prevention (clinical and angiographic endpoints). According to a recommendation by the American Heart Association (AHA) published in 2001, patients with CHD should not receive HRT for secondary prevention (Grady and

Hulley, 2001; Mosca et al., 2001a; Table 2). This recommendation should probably now be extended to primary prevention.

The use of selective modulators of estrogen receptors may be an alternative to HRT using estrogen and gestagens (Haynes and Dowsett, 1999). A tissue-dependent estrogen agonist or antagonist for the treatment of osteoporosis and cardiovascular disease in postmenopausal women has been developed. Estrogen-antagonistic effects may, in addition, protect against breast cancer. Tamoxifen reduces serum cholesterol levels and stabilizes bone density. However, it is associated with an increased risk for endometrium carcinoma, deep vein thrombosis and pulmonal embolism (Meier and Jick, 1998), This finally had led to the development of selective modulators of estrogen receptors not having the side-effects of Tamoxifen (Ma et al., 2000). The *Multiple Outcomes of Raloxifene Evaluation (MORE)* study was a randomized double-blind placebo-controlled trial for the prevention of osteoporosis using 2 dosages of raloxifen as a selective modulator of estrogen receptors. Although cardiovascular events were not the original endpoints of the trial, secondary analysis of 7,705 postmenopausal women with osteoporosis (mean age 67 years) with additional multiple cardiovascular risk factors or previous cornary events or revascularizations, was performed. Evaluation of primary prevention for patients at risk and secondary prevention was conducted. Endpoints were coronary and cerebrovascular events during a follow-up period of 4 years. There was no change in overall cardiovascular events, although there was a reduction of events in women with increased cardiovascular risk. The confirmation of results by a trial with cardiovascular primary endpoints was recommended by investigators (Barrett-Connor et al., 2002). The ongoing *Raloxifene Use for The Heart (RUTH)* study is a randomized double-blind trial for secondary prevention using raloxifene versus placebo with 10,101 postmenopausal women >/= 55 years with documented CHD, peripheral vascular disease (PVD) or multiple cardiovascular risk factors for CHD. The primary endpoints are MI, cardiac death and a secondary endpoint is breast cancer. The follow-up period will be 6 years or disruption as soon as soon as 1,670 participants have reached one of the coronary endpoints (Mosca et al. 2001).

So far HRT should only be administrated for non-cardiovascular indications (which are still the only indications approved), and even in this case, potential risks have to be taken into account. Increased risk concerns women with CHD or following stroke, thromboembolism or breast cancer. If HRT is restricted to a relatively short period during climacterium, women are still young at this point in time, thus, per se at a much lower risk. In addition, if HRT is given only during those few years of climateric symptoms, overall risk will remain low. Nevertheless, the National Institutes of Health (NIH) do recommend low dose medications. Moreover, the Food and Drug Administration (FDA) recommends alternative therapy, if possible, for the remaining 3 indications of HRT: 1) medium to severe vasomotor disfunctions (hot flashes, incontinence), 2) medium to severe symptoms due to atrophy of the vulva (dryness, irritations) due to menopause (here FDA the recommends use of local hormone therapy), and 3) prevention of postmenopausal osteoporosis (FDA recommends a preference of non-estrogen therapy) (www.theheart.org, Heartwire 8.Jan. 2003).

Statines

So far, of important 19 statine studies for primary (90%) and for secondary (77%) prevention were exclusively performed on male probants. In addition, in none of the studies were persons older than 75 years included, although women especially pass frequently this age-limit these days. Therefore, the validity of the data available is for women considerably restricted by sex and age bias. There are hints that women undergoing statine therapy may receive less benefit regarding saved years of life compared to men. On the other hand, costs are increased because of their higher life expectancy (Grover et al., 1999).

Betablockers

The same dose of metoprolol reaches 2-fold increased plasma concentrations in women compared with men (Luzier et al., 1999). Thus, dosing of other betablockers should also be undertaken in a careful manner.

ACE Inhibitors

One of the major risk factors during post-menopause is an increase of blood pressure, which is frequently the underlying cause of cardiac failure in women. At the same time, during post-menopause there is an increase of angiotensin type I receptors and circulating markers of inflammation. Ongoing research is evaluating apparent differences in the pathophysiology of hypertension which may have an impact on therapeutic schemes for the gender-specific pharmacotherapy of hypertension. Multicenter studies like *Heart Outcomes Prevention Evaluation* (HOPE) (Yusuf et al., 2000) and *Acute Infarction Ramipril Efficacy* (AIRE) (The *Acute Infarction Ramipril Efficacy (AIRE)* Study Investigators, 1993) demonstrated a risk reduction in women comparable to that in men. However, ACE inhibitor-induced side effects such as chronic cough was found in women far more often than in men. In contrast, angiotensin-receptor blockers, which are another group of agents which interfere with the renin angiotensin system, seem to have equally beneficial effects on both sexes. This was demonstrated by the *Losartan Intervention For Endpoint Reduction (LIFE)* study with 54% female probants (Oikarinen et al., 2003) and by the *Valsartan Heart Failure Trial* (Val-HEFT) (Cohn and Tognoni, 2001).

Conclusion

There are epidemiological and pathophysiological gender-specific differences for risk for venous or arterial thromboembolism. In premenopausal women, hereditary thrombophilias play an important role whereas acquired conditions determine postmenopausal initialization and course of disease. For the development of arteriosclerosis, metabolic risk factors are more important in women compared to men. The role of estrogen is well-known.

Improvements are still necessary in diagnostic techniques of cardiovascular disease in women, particularly coronary heart disease, as well as the development of guidelines safely pplicable to women. Randomized trials are required for the treatment of thromboembolism and coronary heart disease in sufficiently large female cohorts necessary in order to obtain the data required for such guidelines. The NIH have already regulated the way clinical trials are being conducted in this regard and prohibit trials solely conducted in men.

Acknowledgments

We would like to thank Mrs. Bien-Hung Pham for her editorial help.

References

Alexander KP, Newby K, Hellkamp AS et al. Initiation of hormone replacement therapy after acute myocardial infarction is asscociated with more cardiac events during follow-up. *J Am Coll Cardiol.* 2001;38:1-7.

Arslanian-Engoren C. Gender and age bias in triage decisions. *J Emerg Nurs.* 2000;26:117 124.

Bairey Merz CN, Olson MB, Johnson BD et al. Cholesterol-lowering medication, cholesterol level, and reproductive hormones in women: the Women's Ischemia Syndrome Evaluation (WISE). *Am J Med.* 2002;113:723-727.

Barakat K, Eilkinson P, Suliman A, Randjadayalan K, Timmis A. Acute myocardial infarction in women: contribution of treatment variables to adverse outcome. *Am Heart J.* 2000;140:740-746.

Baranovskaya S, Kudinov S, Fomicheva E et al. Age as a risk factor for myocardial infarction in Leiden mutation carriers. *Mol Genet Metab.* 1998;63: 155-157.

Barrett-Connor E, Grady D, Sashegyi A et al. Raloxifene and cardiovascular events in osteoporotic postmenopausal women: four-year results from the MORE (Multiple Outcomes of Raloxifene Evaluation) randomized trial. *JAMA.* 2002;287:847-857.

Berg M. Gender-related health issues: Stockholm, Sweden: 55th *World Congress of Pharmacy and Pharmaceutical Sciences.* 1995.

Beta-blocker Heart Attack Trial Research Group. A randomized trial of propranolol in patients with acute myocardial infarction. I. Mortality results. *JAMA.*1982;247:1707-1714.

Cherry N, Gilmour K, Hannaford P et al. Oestrogen therapy for prevention of reinfarction in postmenopausal women: a randomised placebo controlled trial. *Lancet.* 2002;360:2001-2008.

Clarke S, Kelleher J, Lloyd-Jones H et al. Transdermal hormone replacement therapy for secondary prevention of coronary artery disease in postmenopausal women. *Eur Heart J.* 2000; 21(Abstr. Suppl.): 212.

Cohn JN, Tognoni G. A randomized trial of the angiotensin-receptor blocker valsartan in chronic Heart failure. *N Engl J Med.* 2001;345:1667-1675. Colditz GA, Hankinson SE, Hunter DJ et al. The use of estrogens and progestins and the risk of breast cancer in postmenopausal women. *N Engl J Med.* 1995;332:1589-1593.

Collins P. Clinical cardiovascular studies of hormone replacement therapy. *Am J Cardiol.* 2002;90: 30F-34F.

Coumadin Aspirin Reinfarction Study (CARS) Investigators. Randomised double-blind trial of fixed low-dose warfarin with aspirin after myocardial infarction. *Lancet.* 1997;350:389-396.

Degre S. Is the exercise test of use in post-menopausal women with unstable coronary artery disease? *Eur Heart J.* 2000;21:175-176.

Doggen CJM, Cats VM, Bertina RM, Rosendaal FR. Interaction of coagulation defects and cardiovascular risk factors – increased risk of myocardial infarction associated with factor V Leiden or prothrombin 20210A. *Circulation.* 1998;97:1037-1041.

Drici MD, Burklow TR, Haridasse V, Glazer RI, Woosley RL. Sex hormones proplong the QT interval and down regulate potassium channel expression in the rabbit heart. *Circulation.* 1996;94:1471-1474.

Dries DL, Rosenberg YD, Waclawiw MA, Domanski MJ. Ejection fraction and risk of thromboembolic events in patients with systolic dysfunction and sinus rhythm: evidence for gender differences in the studies of left ventricular dysfunction trials. *J Am Coll Cardiol.* 1997;29:1074-1080.

Emmerich J, Poirier O, Evans A et al. Myocardial infarction, Arg 506 to Gln factor V mutation, and activated protein C resistance. *Lancet.* 1995;345:321.

Fiebach NH, Viscoli CM, Horwitz RI. Differences between women and men in survival after myocardial infarction. Biology or methodology? *JAMA.* 1990;263:1092-1096.

Foussas SG, Adamopoulou EN, Kafaltis NA et al. Clinical characteristics and follow-up of patients with chest pain and normal coronary arteries. *Angiology.* 1998;49:349-354.

Furberg CD, Vittinghoff E, Davidson M et al. Subgroup interactions in the Heart and Estrogen/Progestin Replacement Study: lessons learned. Circulation. 2002;105:917-922.

Giardina EG. Heart disease in women. *Int J Fertil Womens Med.* 2000;45:350-357.

Grady D, Rubin SM, Petitti DB et al. Hormone therapy to prevent disease and prolong life in postmenopausal women. *Ann Intern Med.* 1992;117:1016-1037.

Grady D, Hulley SB. Postmenopausal hormones and heart disease. *J Am Coll Cardiol.* 2001;38:8-10.

Grady D, Herrington D, Bittner V et al. Cardiovascular disease outcomes during 6.8 years of hormone therapy: Heart and Estrogen/progestin Replacement Study follow-up (HERS II). *JAMA.* 2002a;288:49-57.

Grady D, Yaffe K, Kristof M, Lin F, Richards C, Barrett-Connor E. Effect of postmenopausal hormone therapy on cognitive function: the Heart and Estrogen/progestin Replacement Study. *Am J Med.* 2002b; 113:543-548.

Grady D. Postmenopausal hormones--therapy for symptoms only. *N Engl J Med.* 2003;348:1835-1837.

Greiser E. Rechnung mit Unbekannten: Gemeinsame Stellungnahme der Fachgesellschaften zu dem Beitrag von Klaus Koch im Deutschen Ärzteblatt 18 August. *Deutsches Ärzteblatt.* 2000;97:B2145-2148.

Grodstein F, Stampfer MJ, Goldhaber SZ et al. Prospective study of exogenous hormones and risk of pulmonary embolism in women. *Lancet.* 1996a;348:983-987.

Grodstein F, Stampfer MJ, Manson JE et al. Postmenopausal estrogen and progestin use and the risk of cardiovascular disease. *N Engl J Med.* 1996b;335:453-461.

Grodstein F, Manson JE, Stampfer MJ. Postmenopausal hormone use and secondary prevention of coronary events in the nurses' health study. a prospective, observational study. *Ann Intern Med.* 2001;135:1-8.

Grover SA, Coupal L, Paquet S, Zowall H. Cost-effectiveness of 3-hydroxy-3methylglutaryl-coenzyme A reductase inhibitors in the secondary prevention of cardiovascular disease: forecasting the incremental benefits of preventing coronary and cerebrovascular events. *Arch Intern Med.* 1999;159:593-600.

Hachamovitch R, Berman DS, Kiat H et al. Effective risk stratification using exercise myocardial perfusion SPECT in women: gender-related differences in prognostic nuclear testing. *J Am Coll Cardiol.* 1996;28:34-44.

Hajjar K. Factor V Leiden - an unselfish gene? *New Engl J Med.* 1994;331:1585-1587.

Harris DJ, Douglas PS. Enrollment of women in cardiovascular clinical trials funded by the National Heart, Lung, and Blood Institute. *N Engl J Med.* 2000;343:475-480.

Harris RZ, Benet LZ, Schartz JB. Gender effects in pharmacokinetics and pharmacodynamics, *Drugs.* 1995;50:222-239.

Haynes B, Dowsett M. Clinical pharmacology of selective estrogen receptor modulators. *Drugs Aging.* 1999;14:323-336.

Hays J, Ockene JK, Brunner RL et al. Effects of estrogen plus progestin on health-related quality of life. *N Engl J Med.* 2003;348:1839-1854.

Heartwire 8.Jan. 2003. Available at: *www.theheart.org.*

Hernandez I, Delgado JL, Diaz J et al. 17beta-estradiol prevents oxidative stress and decreases blood pressure in ovariectomized rats. *Am J Physiol Regul Integr Comp Physiol.* 2000;279:R1599-1605.

Herrington DM, Reboussin DM, Brosnihan KB. Effects of estrogen replacement on the progression of coronary-artery atherosclerosis. *N Engl. J Med.* 2000;343:522-529.

Herrington DM, Vittinghoff E, Lin F et al. Statin therapy, cardiovascular events, and total mortality in the Heart and Estrogen/Progestin Replacement Study (HERS). *Circulation.* 2002;105:2962-2967.

Hoibraaten E, Qvigstad E, Arnesen H, Larsen S, Wickstrom E, Sandset PM. Increased risk of recurrent venous thrmboembolism during hormone replacement therapy – results of the randomized, double-blind, placebo-controlled etsrogen in venous thromboembolism trial (EVTET). *Thromb Haemost.* 2000;84:961-967.

Holm J, Zöller B, Svensson PJ, Berntorp E, Erhardt L, Dahlbäck B. Myocardial infarction associated with homozygous resistance to activated protein C. *Lancet.* 1994;344:952 953.

Hulley S, Grady D, Bush T et al. Randomized trial of estrogen plus progestin for secondary prevention of coronary heart disease in postmenopausal women. Heart and Estrogen/progestin Replacement Study (HERS) Research Group. *JAMA.* 1998;280:605-613.

Hulley S, Furberg C, Barrett-Connor E et al. Noncardiovascular disease outcomes during 6.8 years of hormone therapy: Heart and Estrogen/progestin Replacement Study follow-up (HERS II). *JAMA.* 2002;288:58-66.

Inbal A, Freimark D, Modan B et al. Synergistic effects of prothrombotic polymorphisms and atherogenic factors on the risk of myocardial infarction in young males. *Blood.* 1999;93:2186-2190.

Kannel WB, Feinleib M. Natural history of angina pectoris in the Framingham study. *Am J*

Cardiol. 1972;29:154-163.

Keating NL, Cleary PD, Rossi AS, Zaslavsky AM, Ayanian JZ. Use of hormone replacement therapy by postmenopausal women in the United States. *Ann Intern Med.* 1999;130:545-553. Keller KB, Lemberg L. Gender differences in acute coronary events. *Am J Crit Care.* 2000;9:207-209. Khan MA, Heagerty AM, Kitchener H, McNamee R, Cherry NM, Hannaford P. Oestrogen and women's heart disease: ESPRIT-UK. *QJM.* 2000;93:699-700. Kiechl S, Muigg A, Santer P et al. Poor response to activated protein C as a prominent risk predictor of advanced atherosclerosis and arterial disease. *Circulation.* 1999;99:614-619. Kirchgatterer A, Weber T, Auer J et al. Analyse der Zuweisungsdiagnosen bei Patienten mit unauffälligem Koronarangiogramm. *Wien-Klin-Wochenschr.* 1999;111:434-438.

Koch K. Rechnung mit Unbekannten: Nach einer aktuellen epidemiologischen Berechnung ist die Hormonersatztherapie bei Frauen mit einem hohen Karzinomrisiko behaftet. *Deutsches Aezteblatt.* 2000;97:B1823-1824.

Kreling D, Mott D, Wiederholt J, Lundy J, Levitt L. *Prescription drug trend: a chartbook update.* Menlo Park, California: Kaiser Family Foundation; 2001.

Lazzara R. Mechanisms and management of congenital and aquired long QT syndromes. *Arch Mal Coeur Vaiss.* 1996;89 Spec No1:51-55.

Lee PY, Alexander KP, Hammill BG, Pasquali SK, Peterson ED. Representation of elderly persons and women in published randomized trials of acute coronary syndromes. *JAMA.* 2001;286:708-713.

Lerner DJ, Kannel WB. Patterns of coronary heart disease morbidity and mortality in the sexes: a 26-year follow-up of the Framingham population. *Am Heart J.* 1986;111:383 390.

Lowe GDO, Rumley A, Woodward M, Reid E, Rumley J. Activated protein C resistance and the FV:R^{506} Q mutation in a random population sample – Associations with cardiovascular risk factors and coagulation variables. *Thromb Haemost.* 1999;81:918 924.

Luzier AB, Killian A, Wilton JH, Wilson MF, Forrest A, Kazierad DJ. Gender-related effects on metoprolol pharmacokinetics and pharmacodynamics in healthy volunteers. *Clin Pharmacol Ther.* 1999;66:594-601.

Ma KL, Gao F, Yao CL et al. Nitric oxide stimulatory and endothelial protective effects of idoxifene, a selective estrogen receptor m,odulator, in the splanchnic artery of trhe ovariectomized rat. *J Pharmacol Exp Ther.* 2000;295:786-792.

Majerus PW. Bad blood by mutation. *Nature.* 1994;369:14-15.

Makkar RR, Fromm BS, Steinman RT, Meissner MD, Lehmann MH (1993) Female gender as a risk factor for torsades de pointes associated with cardiovascular drugs. *JAMA.* 270: 2590-2597.

Malenka DJ, O'Rourke D, Miller MA et al. Cause of in-hospital death in 12.232 consecutive patients undergoing percutaneous transluminal coronary angioplasty. The Northern New England cardiovascular Disease Study Group. *Am Heart J.* 1999;137:632-638.

Meier CR, Jick H. Tamoxifen and trisk of idiopathic venous thromboembolism. *Br J Clin Pharmacol.* 1998;45:608-612.

Michelena HI, Ezekowitz MD. Atrial fibrillation: are there gender differences? *J Gend Specif*

Med. 2000;3:44-46.

Middendorf K, Göhring P, Huehns TY, Seidel D, Steinbeck G,. Nikol S. Prevalence of resistance against activated protein C resulting from factor V Leiden is significantly increased in myocardial infarction:Investigation of 507 patients with myocardial infarction. *American Heart Journal.* in press.

Miners JO, Grgurinovich N, Whitehead AG, Robson RA, Birkett DJ. Influence of gender and oral contraceptive steroids on the metabolism of salicylic acid and acetylsalicylic acid. Br *J Clin Pharmacol.* 1986;22:135-142.

Mosca L, Collins P, Herrington DM et al. Hormone replacement therapy and cardiovascular diesease: a statement for healthcare professionals from the American Heart Association. *Circulation.* 2001;104:499-503.

Mosca L, Barrett-Connor E, Wenger NK et al. Design and methods of the Raloxifene Use for The Heart (RUTH) study. *Am J Cardiol.* 2001;88:392-395.

Moulin T, Tatu L, Crepin-Leblond T, Chavot D, Berges S, Rumbach T. The Besancon Stroke Registry: an acute stroke registry of 2.500 consecutive patients. *Eur Neurol.* 1997;38:10 20.

Murabito JM, Evans JC, Larson MG, Levy D. Prognosis after the onset of coronary heart disease. An investigation of differences in outcome between the sexes according to initial coronatry disease presentation. *Circulation.* 1993;88:2548-2555.

Nyman I, Wallentin L, Areskog M, Areskog N, Swahn E. Risk stratification by early exercise testing after an episode of unstabel coronary artery disease.The RISC Study Group. *Int J Cardiol.* 1993;39:131-142.

O'Brien JE, Peterson ED, Keeler GP et al. Relation between estrogen replacement therapy and restenosis after percutaneous coronary interventions. *J Am Coll Cardiol.* 1996;28:1111-1118.

Oger E, Scarabin PY. Assessment of the risk for venous thromboembolism among users of hormone replacement therapy. *Drugs Aging.* 1999;14:55-61.

Oikarinen L, Nieminen MS, Toivonen L et al. Relation of QT interval and QT dispersion to regression of echocardiographic and electrocardiographic left ventricular hypertrophy in hypertensive patients: the Losartan Intervention For Endpoint Reduction (LIFE) study. *Am Heart J.* 2003;145:919-925.

Parkin L, Skeeg DC, Wilson M, Herbison GP, Paul C. Oral contraception and fatal pulmonary embolism. *Lancet.* 2000;355:2133-2134. Peters HW, Westendorf ICD, Hak AE et al. Menopausal status and risk factors for cardiovascular disease. *J Intern Med.* 1999;246:521-528. Rathore SS, Wang Y, Krumholz HM. Sex-based differences in the effect of gigoxin for the treastment of heart failure. *N Engl J Med.* 2002;347:1403-1411.

Rees DC, Cox M, Clegg JB. World distribution of factor V Leiden. *Lancet.* 1995;346:1113-1134.

Ridker PM, Hennekens CH, Lindpaintner K, Stampfer MJ, Eisenberg PR, Miletich JP. Mutation in the gene coding for coagulation factor V and the risk of myocardial infarction, stroke, and venous thrombosis in apparently healthy men. *New Engl J Med.* 1995;332:912-917.

Rosano GM, Leonardo F, Sarrel PM, Beale CM De Luca F, Collins P. Cyclical variation in paroxysmal supraventricular tachycardia in women. *Lancet.* 1996;347:786-788.

Rosendaal FR, Siscovick DS, Schwartz SM et al. Factor V Leiden (resistance to activated protein C) increases the risk of myocardial infarction in young women. *Blood.* 1997a;89:2817-2821.

Rosendaal FR, Siscovick DS, Schwartz SM, Psaty BM, Raghunathan TE, Vos HL.A common prothrombin variant (20210 G to A) increases the risk of myocardial infarction in young women. *Blood.* 1997b; 90:1747-1750.

Rossouw JE, Anderson GL, Prentice RL et al. Risks and benefits of estrogen plus progestin in healthy postmenopausal women: principal results from the Women's Health Initiative randomized controlled trial. *JAMA.* 2002;288:321-333.

Samsioe G. Cardiovascular disease in postmenopausal women. Maturitas. 1998;30:11-18.

Schenck-Gustafsson K. Risk factors for cardiovascular disease in women: assessment and management. *Eur Heart J.* 1996;17(Supplement D):2-8.

Severi S, Orsini F, Marraccini C, L'Abbate A. A basal electrocardiogram and the exercise stress test in asessing prognosis in patients with unstable angina. *Eur Heart J.* 1988;9:441-446.

Shumaker SA, Legault C, Thal L et al. Estrogen plus progestin and the incidence of dementia and mild cognitive impairment in postmeopausal women: The Women's Health Initiative Memory Study: A randomized controlled trial. *JAMA.* 2003;289:2651-2662.

Shlipak MG, Simon JA, Vittinghoff E et al. Estrogen and progestin, lipoprotein(a), and the risk of recurrent coronary heart disease events after menopause. *JAMA.* 2000;283:1845-1852.

Spranger M, Aspey BS, Harrison MJ. Sex difference in antithrombotic effect of aspirin. *Stroke.* 1989;20:34-37.

Stampfer MJ, Colditz GA, Willett WC et al. Postmenopausal estrogen therapy and cardiovascular disease. Ten-year nurses' health study. *N Engl J Med.* 1991a;325:756-762.

Stampfer MJ, Colditz GA. Estrogen replacement therapy and coronary heart disease: a quantitative assessment of the epidemiologic evidence. *Prev Med.* 1991b;20:47-63.

Stein PD, Huang HI, Afzal A, Noor HA. Incidence of acute pulmonary embolism in a general hospital: relation to age, sex and race. *Chest.* 1999;116:909-913.

Stumpf WE. Steroid hormones and the cardiovascular system: Direct actions of estradiol, progesterone, testosterone, gluco- and mineralcorticoids, and soltriol (vitamin D) on central nervous regulatory and peripheral tissues. *Experientia.* 1990;46:13-25.

Sullivan AK, Holdright DR, Wright CA, Sparrow JL, Cunningham D, Fox KM. Chest pain in women: clinical, investigative, and prognostic features. *BMJ.* 1994;308:883-836.

Sullivan JM, Vander Zwaag R, Hughes JP et al. Estrogen replacement and coronary artery disease. Effect on survival in postmenopausal women. *Arch Intern Med.* 1990;150:2557-2562.

Sytkowski PA, Kannel WB, D'Agostino RB. Changes in risk factors and the decline in mortality from cardiovascular disease - The Framingham Heart Study. *New Engl J Med.* 1990;322:1635-1641.

Takeuchi M, Sonoda S, Miura Y, Kuroiwa A. Comparative diagnostic value of dobutamine stress echocardiography and stress thallium-201 single-photon-emission computed tomography for detecting coronary artery disease in women. *Coron Artery Dis.* 1996;7:831-835.

Taubert HD. *Geschlechtsspezifische Entwicklung der Frau und ihre Störungen*. In: Schmidt-Matthiesen H, Hepp H (Eds.). *Gynäkologie und Geburtshilfe*. 9. Edition, Stuttgart - New York: Schattauer Verlag; 1998.

The Acute Infarction Ramipril Efficacy (AIRE) Study Investigators. Effect of ramipril on mortality and morbidity of survisors of acute myocardial infarction with clinical evidence of heart failure. *Lancet*. 1993;342:821-828.

The Writing Group for the PEPI Trial. Effects of estrogen or estrogen/progestin regimens on heart disease risk factors in postmenopausal women. The Postmenopausal Estrogen/Progestin Interventions (PEPI) Trial. *JAMA*. 1995;273:199-208.

Vickers MR, Meade TW, Wilkes HC. Hormone replacement therapy and cardiovascular disease: the case for a randomized controlled trial. *Ciba Found Symp*. 1995;191:150-60; discussion 160-4.

Viscoli CM, Brass LM, Kernan WN, Sarrel PM, Suissa S, Horwitz RI. A clinical trial of estrogen-replacement therapy after ischemic stroke. *N Engl J Med*. 2001;345:1243-1249.

Vogels EA, Largo-Janssen ALM, Van Weel C. Sex differences in cardiovascular disease: are women with low socioeconomic status at high risk? *Brit J Gen Pract*. 1999;49:963-966.

Walle T, Walle UK, Cowart TD, Conradi EC. Pathway-selective sex differences in the metabolic clearance of propranolol in human subjects. *Clin Pharmacol Ther*.1989;46:257-263.

Waters DD, Alderman EL, Hsia J et al. Effects of hormone replacement therapy and antioxidant vitamin supplements on coronary atherosclerosis in postmenopausal women: a randomized controlled trial. *JAMA*. 2002;288:2432-2440.

Winkler UH. Thrombophilie und antithrombotische Prävention in Gynäkologie und Geburtshilfe. *Internist*. 1997;38:650-657.

Wyller TB. Stroke and gender. *J Gend Specif Med*. 1999;2:41-45.

Yarzebski J, Col N, Pagley P, Savageau J, Gore J, Goldberg R. Gender differences and factors associated with the receipt of thrombolytic therapy in patients with acute myocardial infarction: a community-wide perspective. *Am Heart J*. 1996;131:43-50.

Yusuf S, Sleight P, Pogue J, Bosch J, Davies R, Dagenais G. Effects of an angiotensin-converting-enzyme inhibitor, ramipril, on cardiovascular events in high-risk patients. The Heart Outcomes Prevention Evaluation Study Investigators. *N Engl J Med*. 2000; 342:145-153.

In: Heart Disease in Women
Editor: B. V. Larner and H. R. Pennelton

ISBN 978-1-60692-066-4
© 2009 Nova Science Publishers, Inc.

Chapter VIII

Aging Women and Coronary Heart Disease

*Marek A. Kosmicki** *and Hanna Szwed*

II Department of Coronary Artery Disease, Institute of Cardiology, Warsaw, Poland

Abstract

Aging, a natural process in human life, begins at conception, continues with growth and development and finishes with dysfunction of various organs towards the end of life. Coronary heart disease (CHD) is one of the most common cardiovascular diseases, leading to death in women and is responsible for more deaths each year than all other diseases together. The incidence of myocardial infarction (MI) in women, although lower than in men, increases dramatically after the menopause. This increase is at least partly due to aging, although men also have a progressive increase in MI with age. The role of the menopause itself is not very clear. The evaluation of chest pain, the main symptom of CHD, is less straightforward in women than in men, because the language used to describe symptoms differs between the sexes. In fact, symptoms in women are slightly different from those in men. Until now, medical data published in literature was based on research done on male patients. However, there are numerous differences in the epidemiology and primary manifestation of CHD in women and men. In addition, the diagnosis of angina pectoris in women is more difficult than in men for several reasons, which are mentioned later in this chapter. The clinical usefulness of some non-invasive tests is lower in women than in men. A number of studies have shown gender-based differences in frequency rates of coronary angiography and revascularization, even among those with acute MI. It should be stressed that women with angina are much more likely than men to have normal coronary arteries on angiography. On the other hand, the risk of complications after coronary angiography in women is higher than in men. This

* Author correspondence information: II Department of Coronary Artery Disease, Institute of Cardiology; ul. Spartanska 1; PL.02-637 Warszawa, Poland; Tel. (+4822) 3434016; -3434050; Fax (+4822) 8449510; E-mail: mkosmicki@ikard.pl

may explain why physicians fail to refer women for subsequent invasive tests. Several case reports included in this paper show the difficulties in diagnosis and treatment of women with CHD.

In conclusion, it could be said that difficulties in diagnosis and limited data on the treatment of CHD in women, have led to a situation in which women with CHD often remain under-investigated and under-treated.

Abbreviations and Acronyms

ACC	American College of Cardiology
ACE inhibitor	angiotensin converting enzyme inhibitor
ACS	acute coronary syndrome
ACOG	American College of Obstetricians and Gynecologists
AHA	American Heart Association
ALLHAT	Antihypertensive and Lipid-Lowering Treatment to Prevent Heart Attack Trial
ARB	angiotensin II receptor blocker
BMI	body mass index
BMS	bare-metal stent
bpm	beats per minute
CABG	coronary artery bypass grafting
CAD	coronary artery disease
CARE	Cholesterol and Recurrent Events trial
CASS	Coronary Artery Surgery Study
CHD	coronary heart disease
CVD	cardiovascular disease
DES	drug-eluting stents
ECG	electrocardiogram
4S	Scandinavian Simvastatin Survival Study
GP IIb/IIIa inhibitors	glycoprotein IIb/IIIa inhibitors
GUSTO-I	Global Utilization of Streptokinase and Tissue Plasminogen Activator for occluded coronary arteries trial
HDL	high density lipoproteins
HERS-I and HERS-II	Heart and Estrogen/Progestin Replacement Study I and –II
HPS	Heart Protection Study
HOPE	Heart Outcomes Prevention Evaluation Study
HR	hazard ratios
HRT	hormone replacement therapy
IFG	impaired fasting glucose
LAD	left anterior descending artery
LCx	left circumflex artery
LDL	low density lipoproteins

LVH	left ventricular hypertrophy
METS	units of metabolic equivalent
MI	myocardial infarction
MPI	myocardial perfusion imaging
NCEP	the National Cholesterol Education Program
NHANES	the National Health and Nutrition Examination Survey
NHEFS	National Health Epidemiologic Followup Study
NSTEMI	myocardial infarction without ST segment elevation, non-ST elevation (non-Q wave)
OC	oral contraceptive
OPCAB	Off Pump Coronary Artery Bypass
PCI	percutaneous coronary intervention
PTCA	percutaneous transluminal angioplasty
RCA	right coronary artery
RCGP	Royal College of General Practitioners study
STEMI	myocardial infarction with ST segment elevation (Q wave)
Tc-99m	technetium-99m
Tl-201	thallium-201
UA	unstable angina
WHI	Women's Health Initiative study
WHO	World Health Organization
WISE	Women's Ischemia Syndrome Evaluation study

Introduction

Aging is any change in an organism over time and is a natural process in human life. It begins at conception, continues with growth and development and finishes with dysfunction of various organs towards the end of life. Some dimensions of aging grow and expand over time, while others decline. Reaction time, for example, may slow with age, while knowledge of world events and wisdom may expand. A human life is often divided into various ages. Because biological changes are slow moving and vary from person to person, arbitrary dates are usually set to mark periods of human life. In some cultures the divisions given below are quite varied. In the USA, adulthood legally begins at the age of eighteen or nineteen, while old age is considered to begin at the age of legal retirement (approximately 65).

Aging is an important part of all human societies reflecting the biological changes that occur, but also reflects cultural and social conventions. Population aging refers to the increase in the number and proportion of older people in society. Population aging has three possible causes: migration, longer life expectancy (decreased death rate), and decreased birth rate. Many societies in the developed world, i.e. Western Europe and Japan, have aging populations. While the effects on society are complex, there is a concern about the impact on health care demand.

The Second World Assembly on Aging, organized by the United Nations in Madrid (2002), stated in its report that the twentieth century saw a revolution in longevity. Since

1950 average life expectancy at birth has increased by 20 years to 66 years and is expected to extend a further 10 years by 2050. This demographic triumph and the fast growth of the population in the first half of the twenty-first century mean that the number of persons over 60 will increase from about 600 million in 2000 to almost 2 billion in 2050 and the proportion of persons defined as older is projected to increase globally from 10 per cent in 1998 to 15 per cent in 2025. The increase will be greatest and most rapid in developing countries, where the older population is expected to quadruple during the next 50 years (fig 1).

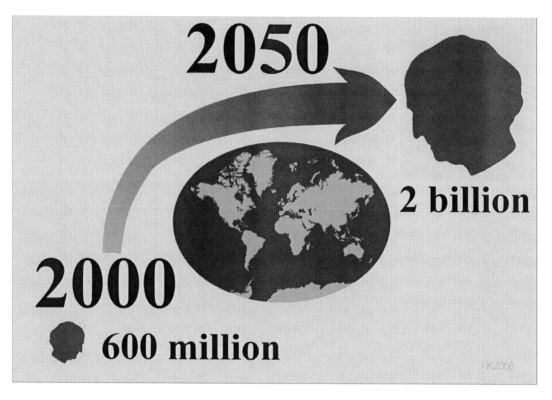

Figure 1. The Second World Assembly on Aging, Madrid 2002, stated that in the first half of the twenty-first century the number of persons over 60 will increase from about 600 million in 2000 to almost 2 billion in 2050 [1]

The sociological effects of age are great. Young people tend to commit most crimes, they are more likely to push for political and social change, to develop and adopt new technologies, and to need education. Older people have different requirements from society and government as opposed to young people, and frequently differing values as well. Older people are also far more likely to vote, and in many countries the young are forbidden from voting, and thus the aged have comparatively more political influence.

Organism aging is generally characterized by the declining ability to respond to stress, increasing homeostatic imbalance and increased risk of disease. Because of this, death is the ultimate consequence of aging. Increased risk of disease means especially the risk of developing of atherosclerotic changes in the arteries, which is one of the most common processes during aging. Atherosclerosis or arteriosclerosis of coronary arteries, the blood vessels which feed the heart, leads to the development of plaques, a combination of cholesterol and other fats, calcium and other elements carried in the blood, and builds up in the walls of these vessels. Arteriosclerosis of coronary arteries is responsible for coronary artery disease (CAD) or coronary heart disease (CHD).

In the United States, about 1 out of 6 people aged 65 and over has CHD. After age 65, the likelihood that a person will develop CHD increases with each passing year. In older men and women, CHD is the most common cause of death.

CHD and other cardiovascular disease (CVD) is the leading cause of death in women in all groups of age, responsible for more deaths each year than all other causes combined [2-4]. The incidence of myocardial infarction (MI) in women, although lower than in men, increases dramatically after the menopause. The increase is at least in part due to increasing age, since men also have a progressive increase in MI with age [5]. The role of menopause itself is not so clear.

CHD mortality is higher in women compared to men, an effect that is largely due to comorbidities, such as older age [6]. Risk factors such as smoking and dyslipidemia may be particularly important [7].

Risk factor reduction may have contributed to the decline in CHD in women that has occurred in recent years. The magnitude of change was illustrated in a report from the Nurses' Health Study of 85,941 women who were followed for 14 years [8]. There was a 31 percent reduction in the incidence of CHD in 1992 to 1994 compared to 1980 to 1982. The overall risk and the magnitude of reduction were greatest in women greater than or equal to 65 years of age.

During this time period, the number of subjects who smoked decreased by 41 percent, the use of hormone replacement therapy (HRT) increased by 175 percent, and the number who were overweight increased by 38 percent. It was concluded that the reduction in smoking accounted for a 13 percent decline in CHD and an improvement in diet explained a 16 percent decline, while the increase in weight accounted for an 8 percent increase in CHD. It was thought that HRT was beneficial but this no longer seems to be correct.

The epidemiology and prognosis; clinical manifestations and diagnosis of CHD; determinants and general management of cardiovascular risk in women, and also the management of women with CHD will be reviewed here.

Epidemiology and Prognosis of CHD in Women

The Framingham Study provides good insight into the clinical spectrum and prognosis of the CHD disease because data collection began in 1949, at a time when there was initially little effective therapy available; later, there was underutilization of what therapy existed. A substantial part of CHD progresses abruptly from inapparent disease to a MI and possible death. Much of this premature mortality occurs in a subset of the population that is prone to accelerated atherogenesis caused by a growing number of modifiable predisposing risk factors.

Advanced occlusive coronary disease often exists with few symptoms or overt clinical manifestations. Silent ischemia, which is thought to account for 75 percent of all ischemic episodes [9], may be brought to light by electrocardiographic changes (ST segment depression) on an exercise test, ambulatory 24 hour electrocardiographic recording, or periodic routine electrocardiogram (ECG).

MIs that are detected by routine ECG examination often occur without symptoms and certain common abnormalities on the resting ECG in persons with an adverse coronary risk profile may signify ischemic myocardial involvement [10].

For these reasons, data from the National Health and Nutrition Surveys (NHANES) that rely on self-reported MI and angina from health interviews probably underestimate the actual prevalence of advanced CHD. These data suggest that 13.7 million persons in the United States have CHD, half of whom have MIs and half angina [11]. For men, the reported prevalence increases with age from 7 percent at ages 40 to 49 years to 13 percent at 50 to 59 years, 16 percent at 60 to 69 years, and 22 percent at 70 to 79 years. The corresponding estimates for women are substantially lower than for men: 5, 8, 11, and 14 percent, respectively.

Autopsy data have documented a reduced prevalence of anatomic CHD since 1979. In a report of 2562 autopsies performed between 1979 and 1994, the prevalence of significant anatomic coronary disease in subjects aged 20 to 59 years fell from 42 to 32 percent in men and 29 to 16 percent in women when the periods 1979 to 1983 and 1990 to 1994 were compared [12]. There was no significant change in prevalence in those greater than or equal to 60 years of age.

Atherosclerotic cardiovascular disease is a diffuse condition that involves the arterial circulation of the heart, brain, kidneys, and limbs. The presence of clinical atherosclerosis in one vascular territory generally indicates an increased likelihood that it exists elsewhere since the risk factors are generally the same [13,14].

Below age 65, all the major risk factors (eg, smoking, hypertension, diabetes mellitus, dyslipidemia) impact significantly on the rate of development of coronary and peripheral artery disease. For atherothrombotic brain infarction, all but dyslipidemia have been considered important. However, data from lipid lowering trials in patients with CHD have shown a concomitant 24 to 29 percent reduction in stroke (4.1 versus 5.6 percent for placebo) that is primarily the result of a significant reduction in nonfatal stroke [15,16]. Over the age of 65 years, the serum total cholesterol predicts less well than the total/HDL cholesterol ratio.

Data from 44 years of follow-up in the original Framingham Study cohort and 20 years of surveillance of their offspring has allowed ascertainment of the incidence of initial coronary events including both recognized and clinically unrecognized MI, angina pectoris, unstable angina, and sudden and non-sudden coronary deaths [17-19]. The following observations were noted:

For persons aged 40 years, the lifetime risk of developing CHD is 49 percent in men and 32 percent in women. For those reaching age 70 years, the lifetime risk is 35 percent in men and 24 percent in women.

For total coronary events, the incidence rises steeply with age, with women lagging behind men by 10 years. For the more serious manifestations of coronary disease, such as MI and sudden death, women lag behind men in incidence by 20 years, but the sex ratio for incidence narrows progressively with advancing age. The incidence at ages 65 to 94 compared to ages 35 to 64 more than doubles in men and triples in women.

In premenopausal women, serious manifestations of coronary disease, such as MI and sudden death, are relatively rare. Beyond the menopause, the incidence and severity of coronary disease increases abruptly, with rates three times those of women the same age who remain premenopausal [17].

Below age 65 years, the annual incidence of all coronary events in men (12 per 1000) more than equals the rate of all the other atherosclerotic cardiovascular events combined (7 per 1000); in women, it equals the rate of the other events (5 per 1000). Beyond age 65 years, coronary disease still predominates. Coronary events comprise 33 to 65 percent of atherosclerotic cardiovascular events in men and 28 to 58 percent in women.

The male predominance of CHD is least striking for angina pectoris. Under age 75, the initial presentation of coronary disease in women is more likely to be angina pectoris than MI [5]. Furthermore, angina in women is more likely to be uncomplicated (80 percent), while angina in men often occurs after a MI (66 percent). Infarction predominates at virtually all ages in men in whom only 20 percent of infarctions are preceded by long-standing angina; the percentage is even lower if the MI is silent or unrecognized [5,18].

The incidence of CHD has decreased over time. This trend illustrate an analysis from the National Health and Nutrition Examination Survey (NHANES) I Epidemiologic Follow-up study [20], and a report from the Mayo Clinic examined the incidence of CHD over time in Olmsted County, Minnesota [21].

The overall incidence of MI has not changed significantly [20]. In the past, ST elevation (Q wave) MI (STEMI) was thought to be transmural and non-ST elevation (non-Q wave) MI (NSTEMI) subendocardial. However, there is little autopsy evidence to support this contention; Q waves are neither sensitive nor specific as markers for transmural MI [22-26]. The incidence of STEMI has decreased over time [27]. In contrast, the incidence of an NSTEMI MI increased. The net effect is that the relative frequency of NSTEMI has increased from 45 percent in 1994 to 63 percent in 1999 [28].

CHD is the leading cause of death in adults in the United States, accounting for about one-third of all deaths in subjects over age 35 [29]. The death rate is higher in men than in women (three times higher at ages 25 to 34, falling to 1.6 times at ages 75 to 84) and in blacks compared to whites, an excess that disappears by age 75. Among the Hispanic population, coronary mortality is not as high as it is among blacks and whites.

Mortality rates for cardiovascular disease and CHD in men and women and in blacks and whites have fallen in most developed countries by 24 to 28 percent since 1975, although the decline has slowed since 1990 [20,30-36].

The decline in CHD mortality in recent decades is significant for both sudden and nonsudden cardiac death. In an analysis from the Framingham study from 1950 to 1999, overall CHD death rates decreased by 59 percent [37]. Nonsudden cardiac death rates decreased by 64 percent, while sudden death rates decreased by 49 percent. Approximately 45 percent of the reduction in CHD mortality is attributable to improvement in medical therapies for coronary disease [32,33]. The remaining 55 percent is due to risk factor reduction, particularly a decline in smoking and treatment of hypertension.

Similar trends toward an improvement in outcome in developed countries have been described in an analysis of death certificates from the World Health Organization database [38].

Between 1965-69 and 1995-97, in the United States, CHD mortality fell by 63 percent in men (331 to 121 per 100,000) and by 60 percent in women (166 to 67 per 100,000). In the same periods of time in the European Union, CHD mortality fell by 32 percent in men (146 to 100 per 100,000) and by 30 percent in women (64 to 45 per 100,000).

However, in eastern Europe the results were variable, with some countries showing an increase in CHD mortality in the early 1990s followed by a subsequent decline (Poland and the Czech Republic). The highest CHD mortality was noted in the Russian Federation (330 and 154 per 100,000 in men and women, respectively, from 1995-98). These values were similar to those in 1985-89.

In Japan, CHD mortality was much lower than in the United States and Europe and fell by 29 percent in men (50 to 36 per 100,000) and by 36 percent in women (28 to 18 per 100,000).

In contrast to the above data, mortality from CHD is expected to increase in developing countries (including China, India, sub-Saharan Africa, Latin America, and the Middle East), from an estimated 9 million in 1990 to a projected 19 million by 2020 [39,40]. This projected increase is thought to be a consequence of social and economic changes in non-Western countries, leading to increased life expectancy, Westernized diets, physical inactivity, and increases in cigarette smoking [41].

Menopause

CHD is unusual in premenopausal women, particularly in the absence of other risk factors [5]. In comparison, the National Cholesterol Education Program (NCEP) recognizes the postmenopausal state as a risk factor for CHD, assigning it the same weight as male sex [42]. Hormonal status may also influence CHD risk in males; men with a common variant in the estrogen receptor alpha gene have an increased risk of MI compared to those without the variant [43].

Early natural menopause (less than or equal to 44 years of age) has been associated with an increase in the risk of cardiovascular disease in two large epidemiologic studies [44,45]. In one, this effect was limited to current smokers [44], while the second study only included women who never smoked [45].

Data are conflicting on whether the type of menopause (surgical or natural) affects cardiovascular risk. In a 1987 report from the Nurses' Health Study, bilateral oophorectomy, but not natural menopause, was associated with an excess risk of cardiovascular disease [46]. However, adjustments were only made for age and smoking, not for other major cardiovascular risk factors. Furthermore, a later study of healthy, postmenopausal women (age 46 to 81) who were not on hormone therapy found that carotid artery intima-media thickness, a marker of subclinical atherosclerosis, was positively associated with years since menopause, but not with the type of menopause (natural versus oophorectomy) [47].

These observations do not prove that menopause itself is a risk factor for CHD. Although the incidence rises dramatically over time after menopause, there is also a marked increase in men with age [5]. An important contributing factor is that postmenopausal women who develop CHD have an increased burden of cardiovascular risk factors compared to those who do not [48].

Consistent with this hypothesis is the observation that postmenopausal endogenous hormone concentrations may not be a significant risk factor after adjustment for other variables. This was suggested by an analysis from the Women's Health Study in which 200 postmenopausal women who had CHD were matched with controls who remained free of CHD [49]. Among women who were not taking hormone replacement therapy (HRT), those with a low serum sex hormone binding globulin concentration or a high free androgen index were at increased risk of cardiac events. However, this correlation was not significant after adjustment for body mass index and other cardiovascular risk factors.

A second finding consistent with menopause not being directly responsible for the increase in CHD risk after menopause is the lack of benefit from HRT in the Women's Health Initiative (WHI), mostly of primary prevention, and in the HERS trials of secondary prevention [50-52]. Estrogen-progestin replacement had no cardioprotective effect and may have produced harm. As a result, HRT cannot be recommended to reduce CHD risk (see below).

Cardiovascular Risk Factors in Women

Risk factor reduction may have contributed to the decline in CHD in women that has occurred in recent years. The magnitude of change was illustrated in a report from the Nurses' Health Study of 85,941 women who were followed for 14 years [8]. There was a 31 percent reduction in the incidence of CHD in 1992 to 1994 compared to 1980 to 1982. The overall risk and the magnitude of reduction were greatest in women greater than or equal to 65 years of age.

During this time period, the number of subjects who smoked decreased by 41 percent, the use of hormone replacement therapy (HRT) increased by 175 percent, and the number who were overweight increased by 38 percent. It was concluded that the reduction in smoking accounted for a 13 percent decline in CHD and an improvement in diet explained a 16 percent decline, while the increase in weight accounted for an 8 percent increase in CHD. It was thought that HRT was beneficial but this no longer seems to be correct (see below).

According to the guidelines of the NCEP [53] and a scientific statement from the American Heart Association (AHA) and American College of Cardiology (ACC) [54], the following are the primary cardiovascular risk factors in women, and their assessment should be an important component of periodic health examinations (see table 1):

Elevated triglycerides, obesity, and a sedentary lifestyle, while not considered primary risk factors in the NCEP guidelines, are also highly associated with coronary risk and assessment is recommended by the AHA/ACC guidelines [54]. These cardiovascular risk factors are more frequent among ethnic minority women than among white women [55]. Central obesity and elevated triglycerides, along with hypertension, glucose intolerance and a low HDL, are diagnostic elements of the metabolic syndrome.

Table 1. The primary cardiovascular risk factors in women, which assessment should be an important component of periodic health examinations – according to the guidelines of the NCEP [53] and a scientific statement from the American Heart Association (AHA) and American College of Cardiology (ACC) [54]

1. Personal history of CHD
2. Age over 55
3. Family history of premature CHD (first degree male relative under age 55 or a female under age 65)
4. Dyslipidemia: high LDL and/or low HDL
5. Diabetes mellitus
6. Smoking
7. Hypertension
8. Peripheral vascular disease

A similar set of risk factors predicts subsequent MI or death from CHD among women who are already known to have CHD. In the HERS trial of 2763 postmenopausal women with CHD, 361 had an MI or CHD death at 4.1 years of follow-up, an average annual rate of 3.4 percent [56]. The annual rate of MI or death from CHD was significantly lower for women with no risk factors than for women with five or more risk factors (1.3 versus 8.7 percent).

A family history of premature CHD is an independent predictor of coronary risk in women. It is also found more commonly in women than in men with CHD [57].

The incidence of MI in women increases dramatically after the menopause. Although **the role of menopause itself is not so clear**, this increase is at least in part due to increasing age [5]. CHD mortality is higher in women compared to men, an effect that is largely due to comorbidities, such as older age [6].

The lipoprotein risk factors for CHD are somewhat different in women compared to men, which shows table 2 [42,58-61].

Table 2. The lipoprotein risk factors for CHD – comparison between women and men, according to [42,58-61]

1. Low HDL, rather than high LDL cholesterol, is more predictive of coronary risk in women [58,59].
2. Lipoprotein(a) is a determinant of CHD (manifested as angina or MI) in premenopausal women and postmenopausal women under age 66 (odds ratio 5.1 and 2.4, respectively) [60].
3. The total cholesterol concentration appears to be associated with CHD only in premenopausal women or at very high levels (>265 mg/dL [6.9 mmol/L]) [42,60].
4. Triglycerides appear to uniquely influence coronary risk in older women [58,59,61], especially at levels above 400 mg/dL (4.5 mmol/L).

The relative predictive value of the different lipid parameters was evaluated in a prospective analysis from the Women's Health Study of over 15,600 initially healthy women greater than or equal to 45 years of age who were followed over a 10 year period [62]. The total cholesterol to HDL-C ratio was most highly predictive of cardiovascular events [62]. It is therefore recommended that every woman over age 20 should have a fasting lipid profile measured [53]. Lipoprotein(a) and apolipoprotein B and A-I levels should be measured if the standard profile is normal in women with premature CHD (less than 60 years of age).

Although data from prospective primary prevention studies are lacking in women, current practice is to treat high-risk women in the same fashion as men. Meta-analysis of the clinical studies which have included women has shown that lipid-altering medications have similar effects in women and men on both the lipid profiles and the reduction in CHD [63].

Secondary intervention trials aimed at regression of CHD have shown that, compared to men, women may have increased regression of coronary lesions and a similar improvement in survival with intensive lipid-lowering [64-68].

Diabetes mellitus is an important predictor of CHD risk and prognosis in women and men [57,58,69-72]. In a study from Finland, patients with type 2 diabetes without a prior infarction were at the same risk for myocardial infarction (20 and 19 percent, respectively) and coronary mortality (15 versus 16 percent) as nondiabetic patients with a prior MI [73]. The risk of infarction was greatest in diabetics with a prior MI and lowest in nondiabetic patients without a prior MI (45 and 4 percent, respectively). These findings were independent of other risk factors such as total cholesterol, hypertension, and smoking.

Based upon such observations, diabetes was considered a CHD equivalent for both men and women in the 2002 National Cholesterol Education Program report, thereby elevating it to the highest risk category [53].

The increase in CHD risk in patients with diabetes is greater in women than in men [69,71,72]. The magnitude of this effect was illustrated in a meta-analysis of 37 studies of almost 450,000 patients with type 2 diabetes: the summary relative risk for fatal CHD in patients with diabetes was 3.5 in women and 2.1 in men [71]. The excess risk is at least in part due to diabetes being more commonly accompanied by other cardiovascular risk factors in women [69].

Diabetes appears to confer greater prognostic information in women than any of the other traditional cardiac risk factors. In a study of women presenting with chest pain, for example, diabetes was the only risk factor that distinguished between those with and those without angiographic CHD [74].

In addition to the risk associated with overt diabetes, there appears to be a graded rise in cardiovascular risk with increasing degrees of **glucose intolerance below the definition of overt diabetes**, as well as with increasing levels of hemoglobin A1c (HbA1c) [75,76].

In contrast to these observations for new onset cardiovascular disease, impaired glucose tolerance may not be a risk factor for adverse cardiovascular outcomes in postmenopausal women with known CHD. This was illustrated in a report from the HERS trial of 2763 such women who were followed for 6.8 years; outcomes were assessed according to the presence or absence of impaired fasting glucose (IFG) at baseline [70]. Using the 2003 definition (IFG 100 to 125 mg/dL [5.6 to 6.0 mmol/L]), IFG was not predictive of risk of CHD, stroke, transient ischemic attack, and heart failure.

Smoking has been associated with one-half of all coronary events in women [77,78]. Furthermore, coronary risk is elevated even in women with minimal use (relative risk 2.4 for 1.4 cigarettes/day) [58,78].

Cessation of smoking in women is associated with a rapid reduction in the risk of MI. In a case control study of 910 patients with a first episode of myocardial infarction, for example, the relative risk was 3.6 among current smokers versus 1.2 in ex-smokers [79]. Most of the increased risk induced by smoking dissipates within two to three years of cessation of smoking. The relative risk in women who had not smoked for three or more years was indistinguishable from that in women who had never smoked.

The prevalence of **hypertension** reaches 70 to 80 percent in women above age 70 [79]. Although the incidence of hypertensive complications is generally lower in women than in men, hypertension is still a strong predictor of cardiovascular risk. Among the elderly, for example, hypertension in women (compared to men) is both a stronger predictor of coronary risk and is more commonly seen in those with CHD [57,58]. This increase in risk is also seen in premenopausal women in whom the presence of hypertension is associated with up to a 10 fold increase in coronary mortality [80,81]. Hypertension also increases the risk of cardiovascular events in women who have known CHD [82].

Initial therapy in hypertensive women is similar to that in men and should begin with lifestyle modification followed, if necessary, by the administration of antihypertensive drugs. Based in part upon results from the ALLHAT trial [83], a low-dose thiazide diuretic is usually recommended as first-line therapy with an angiotensin converting enzyme inhibitor (ACE inhibitor) or angiotensin II receptor blocker (ARB) added if further therapy is needed. Some patients, however, have specific indications or contraindications to the use of particular drugs.

The importance of **obesity as a coronary risk factor** was demonstrated in the prospective cohort Nurses' Health Study of over 115,000 middle-aged women followed for eight years [84,85]. Body weight and mortality were directly related with a relative risk of death from CHD of 4.1 and from all causes of 2.2 in women with a body mass index (BMI) greater than or equal to 32 kg/m^2 compared to lean women with a body mass index below 20 kg/m^2 [85]. The increase in risk associated with obesity was independent of diabetes, although the two disorders may be closely linked in individual patients [58]. Abdominal or central obesity (waist-hip ratio of above 0.9) is more predictive than simple body mass [58,86,87]. The increase in risk is also seen with increasing weight within the "normal" range, but is most pronounced with obesity [85,87,88]. The effect of weight gain is independent of the risk associated with physical inactivity [87].

Although obesity is associated with an increased cardiac mortality and weight loss is beneficial, weight cycling (repeated weight loss and weight gain) increases the risk of CHD death [90,91]. The mechanism for the increase in mortality may be related, in part, to a significant reduction in HDL cholesterol concentration with each cycle [92].

Although it has been recommended that **a low-fat, high carbohydrate diet or a low-fat, vegetarian diet** is a way to reduce the risk for CHD by reducing serum concentrations of LDL, such a diet also reduces the concentration of HDL and raises that of triglycerides [93]. It is likely that specific types of fat may be of importance [94-96].

It was estimated that the risk of CHD would be reduced by 42 percent if 5 percent of energy from saturated fat were replaced with energy from unsaturated fats and by 53 percent if 2 percent of energy from trans fat was replaced by energy from unhydrogenated, unsaturated fat.

Although a low intake of saturated fat appears to reduce CHD risk, such a diet may be associated with an increased risk of intraparenchymal hemorrhagic stroke, primarily in hypertensive women (relative risk 3.66 compared to those with higher saturated fat intake in the Nurses' Health Study); there was no relationship with other stroke subtypes [97].

Alcohol intake above two drinks per day is associated with an increase in the incidence of hypertension. In comparison, mild to moderate alcohol intake may have a cardioprotective effect in men. However, the issue is complicated in women by a potential increase in the risk for breast cancer. The benefit associated with light to moderate drinking was most apparent among women with risk factors for CHD and those 50 years of age or older [98]. In a Nurses' Health Study report, the benefit of moderate drinking was most pronounced in women who also had a high intake of folate [99].

Metabolic syndrome - visceral or abdominal obesity - is associated with insulin resistance and an array of metabolic and hemodynamic disorders, including hyperinsulinemia, atherogenic blood lipid changes, hypertension, and type 2 diabetes. This constellation of findings has been called the metabolic syndrome, insulin resistance syndrome, or syndrome X. Guidelines from the 2001 National Cholesterol Education Program (Adult Treatment Panel [ATP] III) suggest that the clinical identification of the metabolic syndrome should be based upon the presence of any three of the following traits [100]:

- Central obesity as measured by waist circumference (men — greater than 40 inches [102 cm]; women — greater than 35 inches [89 cm])
- Fasting blood triglycerides greater than or equal to 150 mg/dL
- Low blood HDL cholesterol (men — less than 40 mg/dL [1.04 mmol/L]; women — less than 50 mg/dL [1.30 mmol/L])
- Blood pressure greater than or equal to 130/85 mmHg
- Fasting glucose greater than or equal to 110 mg/dL (6.1 mmol/L)

The metabolic syndrome is associated with a significant increase in the subsequent risk of cardiovascular events in both men and women. The largest analysis of this association was performed on data from NHANES III [101]. Of 15,922 participants, 1098 (6.9 percent) had a history of MI or stroke. After adjusting for race, age, and history of cigarette smoking, there was a significant association between the metabolic syndrome and MI or stroke (odds ratio [OR] 2.1) which was comparable for both men (OR 1.9) and women (OR 2.2).

An analysis of the cardiovascular risk of the metabolic syndrome in women was also performed using data from the Women's Ischemia Syndrome Evaluation (WISE) study [102]. Among 755 women referred for coronary angiography, 25 percent had the metabolic syndrome at study entry. At four years of follow-up, women with the metabolic syndrome had a significantly lower rate of survival (94 versus 98 percent) and freedom from major adverse cardiovascular events (88 versus 94 percent). In another analysis from the WISE study, the metabolic syndrome, but not BMI alone, was significantly associated with the subsequent three-year risk of death or major adverse cardiovascular events [103].

Sedentary lifestyle depends, both in women and men, to cardiovascular risk factors, which could be modified. Although women tend to be less physically active than men, higher fitness and activity levels in women as in men are predictive of freedom from all causes of mortality, CHD, and stroke. In addition, healthy women also benefit from light to moderate exercise.

Oral contraceptives (OCs) — although there is no evidence that low-dose OC use increases the risk of CVD in women under age 30 or in nonsmoking women without other risk factors, the cardiovascular effects of OCs should be described in detail. Concern about toxicity (such as thromboembolic events and CVD) initially limited the long-term use of these drugs. However, the decrease in both estrogen and progestin content in the last decade has led to a reduction in both side effects and cardiovascular complications (with the possible exception of venous thrombosis) [104].

While the Food and Drug Administration had previously set upper age limits for OC use as 35 years for smokers and 40 years for nonsmokers, the age limit was removed in 1989 for healthy, nonsmoking women. Thus, OCs can be given until the menopause in such women. Caution is still needed in prescribing OCs for women who smoke, and an effort to induce smoking cessation should be made first.

The greatest concern surrounding the use of OCs has been the increase in cardiovascular morbidity and mortality that occurred with the early high-dose pills. However, the reduction in estrogen content (most pills now contain 30 to 35 mcg of ethinyl estradiol) has increased safety substantially. Some studies suggest that low-dose OCs may be associated with an overall increased risk of CVD. However, because MI is an extremely rare event in otherwise healthy women of reproductive age, even a doubling of the risk would result in an extremely low attributable risk. On the other hand, risk in older women who smoke outweighs the risk of an unwanted pregnancy [105].

Much of what is known about the potential risks of OCs comes from four large cohort studies: the Royal College of General Practitioners (RCGP) study, the Oxford Family Planning Association study, the Walnut Creek Contraceptive Drug Study, and the Group Health Cooperative of Puget Sound study [106,107].

The RCGP reported no increase in CHD mortality of women currently taking an OC, with the exception of women over age 35 years who smoked [108]. Similarly, any increased risk of MI (thought to be related to a thrombotic mechanism rather than the development of atherosclerotic plaques) was also confined to older women who smoked. Heavy smokers (15 or more cigarettes per day) were at particularly high risk as compared with light smokers (fewer than 15 cigarettes per day).

A second study in OC users confirmed the importance of the number of cigarettes smoked per day on MI risk. A significant increase in risk was seen in current pill users smoking 25 or more cigarettes per day (OR 2.5), but not in nonsmokers or women smoking 1 to 24 cigarettes per day (OR 1.3 and 0.8, respectively) [109].

Other studies have confirmed the relationship between OC use and smoking and the risk of CHD [110,111]. In a large case-control study from the World Health Organization, combined OCs in current use (1989-1995) were associated with acute MI only in women who either smoked or had hypertension; the risk was substantial (400/million woman-years) only in older women who smoked [110].

These studies included women who used both high and low-dose OCs. It has been suggested that low-dose OCs may not increase the risk for acute MI, even in smokers [112]. On the other hand, one review of low-dose OC use found that women over the age of 35 years who smoked 25 cigarettes or more per day had a higher mortality rate than that of pregnant women [113]. The relationship between smoking, OC use, and cardiovascular disease may be related to high plasma fibrinogen concentrations and intravascular fibrin deposition [114], and enhanced monocyte tissue factor expression [115].

Newer "third-generation" OCs (eg, those containing desogestrel, norgestimate, or gestodene) have more favorable effects on the lipid profile than second generation preparations, but this did not translate into a lower risk of myocardial infarction in two case-control studies [116,117]. However, in a third case-control study, the risk of MI appeared to be lower in women using third rather than second generation Ocs, although the difference was not statistically significant [118]. Surprisingly, the risk of MI was the same in women with or without a prothrombotic mutation. A meta-analysis of 10 studies calculated a similar overall doubling of risk in women using OCs with less than 50 mcg ethinyl estradiol [119].

Theoretically, the increase in risk may be more clinically relevant in women with polycystic ovary syndrome (who are thought to be at higher risk of CVD) [119]. However, there are no clinical data on the risk of MI with OC use in this group of patients.

A consensus panel reviewing the issue of OCs and smoking suggested that OCs can be considered for fertile women over the age of 35 years who are light smokers (fewer than 15 cigarettes per day) [120]. They cautioned, however, that women may underreport the number of cigarettes smoked per day and that it should be documented that these women have been warned of the risks associated with combined OC use and smoking. The panel also concluded that OCs should not be prescribed for women over age 35 years who smoke more than 15 cigarettes per day. On the other hand, for younger women, OCs could be prescribed, even for heavy smokers, as long as there is no family history of thromboembolic disease. Women who have taken an OC are not at increased risk for coronary heart disease later in life [121,122].

Therefore, it could be repeated that some, but not all, studies report that OCs may be associated with an increased risk of MI. However, because MI is an extremely rare event in otherwise healthy women of reproductive age, even a doubling of the risk would result in an extremely low attributable risk. Risk in older women who smoke outweighs the risk of an unwanted pregnancy. Recommendations from two expert groups: the American College of Obstetricians and Gynecologists (ACOG) and World Health Organization (WHO) are summarized [104] in table 3.

Psychosocial and behavioral factors are associated with an increased risk and a worse prognosis of CHD in women [123]. Lower socioeconomic status in men and particularly in women has consistently been associated with increased cardiovascular morbidity and mortality, but most of the increased risk appears to be due to psychosocial stress and lifestyle factors and, to a lesser extent, traditional risk factors of hypertension and hyperlipidemia [124].

Table 3. Summary of guidelines for the use of combination estrogen-progestin oral contraceptives, according to Petitti 2003 [104].

Variable	ACOG* guidelines	WHO** guidelines
Smoker, >35 yr of age		
<15 cigarettes/day	Risk unacceptable	Risk usually outweighs benefit
15 cigarettes/day	Risk unacceptable	Risk unacceptable
Hypertension		
Blood pressure controlled	Risk acceptable; no definition of blood-pressure control	Risk usually outweighs benefit if systolic blood pressure is 140-159 mmHg and diastolic blood pressure is 90-99 mmHg
Blood pressure uncontrolled	Risk unacceptable; no definition of uncontrolled blood pressure	Risk unacceptable if systolic blood pressure is 160 mmHg or diastolic blood pressure is 100 mmHg
History of stroke, ischemic heart disease, or venous thromboembolism	Risk unacceptable	Risk unacceptable
Diabetes	Risk acceptable if no other cardiovascular risk factors and no end-organ damage	Benefit outweighs risk if no end-organ damage and diabetes is of ≤20 yr duration
Hypercholesterolemia	Risk acceptable if LDL cholesterol <160 mg/dL and no other cardivascular risk factors	Benefit-risk ratio is dependent on the presence or absence of other cardiovascular risk factors
Multiple cardiovascular risk factors	Not addressed	Risk usually outweighs benefit or risk unacceptable, depending on risk factors

*ACOG = American College of Obstetricians and Gynecologists; **WHO = World Health Organization

Framingham Risk Score for Women

Assessing the risk of CHD requires the synthesis of multiple risk factors into a multivariable profile. The model most frequently used is that developed by the Framingham Heart Study, which allows the sex-specific calculation of the risk of a coronary event within 10 years (see tables: 4A and 4B) [125]. A validation study found that the Framingham CHD predictor performed well for prediction of CHD events in white men and women and black men and women [126]. The Framingham score may overestimate risk among some other populations.

Table 4A. Framingham risk score for women* -
Part I, according to Wilson et al., 1998 [125]

Age (Years)	Points	Diabetes	Points			
30-34	-9	No	0			
35-39	-4	Yes	4			
40-44	0					
45-49	3	**Smoker**	**Points**			
50-54	6	No	0			
55-59	7	Yes	2			
60-64	8					
65-69	8					
70-74	8					

LDL-C			HDL-C			
mg/dL	Mmol/L	Points	mg/dL	mmol/L	Points	
<100	<2.59	-2	<35	<0.90	5	
100-129	2.60-3.36	0	35-44	0.91-1.16	2	
130-159	3.37-4.14	0	45-49	1.17-1.29	1	
160-190	4.50-4.92	2	50-54	1.30-1.55	0	
>190	>4.92	2	>60	>1.56	-2	

* Framingham risk scoring system for women. Use to calculate the risk of developing clinical coronary heart disease (CHD) in women who do not have known CHD. Clinical CHD includes angina pectoris, recognized or unrecognized myocardial infarction (MI), coronary insufficiency (prolonged chest discomfort associated with transient repolarization abnormalities without criteria for MI), or CHD death.

To calculate the Framingham risk estimate, add points for age (see table 4A), presence of diabetes (table 4A), smoking status (table 4A), LDL-cholesterol (LDL-C) (table 4A), HDL-cholesterol (HDL-C) (table 4A), and blood pressure (table 4B). Find the total point score on the bottom table 4B to determine the 10-year risk of CHD.

Table 4B Framingham risk score for women* -
Part II, according to Wilson et al., 1998 [125]

Systolic blood Pressure	Diastolic <80 mmHg	Diastolic 80-84	Diastolic 85-89	Diastolic 90-99	Diastolic ≥100
(mmHg)					
<120	-3	0	0	2	3
120-129	0	0	0	2	3
130-139	0	0	0	2	3
140-159	2	2	2	2	3
≥160	3	3	3	3	3

Coronary heart disease (CHD) risk

Table 4 B. (Continued)

Total points	10 yr CHD risk percent	Total points	10 yr CHD risk percent	Total point	10 yr risk percent
<-2	1	5	5	12	15
-1	2	6	6	13	17
0	2	7	7	14	20
1	2	8	8	15	24
2	3	9	9	16	27
3	3	10	11	17	32
4	4	11	13		

* Framingham risk scoring system for women. Use to calculate the risk of developing clinical coronary heart disease (CHD) in women who do not have known CHD. Clinical CHD includes angina pectoris, recognized or unrecognized myocardial infarction (MI), coronary insufficiency (prolonged chest discomfort associated with transient repolarization abnormalities without criteria for MI), or CHD death.

To calculate the Framingham risk estimate, add points for age (table 4A), presence of diabetes (table 4A), smoking status (table 4A), LDL-cholesterol (LDL-C) (table 4A), HDL-cholesterol (HDL-C) (table 4A), and blood pressure (table 4B). Find the total point score on the bottom table 4B to determine the 10-year risk of CHD.

Clinical Features (Clinical Manifestations) and Outcome

Women with CHD are generally about 10 years older than men at the time of presentation and carry a greater burden of risk factors [127-129]. They are more likely to initially present with chest pain than a more clearly defined event such as a myocardial infarction. In a 26 year follow-up from the Framingham Study, for example, angina was uncomplicated in 80 percent of women, whereas it evolved out of infarction in 66 percent of men [129].

Chest pain — as in men, the quality of chest pain is an important predictor of angiographic disease in women [130,131]. Women are less likely than men to have typical angina (28 versus 55 percent in a review of over 3100 patients undergoing exercise stress testing) [132]. In addition, the prevalence of significant coronary disease is lower in women presenting with chest pain.

The differences between women and men was illustrated in a review of 38 women and 94 men who, in a prospective study of 907 patients undergoing exercise stress testing with perfusion imaging, had both angina and imaging evidence of ischemia [133]. Women rated their chest pain as more intense, used different terms to describe the pain (more often sharp and burning), had more symptoms unrelated to pain, and more frequently had pain and other sensations in the neck and throat.

Another factor important in the interpretation of chest pain in women is the greater likelihood of angina being induced by rest, sleep, and mental stress [134]. Women who present to the emergency department with new onset chest pain are approached and diagnosed less aggressively than men [135]. On the other hand, such women are more likely to receive controlled substances and anxiolytics in the emergency department, suggesting that they were being treated for psychiatric or psychosomatic complaints.

In a survey from Rochester, Minnesota of patients seen between 1960 and 1979, women with angina pectoris as an initial diagnosis had a longer survival and lower risk of subsequent MI or cardiac death than age-matched men with the same presentation [136]. This difference did not apply to presentations with MI or sudden unexpected death.

The incidence and prevalence of MI increases progressively in older women, especially after the age of 45 [129]. Women presenting with a first symptomatic MI are generally older than men (by six to ten years) [136,137] and more likely to have a history of diabetes, hypertension, hyperlipidemia, heart failure and an unstable anginal pattern than their male counterparts [137].

Noninvasive Tests in the Diagnosis of CHD in Women

The initial evaluation of patients presenting with chest pain and suspected CHD often includes some form of stress testing. The American College of Cardiology/American Heart Association (ACC/AHA) has issued guidelines for the role of exercise testing in such patients that takes into consideration the patient's ability to exercise and the ability to detect the electrocardiographic changes induced by ischemia [138].

However, these general guidelines are not always applicable to women. The underestimation of clinical coronary risk in women and the limited diagnostic accuracy of some noninvasive tests probably contributes to the increased mortality, compared to men, after myocardial infarction or coronary artery bypass surgery. However, increased comorbidity is probably of greater importance.

The pretest likelihood of CHD in a patient depends upon symptoms and other clinical characteristics; it influences the posttest risk of having CHD and therefore the likelihood that the results of a noninvasive test for CHD is accurate.

The features of the chest pain are an important determinant of the pretest likelihood of CHD. The following definitions were used in the Coronary Artery Surgery Study (CASS) [131]:

– Definite or classic angina — Substernal chest discomfort with a characteristic quality and duration, which is provoked by exertion or emotional stress, and relieved by rest or nitroglycerin.
– Probable or atypical angina — Chest pain with two of the three above characteristics.
– Nonanginal or nonischemic chest pain — Chest pain with one or none of the above characteristics.

When patients are divided into subgroups based upon the characteristics of their chest pain, age, and gender, the pretest probability of CHD can vary between 1 and 94 percent with a resulting marked variability in the likelihood of false-positive and false-negative exercise tests (see table 5) [130,131].

Table 5. Pretest probability of coronary heart disease in patients with chest pain according to age, gender, and symptoms. Combined data from Diamond & Forrester, 1979 [130]; and from Weiner et al., 1979 [131]. The probability values are expressed as the percent of patients with significant coronary artery disease on angiography.

Age	Nonanginal pain		Atypical angina		Typical angina	
	Men	Women	Men	Women	Men	Women
30-39	4	2	34	12	76	26
40-49	13	3	51	22	87	55
50-59	20	7	65	31	93	73
60-69	27	14	72	51	94	86

According to the ACC/AHA guidelines, women at intermediate to high pretest probability of CHD are broadly defined as those with classic or atypical angina who are greater than or equal to 50 years of age, and those <50 years of age with classic angina [138]. Women are less likely than men to have classic angina (28 versus 55 percent in a review of over 3100 patients undergoing exercise stress testing) [132].

The importance of pretest probability in assessing the results of noninvasive testing was illustrated in an example published in a report from the 1999 ACC/AHA Task Force on Practice Guidelines (Committee on Management of Patients with Chronic Stable Angina) [139]:

In patients with a low pretest probability of CHD (5 percent), the positive predictive value of an abnormal test (using a sensitivity and specificity of 50 and 90 percent, respectively) is only 21 percent. Thus, if 1000 such patients are tested, 120 will have a positive result, of whom 95 will not have significant CHD. The high likelihood of a false-positive result must be considered before ordering a noninvasive test in such a group of patients.

In patients with a high pretest probability of CHD (90 percent), a positive test increases the probability of disease to 98 percent, while a negative result lowers the probability to only 83 percent. Thus, a noninvasive test may have little diagnostic information to offer since, unless the test is perfectly sensitive, a negative result is likely to be falsely negative and further testing will be necessary.

In patients with an intermediate pretest probability of CHD (50 percent), a positive test result increases the likelihood of disease to 83 percent, while a negative test decreases the likelihood to 36 percent. Thus, it is this group that is most likely to benefit from a noninvasive diagnostic test.

However, pretest CHD probabilities and recognized coronary risk factors have largely been based upon data from men. In addition, women have until recently been underrepresented in studies of coronary risk and CHD prevention [140].

During exercise stress testing, women are less likely than men to have typical angina (28 versus 55 percent in a review of over 3100 patients) [132]. The characteristics of the differences between women and men was illustrated in a review of 38 women and 94 men who, in a prospective study of 907 patients undergoing exercise stress testing with perfusion imaging, had both angina and imaging evidence of ischemia [133]. Women rated their chest pain as more intense, used different terms to describe the pain (more often sharp and burning), had more symptoms unrelated to pain, and more frequently had pain and other sensations in the neck and throat.

Exercise ECG testing is primarily performed in patients who are able to attain a sufficient level of exercise and who do not have baseline ECG abnormalities that can interfere with interpretation. These include preexcitation (Wolff-Parkinson-White) syndrome, a paced ventricular rhythm, more than 1 mm of ST depression at rest, complete left bundle branch block, and patients taking digoxin or with ECG criteria for left ventricular hypertrophy, even if they have less than 1 mm of baseline ST depression. Patients with one or more of these abnormalities should be tested with echocardiography or myocardial perfusion imaging; pharmacologic stress is warranted in patients who are unable to exercise.

Treadmill exercise testing has a lower sensitivity and specificity in women compared to men; furthermore, both positive and negative tests in women have relatively low predictive value [140].

Test accuracy varies with the pretest probability of disease, as illustrated in a report from the CASS of 580 women and 1465 men with chest pain [131]. The CASS examined in part the pretest probability of CHD and the accuracy of exercise testing among patients presenting with complaints of chest pain. The exercise test was considered positive when there was greater than or equal to 1 mm ST segment depression or elevation for at least 0.08 sec compared to the baseline ECG. When patients were divided into subgroups based upon gender and the quality of their chest pain complaints, the pretest probability of CHD (as determined by coronary angiography) varied between 5 and 89 percent and the false positive and negative rates of exercise testing varied between 4 and 94 and 5 and 65 percent, respectively. Positive tests in women, particularly those with nonischemic chest pain and, to a lesser degree, those with probable angina, were likely to be false positives. The higher false positive rate in women compared to men could be explained by the lower prevalence of CHD in women (see table 6).

In CASS, the higher false-positive rate on exercise ECG testing in women compared to men could be explained by the lower prevalence of CHD in women (see table 6) [131]. Other possible contributing factors are a greater prevalence of both mitral valve prolapse and syndrome X (angina with normal coronary arteries) than in men. The magnitude of the latter disparity was illustrated in a report of 886 patients referred for angiographic evaluation of chest pain; normal coronary arteries were found in 41 percent of the women compared to only 8 percent of the men [57].

Table 6. Pretest probability of CHD and accuracy of exercise test in CASS, according to Weiner, et al. [131].

Clinical history	Gender	Prevalence of CHD, percent	False positive, percent	False negative, percent
Definite angina	Male	89	4	65
Definite angina	Female	63	27	23
Probable angina	Male	70	13	44
Probable angina	Female	40	46	22
Nonischemic chest pain	Male	22	91	14
Nonischemic chest pain	Female	5	94	5

Similar limitations to classic signs of ischemia were noted in an analysis from a Lipid Research Clinics study of 2994 asymptomatic women who underwent exercise testing at study entry and were then followed for 20 years [142]. Exercise-induced ST segment depression did not increase the risk of cardiovascular death (age-adjusted hazard ratio 1.02). In contrast, women who were below the median for either exercise capacity or heart rate recovery, both of which were considered measures of fitness, were at increased risk: those below the median for both variables were at highest risk (multivariable-adjusted hazard ratio 3.5 compared to those above the median for both variables).

The predictive value of the stress ECG in women may be improved by use of the **Duke treadmill score** [132]. The former is calculated from the following formula:

Duke prognostic treadmill score = Exercise time (minutes based on the Bruce protocol) - (5 x maximum ST segment deviation in mm) - (4 x exercise angina [0=none, 1=nonlimiting, and 2= exercise limiting])

Patients are classified as low, moderate, or high risk according to the score:

* Low-risk — score greater than or equal to +5
* Moderate-risk — score from -10 to +4
* High-risk — score <-11

The Duke treadmill score appears to perform better in women than men for excluding disease. This was illustrated in the report cited above of 976 women and 2249 men with chest pain and suspected CHD [132]. The following findings were noted (see table 7).

Fewer low risk women had any coronary artery with greater than or equal to 75 percent stenosis (19 versus 47 percent in men) or three vessel or left main disease (3.5 versus 11.4 percent).

The risk of coronary artery disease increased in women with moderate or high risk scores. The values for three vessel or left main disease were 12.4 and 46 percent, respectively.

The treadmill score was of limited value for predicting short-term prognosis. At two years, the mortality rate was 1.0, 2.2, and 3.6 percent in women at low, moderate, and high risk. Comparable values in men were 1.7, 5.8, and 16.6 percent, indicating substantial prognostic stratification.

Table 7. Exercise ECG women v men. Comparison of predictive value of exercise ECG testing in 976 women and 2249 men referred for evaluation of chest pain, data from Alexander et al, 1998 [132].

Finding	Women*	Men*
Baseline characteristics:		
Median age (years)	51	50
Typical angina	28	55
Atypical angina	53	34
Exercise-induced angina	42	54
No coronary stenosis ≥75 percent	68	28
Two-year mortality according to Duke treadmill score		
Low risk	1.0	1.7
Moderate risk	2.2	5.8
High risk	3.6	16.6
Among patients with high risk score:		
≥1 vessel with 75 percent stenosis	89	98
Three vessel or ≥75 percent left main disease	46	72
Among patients with low risk score:		
≥1 vessel with ≥75 percent stenosis	19	47
Three vessel or ≥75 percent left main disease	3.5	11.4

* All values in percent unless noted.

A possible explanation for the inability to identify a high-risk group in women in this study is that the mean age was 51 years, an age at which there is a low frequency of clinically important CHD in women. Only 32 percent of the women had a coronary stenosis greater than or equal to 75 percent, compared to 72 percent of men (see table 7).

The addition of any form of **myocardial perfusion imaging (MPI)** to stress testing greatly increases diagnostic accuracy compared to stress ECG alone in both sexes. This may be particularly true in women, and some have suggested that all women should undergo an imaging stress test (nuclear or echocardiography) as their initial examination [143].

MPI is preferably performed with exercise stress, but can be readily combined with pharmacologic stress (using dipyridamole, adenosine, or dobutamine) in patients who are unable to exercise sufficiently.

Myocardial perfusion images are obtained following the injection of perfusion radiotracers. Areas of absolutely or relatively reduced myocardial blood flow, called "perfusion defects," can be readily recognized on scintigraphic images. The presence and extent of these perfusion defects has both diagnostic and prognostic significance.

In addition to use in the diagnosis of large vessel CHD, imaging can also help establish the diagnosis of chest pain due to microvascular disease in women with normal coronary arteries (also called syndrome X). As noted above, this disorder is substantially more common in women [57].

As noted above, stress testing with MPI should be performed in women at intermediate risk (15 to 85 percent) of CHD, especially if the resting ECG is not normal or a prior false-positive ST segment response is suspected. This approach improves specificity, enhances the accuracy of multivessel CHD detection, and offers an excellent (>99 percent) negative predictive value for CHD exclusion [144].

Stress MPI is also an effective tool for assessment of women with diabetes who may have CHD. This was illustrated in a study of 4755 patients with symptoms of CHD; 20 percent were diabetic and 44 percent were women [145]. The estimated three-year incidence of death or MI among diabetic women without evidence of ischemia on perfusion imaging was significantly lower than for those with single vessel or multivessel ischemia (3 versus 27 and 40 percent).

Most initial studies utilized standard perfusion imaging with **thallium (Tl)-201** as the radiotracer [146]. Exercise thallium testing has the high false-positive rate [147] and the sensitivity for CHD detection is lower than in men [148].

However, Tl-201 has significant drawbacks when used in women. Because of the reduced energy level of Tl-201 and the distance its emitted photons must travel, some myocardial radioactivity may never reach the camera detector. In nuclear imaging terms, the activity becomes "attenuated." The "scatter" and attenuation of Tl-201 photons is accentuated in obese patients and in women with dense or extensive breast tissue. When attenuation is nonuniform, eg, when a woman's left breast partially covers her heart, substantial artifactual image distortion can occur. These artifacts mimic fixed or reversible myocardial perfusion defects and can be wrongly interpreted as representing a positive test.

The importance of breast artifacts was assessed in a report of 840 patients with suspected CHD, almost one-half of whom were women [149]. Diagnostically inadequate Tl-201 imaging due to breast artifact occurred in 11 percent of women compared to 2 percent of men. The use of breast "markers" can improve the specificity, but suboptimal studies still occur [150].

Another factor that may contribute to the lower diagnostic accuracy of Tl-201 imaging in women is a smaller left ventricular chamber size.

The problem of false-positive results with Tl-201 led to the development and clinical validation of **technetium (Tc)-99m** labeled myocardial perfusion agents in both men and women [151]. These are higher energy radio tracers that are better suited for imaging with standard gamma camera systems. Since Tc-99m emits substantially higher levels of energy (140 keV) than Tl-201, photon scattering is less of a problem, and tissue attenuation is reduced by approximately 15 percent.

The technique of Tc-99m perfusion imaging is similar to that of Tl-201 imaging with one important exception: two separate injections of the radiotracer are required to document the perfusion status at rest and at the peak of stress. A one-day imaging protocol has demonstrated high diagnostic accuracy in conditions of both exercise and dipyridamole stress. A two-day high-dose sestamibi (22 to 25 mCi) protocol can optimize imaging in women with significant breast attenuation problems.

A number of studies have evaluated the performance of exercise or pharmacologic **stress echocardiography** in women with chest pain and some have compared the results to exercise ECG testing and stress MPI [143,152]. In a meta-analysis of three studies of at least 50 women who underwent both exercise echocardiography and coronary angiography, the sensitivity and specificity for CHD were 86 and 79 percent, respectively. Comparable values in 19 studies of exercise ECG testing were lower at 61 and 70 percent.

One of the studies in the meta-analysis evaluated 161 women without a previous Q wave myocardial infarction in whom exercise echocardiography was compared to exercise ECG testing; all women also underwent coronary angiography and 59 had greater than or equal to 50 percent diameter narrowing [143]. Among patients with an interpretable ECG, exercise echocardiography was as sensitive as exercise ECG testing (81 versus 77 percent), but significantly more specific (80 versus 56 percent) and accurate (81 versus 64 percent). It also stratified significantly more patients with intermediate pretest probability into a high or low posttest probability group. The authors concluded that, among women with suspected CHD, exercise echocardiography had the best balance between accuracy and cost for the diagnosis of CHD.

The ACC/AHA/ASE guidelines on echocardiography reviewed studies involving a total of almost 1000 women with suspected CHD (usually because of chest pain) [153]. Stress echocardiography, including both exercise and pharmacologic stress, had a weighted mean sensitivity of 81 percent (89 percent with multivessel disease), specificity of 86 percent, and overall accuracy of 84 percent.

Pharmacologic stress echocardiography appears to be as accurate as stress MPI. With both techniques, women have more false-negative (ie, lower sensitivity) [154-156] studies than men. In one series of 2748 patients, 44 percent of whom were women, the sensitivity of adequately performed dobutamine echocardiography was significantly lower in women than in men (78 versus 88 percent) [155].

A contributing factor to false-negative results in women is the greater likelihood of single vessel coronary disease. In one report evaluating dobutamine stress, 10 of 13 women with false-negative echocardiograms and 9 of 13 with false-negative scintigrams had single vessel stenoses [154]. Similar findings were noted in the Women's Ischemia Syndrome Evaluation (WISE) study in which dobutamine echocardiography and quantitative coronary angiography were performed in 92 women with chest pain and risk factors for CHD [156]. The sensitivity of dobutamine echocardiography for multivessel disease was 60 percent overall and 82 percent in those who had an adequate heart rate response; in comparison, the test was negative in nine of ten patients with single vessel disease.

However, the greater likelihood of single vessel disease does not entirely explain the lower sensitivity in women. In the series of 2748 patients cited above, the sensitivity in adequately performed tests was lower in women with multivessel disease (82 versus 93 percent in men) [155]. Another problem with dobutamine echocardiography described in this report was that women had a more rapid increase in heart rate with low dose dobutamine than men, resulting in more frequent test termination at a submaximal dose of dobutamine and less frequent use of atropine.

In addition to its diagnostic value, stress echocardiography also has prognostic value, and this appears to be similar in men and women [157].

Noninvasive stress-testing: conclusion and recommendations – The decision to perform stress testing for suspected CHD in women is based in part upon the estimated pretest probability of disease. The 2002 ACC/AHA guidelines for exercise testing and for chronic stable angina recommend that, for patients who can attain an adequate level of exercise (defined as greater than or equal to 85 of their predicted maximal heart rate), symptom-limited treadmill or bicycle exercise is the preferred form of stress because it provides the most information concerning patient symptoms, cardiovascular function, and the hemodynamic response during usual forms of activity [138,139]. The inability to perform an exercise test is in itself a negative prognostic factor in patients with CHD.

The following sequential approach could be recommended, which is based upon exercise tolerance, the baseline ECG, and the presence of other comorbidities such as diabetes mellitus [158]. This approach is consistent with the 2005 AHA guidelines on noninvasive testing for women with suspected CHD [159]:

The evaluation of a woman with suspected CHD begins with pretest screening. Stress testing for diagnosis is warranted only in women with an intermediate (10 to 90 percent) pretest probability of CHD (table 5 and table 6). Stress testing for diagnosis is of limited value in women at high pretest risk, but may be performed to estimate prognosis and guide therapy. Stress testing is not warranted in women at low risk since almost all positive tests will be false positives (table 6) [131].

Among women at intermediate risk, exercise electrocardiography should be performed, assuming that the patient can exercise and has no baseline ECG abnormalities that would interfere with interpretation of the test. This approach is consistent with the 2002 ACC/AHA guidelines on exercise testing and on chronic stable angina, which concluded that there were insufficient data to justify routine stress imaging tests as the initial stress test for CHD in women [138,139].

No further evaluation is necessary if the maximum stress test is negative and the patient can achieve an adequate work level, although risk factor modification with or without antiischemic therapy is warranted if the clinical history strongly suggests classic angina.

Women with an intermediate risk test (as estimated, for example, from the Duke treadmill score), a negative submaximal test, or those who are unable to exercise or have baseline ECG abnormalities that would interfere with interpretation of exercise ECG testing should undergo stress MPI, ideally with a technetium perfusion radiotracer, or stress echocardiography. Both noninvasive imaging tests appear to have comparable accuracy. Local expertise and test availability should dictate test selection. Women with a moderate to severely abnormal test should go on to coronary angiography if they are a candidate for percutaneous coronary intervention or coronary artery bypass grafting.

Women with a high risk test (as estimated, for example, from the Duke treadmill score) also should be referred for angiography.

Case Report 1. (EC 77 Years Old)

A 77-year-old female (EC), a retired shop assistant with hypercholesterolemia and labile hypertension caused by emotional stress, was referred by her family doctor to our outpatients clinic due to chest pains not directly connected with effort. She was overweight (weight-69 kg, height-152 cm; BMI = 29.86 kg/m2.) and had been a smoker in the past. She had smoked 10 cigarettes a day for 20 years, but had stopped smoking 10 years earlier. On examination heart rate (HR) was 79 bpm and blood pressure (BP) was 120/80 mmHg. Rest ECG did not reveal any significant abnormalities (figure 2).

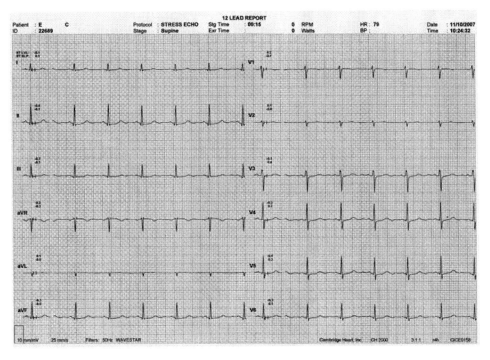

Figure 2. Rest ECG of patient no. 1 (EC). Sinus rhythm 79 bpm. Nonspecific T wave abnormality.

Exercise on a supine cycloergometer (bicycle exercise) was stopped at 75 W because of fatigue without chest pain. Blood pressure during exercise was slightly too high and significant ST depression occurred in 1 lead: V4 –1.3 mm (at rest -0.3 mm). The test was electrocardiographically positive without chest pain (figure 3).

Stress echo during the same exercise did not reveal any abnormalities in the contraction of heart walls (normokinesis in all phases of the test). Stress echo was negative, there was no danger of narrowing in the coronary arteries and the patient was not referred for coronary angiography. She was advised to go on a weight reducing diet, take statin and hypotensive drugs, and to check her blood pressure frequently. A cervical and thoracic X-ray of the spine was recommended and she was also told to come back for further tests if chest pains occurred again.

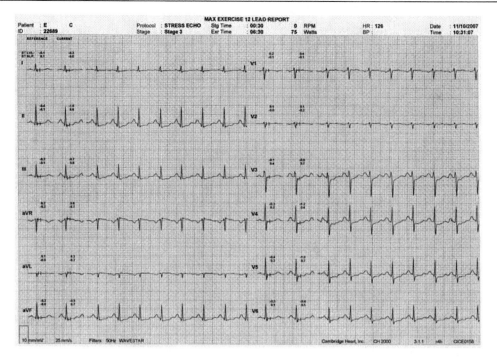

Figure 3. ECG stress test of patient no.1 (EC). Bicycle exercise was stopped at 75 W because of fatigue without chest pain. Bordeline ST depression occurred in 1 lead: V4 –1.2 mm (at rest = -0.3 mm, change = -0.9). Maximal ST depression on V4=-1.3 (significant change = -1.0). Result: test positive without chest pain.

Invasive Diagnostic Procedures (Coronary Angiography)

The prevalence of significant coronary disease is lower in women presenting with chest pain [57]. The magnitude of this difference was illustrated in a report of 886 patients referred for angiographic evaluation of presumed angina, 23 percent of whom were women [57]. Normal coronary arteries were much more common in women (41 versus 8 percent in men).

Myocardial ischemia and/or coronary microvascular dysfunction is present in 20 to 50 percent of women with chest pain and normal coronary arteries [160]. A higher rate of lack of significant coronary stenoses has also been noted in women with a non-ST elevation acute coronary syndrome (unstable angina or non-ST elevation myocardial infarction). In different clinical trials, 12 to 14 percent of such patients have, on coronary angiography, either normal vessels or no vessel with greater than or equal to 50 to 60 percent stenosis. This appears to be more common in women.

Possible mechanisms for the absence of significant coronary disease in these patients include rapid clot lysis, vasospasm, and coronary microvascular disease.

Gender bias in use of coronary angiography — A number of studies have documented gender-based differences in utilization rates of coronary angiography and revascularization, even among those with an acute MI [149]. These differences reflect physicians' failure to refer women with positive exercise tests for subsequent testing, leading to a poorer outcome.

In one report, for example, women with a positive exercise test were more likely to have no further cardiac evaluation than men (62 versus 38 percent), a difference that, at three year follow-up, was associated with a higher incidence of MI or death in women (14.3 versus 6 percent per year in men) [149]. All events occurred in nonrevascularized individuals.

A separate issue is whether gender bias affects the likelihood of revascularization after cardiac catheterization. In a review of over 21,000 patients, women had equal access to revascularization after adjustment for clinical variables (eg, age, diabetes, heart failure, renal insufficiency) and coronary variables (eg, extent of disease, left ventricular ejection fraction) [161] (see below).

Management of Coronary Heart Disease in Women

The success rate of therapy for CHD is similar in women and men; however, the complication rates differ, resulting in a gender specific profile of benefit. The 2002 ACC/AHA Task Force recommended that women with unstable angina or non-ST segment elevation MI be treated in a similar manner to men with the same indications for noninvasive and invasive testing [162].

Recommendations for Management of Cardiovascular Risk in Women

The following lifestyle recommendations for all women, which are in accord with the 2004 AHA guidelines on CVD prevention in women [163] are listed in table 8:

Table 8. The lifestyle recommendations for all women, which are in accord with the 2004 American Heart Association guidelines on CVD prevention in women [163]:

1. Regular physical activity on most days of the week.
2. Avoidance and cessation of smoking.
3. Weight maintenance/reduction to achieve a BMI of 18.5 to 24.9 kg/m^2.
4. Maintenance of a low fat diet.
5. Treatment of hypercholesterolemia to primary prevention targets.
6. Treatment of hypertension.
7. Treatment of diabetes.
8. Avoidance of oral contraceptives in women who smoke.

Table 9. The lifestyle recommendations, according to the 2004 American Heart Association guidelines on CVD prevention in women [163], for women at high risk (Framingham risk score >20 percent [see tables 4A and 4B], established CHD, other vascular disease, diabetes mellitus, or chronic kidney disease), we recommend the following additional measures.

1. Treatment of hypercholesterolemia to secondary prevention targets, which many feel is a goal serum LDL-cholesterol concentration below 80 mg/dL (2.1 mmol/L) that is achieved at least in part with statin therapy.
2. Aspirin therapy at a dose of 75 to 162 mg/day.
3. Beta blocker therapy in all women who have had an MI or who have an acute ischemic syndrome.
4. Treatment of hypertension to achieve a goal blood pressure of less than 130/80 mmHg in women with diabetes or chronic renal failure and 140/90 mmHg (or even less than or equal to130/80 mmHg) in women with established CVD.
5. Folic acid supplementation if hyperhomocysteinemia has been detected.
6. Hormone replacement therapy is not recommended for the primary or secondary prevention of CVD. It has no cardioprotective effect and may produce harm [50-52].

For women at high risk (Framingham risk score >20 percent [see tables 4A and 4B], stablished CHD, other vascular disease, diabetes mellitus, or chronic kidney disease), the 2004 AHA guidelines on CVD prevention in women [163] recommend the following additional management, which shows table 9.

Medical Treatment

A variety of drugs are used in the treatment of CHD. Women are more likely to receive nitrates, calcium channel blockers, diuretics, and sedatives than men, while some studies suggest that women are less likely to receive aspirin, beta blockers and statins [164]. In a review of almost 3800 patients with stable angina in the Euro Heart Survey, women were as likely to be treated with a beta blocker as men, but significantly less likely to be treated with aspirin (73 versus 81 percent) and a statin (45 versus 51 percent) [164]. Hormone replacement therapy is not recommended for cardiac protection in women with CHD since the HERS trials showed no evidence of benefit [51,52] (see below).

When used for secondary prevention of CHD, an overview of randomized trials from the Antiplatelet Trialists' Collaboration found that **aspirin** (75 to 162 mg/day) was beneficial in women [165]. Among patients with an acute coronary syndrome, aspirin (162 to 325 mg) should be part of initial management of all patients, both men and women.

Although not as well studied for primary prevention as in men, aspirin may provide the same benefit in women with at least one risk factor [166]. Aspirin was also studied in women at average risk in the Women's Healthy Study [167]. The data suggested benefit against stroke but not MI, although there was a significant reduction in MI in women greater than or equal to 65 years of age that was similar to the reported benefit in men. Low-dose aspirin in women appears to produce a similar or even greater reduction in platelet reactivity than seen in men [168].

The benefit of **beta blockers** after MI is well demonstrated in women [169].

The benefits of **angiotensin converting enzyme (ACE)** inhibition after acute MI have been demonstrated in a number of trials that included some women [170]. Although efficacy in women has not been specifically studied, the criteria for ACE inhibitor therapy should be the same as in men.

It has also been demonstrated that patients at high risk for cardiovascular disease, as defined by the HOPE trial, have improved survival when treated with an ACE inhibitor. However, it is likely that this benefit is due to blood pressure reduction rather than a specific effect of ACE inhibition.

Analyses of four major trials of lipid lowering for secondary prevention in different patient populations (4S, CARE, HPS & PROVE IT-TIMI 22) support a beneficial effect of **statins** in women with CHD, even in those with borderline elevations in serum cholesterol [171-175].

Management of acute coronary syndrome (ACS): unstable angina (UA) and non-ST elevation MI (NSTEMI). Women with a non-ST elevation ACS tend to be older than men and have more comorbidities such as diabetes and hypertension [176]. Several specific issues have been raised concerning the management of women with these disorders, although women are generally treated the same as men.

A 2002 update from the ACC/AHA task force recommended that women with unstable angina or a non-ST elevation MI should be managed in a manner similar to men [162]. Women, like men, with high risk features benefit from an early invasive strategy within the first 48 hours. They should also receive aspirin and clopidogrel. However, biomarker negative women (ie, those with a negative serum troponin) should not receive a glycoprotein (GP) IIb/IIIa inhibitor.

Despite these general recommendations and the increase in mortality, women with a non-ST elevation ACS are treated less aggressively than men. In a review from the CRUSADE National Quality Improvement Initiative of almost 36,000 such patients (41 percent women) seen at 391 hospitals in the United States between 2000 and 2002, women were treated less aggressively than men [176]. They were significantly less likely to undergo catheterization within 24 hours of admission (42 versus 49 percent in men) and less likely to undergo percutaneous coronary intervention (PCI) within this time (44 versus 52 percent). Women had higher rates of in-hospital mortality, reinfarction, and heart failure but, after adjustment, the rates were similar to those in men.

As in non-ST elevation ACS, several issues have been raised concerning the management of women with **ST elevation MI (STEMI)**, although women are generally treated the same as men. Coronary reperfusion after acute MI can be achieved by thrombolysis or, preferably, primary PCI, usually performed with stenting.

In most studies, women were somewhat less likely to receive **thrombolysis**, even if eligible, and were likely to experience a greater delay in being treated [177]. Although definitive data are not available, it appears that thrombolysis reduces mortality in acute MI by the same proportion in both sexes [81].

Women have a modestly increased risk of bleeding, including hemorrhagic stroke, after thrombolysis. An additional bleeding concern is the use of thrombolytic agents in menstruating women. Data on this issue are limited. Among 12 menstruating women in GUSTO-I, there was no significant increase in severe bleeding compared to nonmenstruating women [178]. A significant increase in moderate bleeding was found that was offset by the benefits of thrombolytic therapy. Thus, menstruating women should not automatically be excluded from thrombolytic therapy.

Case Report 2. (IK 78 Years Old)

A 78-year-old female (IK), a retired secretary, with hypertension and hypercholesterolemia, was admitted to our department for a coronary angiography 4 months after acute coronary syndrome (NSTEMI) treated by percutaneous transluminal angioplasty (PTCA) of the left circumflex artery (LCx) with stent implantation (see figs 6A & 6B). The following drugs had been recommended: acetylsalicylic acid, clopidogrel, beta-blocker, statin and ACE inhibitor. Since the episode the patient had been in good health and had not complained of any chest pain. A further coronary angiography was advised because there was a suspicion that the right coronary artery (RCA) would need intervention. Rest ECG revealed ST segment and T wave abnormality without any significant changes as compared with previous ECGs (fig 4).

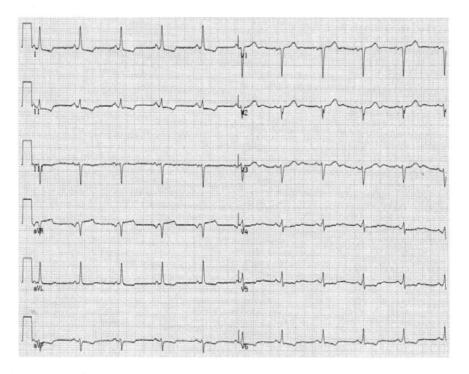

Figure 4. Rest ECG of patient no. 2 (IK). Normal sinus rhythm 61 bpm. ST & T wave abnormality. No significant changes as compared with previous ECGs.

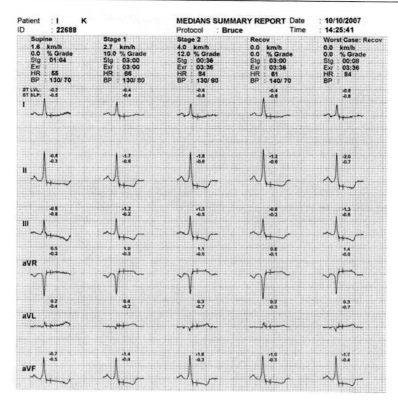

Figure 5. ECG stress test of patient no. 2 (IK). Exercise on treadmill was stopped after 3 minutes 36 seconds, according to the Bruce protocol (5.3 METS), because of fatigue without chest pain. Significant ST depression occurred in 2 leads: II -2.0 (at rest = -0.8, significant change =-1.2) & aVF -1.7 (at rest = -0.7, change -1.0). Result: test positive without chest pain.

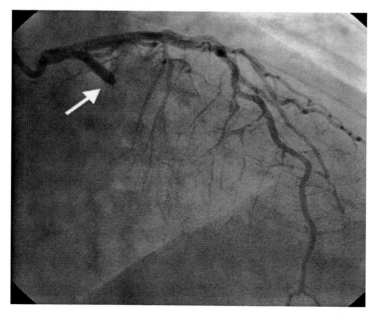

Figure 6A. Coronary angiography of patient no. 2 (IK). Acute coronary syndrome (NSTEMI). Total occlusion of left circumflex artery (LCx) – see arrow.

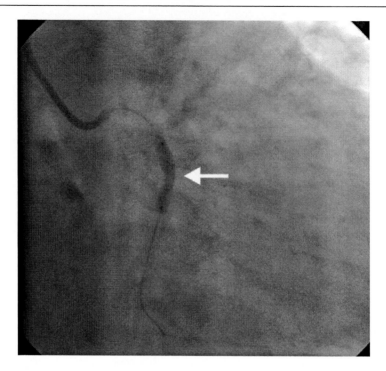

Figure 6B. Percutaneous coronary intervention (PCI) in of patient no. 2 (IK) during acute coronary syndrome (NSTEMI). PTCA with stent implantation of total LCx occlusion (arrow).

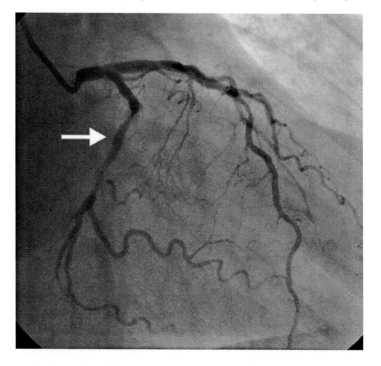

Figure 6C. Coronary angiography (left coronary artery) of patient no. 2 (IK) – 4 months after acute coronary syndrome treated by PTCA with stent implantation of total LCx occlusion. LCx: Nonsignificant (30%) stenosis inside the stent (arrow) & long borderline stenosis (60%) after the stent. Left anterior descending artery (LAD) borderline (60%) stenosis in segment no. 7.

Echocardiography showed akinesis of the basic part of the inferior cardiac wall. ECG stress test was positive without chest pain (fig 5).

A coronary angiography confirmed the effectiveness of PTCA LCx (fig 6C) and only borderline changes in left anterior descending artery (LAD) and RCA. Because the patients had no chest pain, a further coronary intervention was not recommended. The patient was advised to be more active and to continue her diet and medical treatment.

Hormone Replacement Therapy and CHD

Although initial observational studies suggested benefit from HRT for both primary and secondary prevention of CHD, this has not been confirmed in subsequent large trials. The net benefit of estrogen or combined estrogen-progestin replacement therapy in postmenopausal women is still uncertain. It had been thought for many years that estrogen was cardioprotective; as a result, estrogen replacement therapy was routinely prescribed for both primary and secondary prevention of CHD. However, data from the Women's Health Initiative (WHI), the Heart and Estrogen/Progestin Replacement Study (HERS-I and -II), other small controlled trials, and two meta-analyses, do not confirm a protective effect on the heart [51,52,179-182]. In contrast, the WHI unopposed estrogen trial did not report an increase in CHD events, although stroke and venous thromboembolism were increased as was seen in the combined estrogen-progestin trial [183,184].

Based upon the WHI trial results, and consistent with guidelines as well as updated recommendations issued by the American Heart Association (AHA) [182-186], estrogen is still a reasonable therapy when used short-term for menopausal symptoms, but should not be prescribed for either primary or secondary prevention of CHD. The following recommendations are currently accepted for primary prevention:

1. Estrogen-progestin therapy should not be prescribed for primary prevention of CHD.
2. Estrogen-progestin therapy should be discontinued if an acute CHD event occurs, and should not be resumed as a secondary prevention strategy.
3. Unopposed estrogen, although it does not appear to increase CHD risk, should not be prescribed for primary prevention because no reduction in CHD risk was observed in the WHI trial [182].
4. Estrogen or estrogen-progestin therapy should be reserved for perimenopausal women with moderate to severe menopausal symptoms. The lowest estrogen dose that relieves symptoms should be used for the shortest duration possible.

Although some observational and angiographic studies had strongly suggested that women with CHD derive the greatest benefit for prevention of subsequent coronary events and survival, clinical trial data have not confirmed these benefits [51,52,180].

The HERS-I trial (Heart and Estrogen/Progestin Replacement Study) was a randomized, blinded, placebo-controlled secondary prevention trial [51]. In this study, 2763 postmenopausal women under the age of 80 with a history of CHD were randomly assigned to receive the same regimen used in the WHI (0.625 mg of conjugated equine estrogen plus

2.5 mg of medroxyprogesterone acetate daily) or placebo for an average of four years [51]. Findings from this trial included:

There was no significant difference between the two groups in the incidence of CHD events despite a net 11 percent decrease in serum low density lipoprotein (LDL) cholesterol concentrations and 10 percent increase in serum high density lipoprotein (HDL) cholesterol concentrations in the hormone cohort.

More CHD events occurred in the hormone group during the first year of therapy, with a subsequent trend toward a reduction in risk in years four and five.

An extensive post-hoc analysis of HERS-I did not identify any subgroup in which estrogen therapy was beneficial or harmful.

In another post hoc analysis, combined oral estrogen and progestin therapy appeared to reduce the risk of developing type 2 diabetes mellitus. However, this effect is insufficient to recommend HRT as a diabetes prevention strategy in women with CHD.

The HERS-II trial was a continuation of HERS-I in which 93 percent of HERS-I participants enrolled in an unblinded follow-up study for 2.7 years [52]:

The lower rates of CHD events in the estrogen–progestin group in years four and five did not persist in the follow-up years.

Over the 6.8 years of HERS-I and HERS-II, continuous estrogen-progestin therapy did not reduce the risk of CHD events in women with established CHD (HR 0.99, 95 percent CI 0.84 to 1.14).

There were no differences in women taking statins or aspirin.

Other data have confirmed the lack of efficacy of estrogen-progestin therapy for secondary prevention of CHD [184,185].

Although transdermal preparations might be expected to be less thrombogenic than oral preparations, and therefore could be cardioprotective, this may not be true. In the Papworth trial, 255 postmenopausal women with ischemic heart disease were randomly assigned to transdermal preparations (estrogen alone or combined with progestin) or placebo. After an average of 31 months of follow-up, there was a nonsignificant increase in coronary disease-related events in the transdermal hormone therapy group when compared to placebo [184].

Based upon the WHI and HERS trials and other studies, and consistent with guidelines as well as updated recommendations issued by the AHA [185,186], the following recommendations, are currently accepted for secondary prevention:

Estrogen-progestin therapy should not be prescribed for secondary prevention of CHD.

Estrogen-progestin therapy should be discontinued if an acute CHD event occurs, and should not be resumed as a secondary prevention strategy.

Unopposed estrogen therapy should not be prescribed for secondary CHD prevention.

Estrogen or estrogen-progestin therapy should be reserved for perimenopausal women with moderate to severe menopausal symptoms. The lowest estrogen dose that relieves symptoms should be used for the shortest duration possible.

Case Report 3. (ZD 58 Years Old)

A 58-year-old female schoolteacher (ZD) with hypertension and spondylosis was admitted to our department because of unusual pains in the left side of the chest and lower sternum not connected with effort, and changes in rest ECG (figure 7).

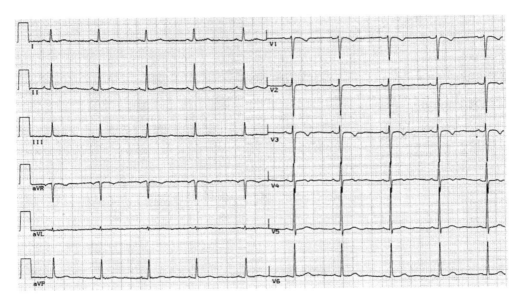

Figure 7. Rest ECG of patient no. 3 (ZD). Sinus bradycardia 58 bpm. Minimal voltage criteria for left ventricular hypertrophy (LVH), may be normal variant. Nonspecific T wave abnormality.

She had had a hysterosalpingo-oophorectomy 7 years earlier. Hipercholesterolemia was found, an exercise stress test proved positive (figure 8) and a rest echocardiogram was normal.

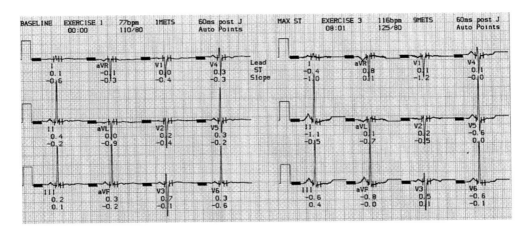

Figure 8. ECG stress test of patient no. 3 (ZD). Rest ECG (BASELINE) – left, and maximal ST changes (MAX ST) – right. The exercise on treadmill was stopped after 8 minutes because of fatigue and pain in the left side of the chest. Effort tolerance was normal (9 METS). On lead II significant ST depression (-1.1 mm), occurred at the same time as chest pain. Test result - positive.

Coronary angiography did not reveal any abnormalities (figures 9A and 9B).

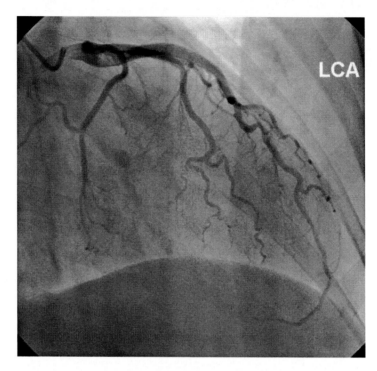

Figure 9A. Normal coronary angiography of patient no. 3 (ZD). Left coronary artery (LCA).

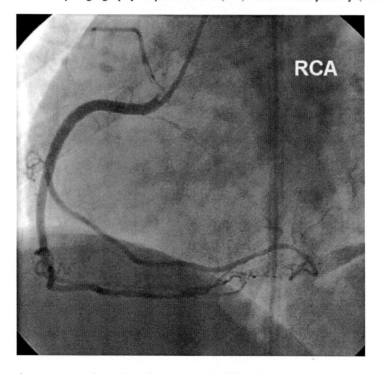

Figure 9B. Normal coronary angiography of patient no. 3 (ZD). Right coronary artery (RCA).

Medical treatment was modified, her blood pressure became normal, and chest pains stopped. The patient has been receiving HRT (transdermal estradiol) since the operation. She has been advised to consult her gynaecologist as to further continuation of HRT. If this treatment is not absolutely essential, estradiol should be gradually withdrawn. She should change her diet and lifestyle, continue medical treatment and also check her blood pressure frequently.

Invasive Procedures

Cardiac catheterization and coronary revascularization in selected patients are fundamental to the management of coronary disease. Some but not all studies have noted decreased utilization of these procedures in women, suggesting possible gender bias [187,188]. However, women often are older and have a greater burden of risk factors than men.

Percutaneous Coronary Intervention

Coronary artery stenting has largely replaced of balloon angioplasty alone or atherectomy as percutaneous treatment for coronary heart disease in both men and women. Women undergoing PCI are older and have a greater burden of risk factors than men [189]. The outcomes in women with PCI have improved over the years. In a study from the NHLBI Registry, the procedural success rate in women was significantly higher in 1997-1998 compared to 1985-1986 (92 versus 79 percent) and the rate of major complications (death, MI, and emergency CABG) was significantly lower (6.0 versus 11.6 percent) [190]. These improvements occurred despite a higher risk profile in the later registry data. The degree to which they were due to increased use of stents (63 percent) and GP IIb/IIIa inhibitors could not be determined.

Data from large national databases suggest that periprocedural mortality after PCI is increased in women compared to men [191,192]. Mortality remained higher after stenting for women with an MI and without an MI. Women also had a higher CABG rate after stenting. Women may have smaller coronary arteries independent of body size, and small coronary artery diameter is associated with worse outcomes after PCI [193].

Stent thrombosis after percutaneous coronary intervention is an uncommon and potentially catastrophic event that might manifest as myocardial infarction and sudden death. Optimization of stent implantation and dual antiplatelet therapy have markedly reduced the occurrence of this complication. Bare-metal stent (BMS) thrombosis occurs in <1% of the cases, usually within the first month after implantation. The advent of drug-eluting stents (DES) has raised concerns regarding later occurrence of stent thrombosis, beyond the traditional 1-month timeframe, especially in complex lesion subsets that were excluded from randomized trials that compared BMS to DES. There is widespread controversy regarding the actual incremental risk associated with DES. Recent studies suggest a 0.5% increased long-term thrombosis risk with DES; however, the clinical significance of these events remains under debate. The degree of protection achieved by dual antiplatelet therapy and optimal duration of treatment are under investigation [194].

The rate of target lesion revascularization at one year after DES implantation was higher in women than men. However, women were older than men and had more comorbidities (diabetes, hypertension, heart failure, renal insufficiency). After adjustment, female gender was not an independent predictor of target lesion revascularization.

The 2005 statement from the AHA on PCI in women concluded that, although mortality rates after PCI with stenting are similar or higher in women compared to men in a broad range of patient and lesion subsets, any differences are due to confounding risk factors, not female sex [195].

Case Report 4. (DG 76 Years Old)

A 76-year-old female (DG), a retired bank employee living alone, with a history of two pharmacologically treated acute coronary syndromes which had occurred two weeks and three months earlier, was transferred from the local hospital to our department due to effort angina. Her typical chest pains were caused by walking about 80 paces along the hospital corridor. She also complained of chest pain in periods of emotional stress, but had no rest angina or nocturnal angina. She was overweight with hypercholesterolemia and hypertension and had been a heavy smoker in the past. Rest ECG showed nonspecific intraventricular conduction disturbances and ST abnormality in infero-lateral leads. Subsequent ECGs did not differ greatly from the first (fig. 10).

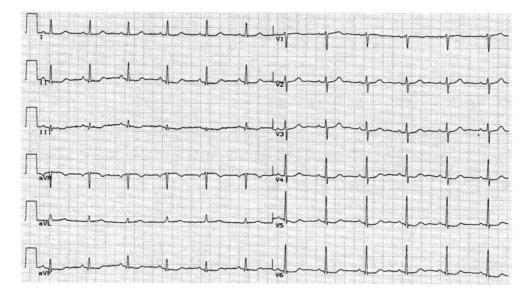

Figure 10. Rest ECG of patient no. 4 (DG). Normal sinus rhythm 70 bpm. Nonspecific intraventricular conduction disturbances and ST abnormality in infero-lateral leads.

An ECG stress test on treadmill revealed significant ST depression in one lead (V6) after the first minute of walking on the treadmill (Bruce protocol). Exercise was stopped after three minutes because of fatigue without typical angina. The test proved positive with severe limitation of effort tolerance (figure 11).

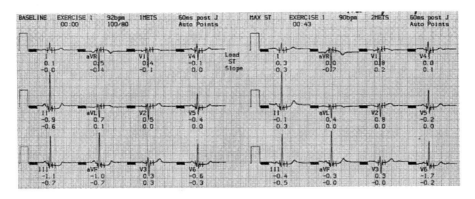

Figure 11. ECG stress test of patient no. 4 (DG). Rest ECG (BASELINE) – left, and maximal ST changes (MAX ST) – right. The exercise on treadmill was stopped after 3 minutes 8 seconds (Bruce protocol) because of fatigue without typical angina. Effort tolerance was significantly limited (4 METS). On lead V6 significant ST depression -1.7 mm (baseline -0.6 mm), occurred at 43 seconds of exercise. Test result – positive with severe limitation of effort tolerance.

Coronary angiography showed one-vessel CHD with changes in the right coronary artery (figure 12).

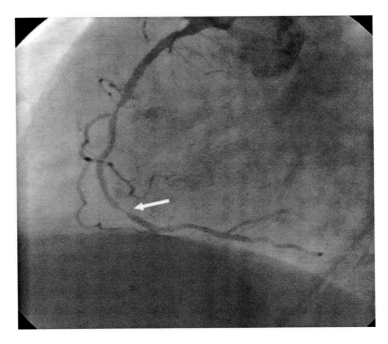

Figure 12. Coronary angiography (right coronary artery) of patient no. 4 (DG): Nonsignificant (50%) stenosis in segment no. 2 & significant (95%) stenosis in segment 2/3 (arrow).

The patient was referred for PTCA in 1-2 months. On discharge from the hospital she was advised to change her diet, continue medical treatment and to reduce effort considerably until PTCA had been carried out.

Bypass Surgery

Bypass surgery — A similarly high burden of comorbidities exists in women undergoing coronary artery bypass grafting (CABG). Although there has been a significant and similar reduction in in-hospital mortality in women and men, women still have a greater likelihood of procedural complications (new neurologic event, heart failure, perioperative infarction, and hemorrhage) and death at 30 days [196].

In an analysis from the Society of Thoracic Surgery national database of 416,347 patients undergoing CABG in 1996 and 1997, women had a higher 30 day mortality than men (5.7 versus 3.5 percent) [197]. The increase in mortality compared to men may be most pronounced in patients under age 50.

The overall increase in short-term mortality in women has been attributed primarily to patient-related factors, including age and coronary risk factors [197]. As noted above with regard to PCI, another factor that may account for increased in-hospital mortality after CABG is smaller body size with consequently smaller coronary artery size [196]. During CABG, smaller vessel size may impose more technical difficulties and may be associated with a higher risk of graft failure.

In contrast to the short-term findings, long-term survival after CABG in women is comparable to, or better than, that for men [198].

Case Report 5. (ZG 81 Years Old)

An 81-year-old female (ZG), a retired office worker with hypertension and typical chest pain occurring after minimal effort (30-40 paces in the corridor), without rest angina or nocturnal angina, was transferred from the local hospital to our department a few days after a stress test which proved positive. Rest ECG did not reveal any significant abnormalities (figure 13).

Echocardiography showed normal dimensions of cardiac cavities with small LVH and moderate mitral insufficiency. Coronary angiography revealed several stenoses in the branches of the left coronary artery, with no significant changes in the right coronary artery (figure 14).

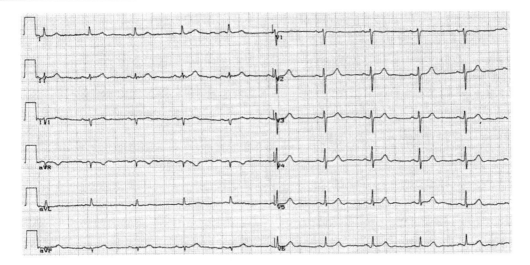

Figure 13. Rest ECG of patient no. 5 (ZG). Normal sinus rhythm 60 bpm. Nonspecific intraventricular conduction disturbances.

The patient was referred for an operation (CABG) and transferred to the Cardiosurgical Department of our institute. The next day she was operated on. The operation OPCAB (Off Pump Coronary Artery Bypass): left internal mammary artery (LIMA) to the left anterior descending artery (LAD) & saphenous vein graft (SVG) to the marginal branch of the left circumflex artery (LCx) was successful with no severe complications. After a few days the patient started walking.

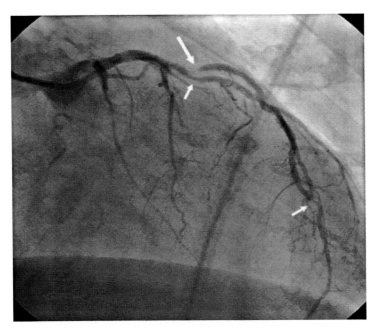

Figure 14. Coronary angiography (left coronary artery) of patient no. 5 (ZG): Left anterior descending artery (LAD): nonsignificant stenosis in segment no. 6 & 2 significant stenoses (2 small arrows): 80% segment no. 7 & 85% segment no. 8. 1st diagonal branch in proximal part severe stenosis 99% (big arrow). Left circumflex (LCx) recessive: 95% stenosis in proximal part.

Pregnancy and CHD

There is limited evidence correlating the number of pregnancies with the risk of CHD. In an analysis of data from the Framingham Heart Study and the NHEFS study, the rates of CHD were higher for multigravid women than for women who had never been pregnant, although this finding was statistically significant only for women with six or more pregnancies (20 versus 32 percent) [199]. Most, although perhaps not all, of this effect may be accounted for by lifestyle risk factors found to be associated with child-rearing, including smoking, physical inactivity, and obesity [200].

In primigravid women, development of early-onset preeclampsia may predict remote cardiovascular events (eg, hypertension, ischemic heart disease, stroke). In contrast, preeclampsia/eclampsia occurring late in gestation in primigravid women does not appear to be associated with remote cardiovascular risk. Review of all of a woman's pregnancies is necessary to define her long-term risk accurately. Those with early onset severe preeclampsia, recurrent preeclampsia, gestational hypertension, or preeclampsia with onset as a multipara appear to be at increased risk of cardiovascular disease later in life.

Since women are delaying childbearing until older age, and the prevalence of CHD in female patients is increasing due to changing lifestyle patterns (eg, cigarette smoking, diabetes and stress) - acute coronary syndrome will more frequently occur during pregnancy. Although rare, acute coronary syndrome during pregnancy often has devastating consequences. It is associated with increased maternal and neonatal mortality and morbidity compared with the nonpregnant situation. Furthermore, it constitutes an important problem for the patient and the treating physician, because the selection of diagnostic and therapeutic approaches is greatly influenced not only by maternal, but also by fetal safety [201].

Conclusion

CHD is one of the most common cardiovascular diseases, leading to death in women and is responsible for more deaths each year than all other diseases together. There are numerous differences in the epidemiology and primary manifestation of CHD in women and men. Stable angina pectoris is most frequent initial manifestation of CHD in women, but MI or sudden death the most frequent initial manifestation in men. The incidence of MI in women increases dramatically after the menopause. This increase is at least partly due to aging and the role of menopause itself is not very clear. The evaluation of chest pain in women is less straightforward than in men at multiple levels, because of gender differences in presentation and disease manifestation and also the preponderance of male-specific data in the published literature. In addition, the clinical usefulness of some non-invasive tests is lower in women than in men. A number of studies have shown gender-based differences in frequency rates of coronary angiography and revascularization, even among those with acute MI. However, it should be stressed that the correlation between symptoms and significant luminal obstruction at coronary angiography is weaker in women than in men. On the other hand, the risk of complications after coronary angiography is higher in women. This may explain why physicians fail to refer women for subsequent invasive tests. Several case reports included in this paper show the difficulties in diagnosis and treatment of women with CHD.

In conclusion, it could be said that difficulties in diagnosis and limited female-specific literature regarding the treatment of angina pectoris, have led to a situation in which women with CHD often remain under-investigated and under-treated.

References

[1]   Second World Assembly on Aging Madrid 02. Report of the Second World Assembly on Ageing Madrid, 8-12 April 2002. New York: United Nations; 2002.

[2]   Eaker, E.D., Chesebro, J.H., Sacks, F.M., Wenger, N.K., Whisnant, J.P. & M Winston, M. (1993). Cardiovascular disease in women. *Circulation, 88,*1999- 2009.

[3]   Higgins, M. & Thom, T. Cardiovascular disease in women as a public health problem. In: Wenger NK, Speroff L & Packard B editors. *Cardiovascular health and disease in women.* Greenwich CT: Le Jacq Communications; 1993; 15-19.

[4]   Mosca, L., Manson, J.E., Sutherland, S.E., Langer R.D., Manolio T. & Barrett-Connor E. (1997). Cardiovascular disease in women: a statement for healthcare professionals from the American Heart Association. *Circulation, 96,* 2468-2482.

[5]   Lerner, D.J. & Kannel, W.B. (1986). Patterns of coronary heart disease morbidity and mortality in the sexes: a 26-year follow-up of the Framingham population. *Am Heart J, 111,* 383-390.

[6]   Roger, V.L., Jacobsen, S.J., Pellikka, P.A., Miller T.D., Bailey K.R. & Gersh B.J. (1998). Gender differences in use of stress testing and coronary heart disease mortality: a population-based study in Olmsted Country, Minnesota. *J Am Coll Cardiol, 32,* 345-352.

[7]   Wang, X.L., Tam, C., McCredie, R.M. & Wilcken, D.E. (1994). Determinants of severity of coronary artery disease in Australian men and women. *Circulation, 89,* 1974-1981.

[8]   Hu, F.B., Stampfer, M.J., Manson, J.E., Grodstein, F., Colditz, G.A., M.D., Speizer, F.E., & Willett, W.C. (2000). Trends in the incidence of coronary heart disease and changes in diet and lifestyle in women. *N Engl J Med., 343,* 530-537.

[9]   Deedwania, P.C. & Carbajal, E.V. (1991). Silent myocardial ischemia: a clinical perspective. *Arch Intern Med., 151,* 2373-2382.

[10]   Kannel, W.B. (1989). Detection and management of patients with silent myocardial ischemia. *Am Heart J, 117,* 221-226.

[11]   American Heart Association. Heart and Stroke Facts: 1995 Statistical Supplement. American Heart Association 1994. Dallas TX 75231. Heart Disease and Stroke Statistics – 2005 update. Dallas TX: American Heart Association; 2005.

[12]   Roger, V.L., Weston, S.A., Killian, J.M., Pfeifer E.A., Belau P.G., Kottke T.E., Frye R.L., Bailey K.R. & Jacobsen S.J. (2001). Time trends in the prevalence of atherosclerosis: a population-based autopsy study. *Am J Med., 110,* 267-273.

[13]   Cupples, L.A., Gagnon, D.R., Wong, N.D., Ostfeld A.M. & Kannel W.B. (1993). Preexisting cardiovascular conditions and long-term prognosis after initial myocardial infarction: the Framingham Study. *Am Heart J, 125*, 863-872.

[14]   Choudhri, A.H., Cleland, J.G., Rowlands, P.L., Tran T.L., McCarthy M. & Al-Kutoubi M.A. (1990). Unsuspected renal artery stenosis in peripheral vascular disease. *BMJ, 301*, 1197-1198.

[15]   Bucher, H.C., Griffith, L.E. & Guyatt, G.H. (1998). Effect of HMGCoA reductase inhibitors on stroke: a meta-analysis of randomized controlled trials. *Ann Intern Med, 128*, 89-95.

[16]   Crouse, J.R., Byington, R.P., Hoen, H.M. & Furberg C.D. (1997). Reductase inhibitor monotherapy and stroke prevention. *Arch Intern Med., 157*, 1305-1310.

[17]   Gordon, T., Kannel, W.B., Hjortland, M.C. & McNamara, P.M. (1978). Menopause and coronary heart disease: the Framingham Study. *Ann Intern Med., 89*, 157-161.

[18]   Kannel, W.B. (1987). Prevalence and clinical aspects of unrecognized myocardial infarction and sudden unexpected death. *Circulation, 75*, II4-115.

[19]   Go, A.S., Iribarren, C., Chandra, M., Lathon P.V., Fortmann S.P., Quertermous T. & Hlatky M.A., for the Atherosclerotic Disease, Vascular Function and Genetic Epidemiology (ADVANCE) Study. (2006). Statin and beta-blocker therapy and the initial presentation of coronary heart disease. *Ann Intern Med., 144*, 229-238.

[20]   Ergin, A., Muntner, P., Sherwin, R. & He, J. (2004). Secular trends in cardiovascular disease mortality, incidence, and case fatality rates in adults in the United States. *Am J Med., 117*, 219-227.

[21]   Arciero, T.J., Jacobsen, S.J, Reeder, G.S., Frye R.L., Weston S.A., Killian J.M., & Roger V.L. (2004). Temporal trends in the incidence of coronary disease. *Am J Med., 117*, 228-233.

[22]   Phibbs, B. (1983). "Transmural" versus "subendocardial" myocardial infarction: an electrocardiographic myth. *J Am Coll Cardiol, 1*, 561-564.

[23]   Liebson, P.R. & Klein, L.W. (1997). The non-Q wave myocardial infarction revisited: 10 years later. *Prog Cardiovasc Dis, 39*, 399-444.

[24]   The TIMI IIIA Investigators. (1993). Early effects of tissue-type plasminogen activator added to conventional therapy on the culprit coronary lesion in patients presenting with ischemic cardiac pain at rest: results of the Thrombolysis in Myocardial Ischemia (TIMI IIIA) Trial. *Circulation, 87*, 38-52.

[25]   Kerensky, R.A., Wade, M., Deedwania, P., Boden W.E. & Pepine C.J. (2002). Revisiting the culprit lesion in non-Q-wave myocardial infarction: results from the VANQWISH trial angiographic core laboratory. *J Am Coll Cardiol, 39*, 1456-1463.

[26]   Wong, G.C., Morrow, D.A., Murphy, S., Kraimer, N., Pai R., James, D., Robertson, D.H., Demopoulos, L.A., DiBattiste, P., Cannon, C.P. & Gibson, M., for the TACTICS-TIMI 18 Study Group. (2002). Elevations in troponin T and I are associated with abnormal tissue level perfusion: a TACTICS-TIMI 18 substudy: treat angina with aggrastat and determine cost of therapy with an invasive or conservative strategy-thrombolysis in myocardial infarction. *Circulation, 106*, 202-207.

[27]   Furman, M.I., Dauerman, H.L., Goldberg, R.J., Yarzebski J., Lessard D. & Gore J.M. (2001). Twenty-two year (1975 to 1997) trends in the incidence, in-hospital and long-

term case fatality rates from initial Q-wave and non-Q-wave myocardial infarction: a multi-hospital, community-wide perspective. *J Am Coll Cardiol, 37*, 1571-1580.

[28]   Rogers, W.J., Canto, J.G., Lambrew, C.T., Tiefenbrunn, A.J., Kinkaid, B., Shoultz, D.A., Frederick, P.D. & Every, N. (2000). Temporal trends in the treatment of over 1.5 million patients with myocardial infarction in the US from 1990 through 1999: the National Registry of Myocardial Infarction 1, 2 and 3. *J Am Coll Cardiol, 36*, 2056-2063.

[29]   Thom, T.J., Kannel, W.B., Silbershatz, S. & D'Agostino, R.B. Incidence, Prevalence, and Mortality of Cardiovascular Diseases in the United States. In: Alexander RW, Schlant RC, Fuster V & Roberts R editors. *Hurst's the Heart, 9th ed.* New York: McGraw Hill; 1998; 3-17.

[30]   Kuulasmaa, K., Tunstall-Pedoe, H., Dobson, A., Fortmann, S., Sans, S., Tolonen, H., Evans, A., Ferrario, M. & Tuomilehto, J. (2000). Estimation of contribution of changes in classic risk factors to trends in coronary-event rates across the WHO MONICA Project populations. *Lancet, 355*, 675-687.

[31]   McGovern, P.G., Pankow, J.S., Shahar, E., Doliszny, K.M., Folsom, A.R., Blackburn, H. & Luepker, R.V. (1996). Recent trends in acute coronary heart disease - mortality, morbidity, medical care, and risk factors: the Minnesota Heart Survey Investigators. *N Engl J Med., 334*, 884-890.

[32]   Capewell, S., Morrison, C.E. & McMurray, J.J. (1999). Contribution of modern cardiovascular treatment and risk factor changes to the decline in coronary heart disease mortality in Scotland between 1975 and 1994. *Heart, 81*, 380-386.

[33]   Capewell, S., Beaglehole, R., Seddon, M. & McMurray, J. (2000). Explanation for the decline in coronary heart disease mortality rates in Auckland, New Zealand, between 1982 and 1993. *Circulation, 102*, 1511-1516.

[34]   Cooper, R., Cutler, J., Desvigne-Nickens, P., Fortmann, S.P., Friedman, L., Havlik, R., Hogelin, G., Marler, J., McGovern, P., Morosco, G., Mosca, L., Pearson, T., Stamler, J., Stryer, D. & Thom, T. (2000). Trends and disparities in coronary heart disease, stroke, and other cardiovascular diseases in the United States: findings of the national conference on cardiovascular disease prevention. *Circulation, 102*, 3137-3147.

[35]   McGovern, P.G., Jacobs, D.R. Jr, Shahar, E., Arnett, D.K., Folsom, A.R., Blackburn, H. & Luepker, R.V. (2001). Trends in acute coronary heart disease mortality, morbidity, and medical care from 1985 through 1997: the Minnesota Heart Survey. *Circulation, 104*, 19-24.

[36]   Rosamond, W.D., Chambless, L.E., Folsom, A.R., Cooper, L.S., Conwill, D.E., Clegg, L., Wang, C.H. & Heiss G. (1998). Trends in the incidence of myocardial infarction and in mortality due to coronary heart disease, 1987 to 1994. *N Engl J Med, 339*, 861-867.

[37]   Fox, C.S., Evans, J.C., Larson, M.G. Kannel, W.B. & Levy, D. (2004). Temporal trends in coronary heart disease mortality and sudden cardiac death from 1950 to 1999: the Framingham Heart Study. *Circulation, 110*, 522-527.

[38] Levi, F., Lucchini, F., Negri, E. & La Vecchia, C. (2002). Trends in mortality from cardiovascular and cerebrovascular diseases in Europe and other areas of the world. *Heart, 88*, 119-124.

[39] Reddy, K.S. (2004). Cardiovascular disease in non-Western countries. N Engl J Med, 350, 2438-2440.

[40] Okrainec, K., Banerjee, D.K. & Eisenberg, M.J. (2004). Coronary artery disease in the developing world. *Am Heart J, 148*, 7-15.

[41] Critchley, J., Liu, J., Zhao, D., Wei, W. & Capewell, S. (2004). Explaining the increase in coronary heart disease mortality in Beijing between 1984 and 1999. *Circulation, 110*, 1236-1244.

[42] Grundy, S.M. (1994). Guidelines for cholesterol management: recommendations of the National Cholesterol Education Program's Adult Treatment Panel II. *Heart Dis Stroke, 3*, 123-127.

[43] Shearman, A.M., Cupples, L.A., Demissie, S., Peter, I. Schmid, C.H., Karas, R.H., Mendelsohn, M.E., Housman, D.E. & Levy, D. (2003). Association between estrogen receptor alpha gene variation and cardiovascular disease. *JAMA, 290*, 2263-2270.

[44] Hu, F.B., Grodstein, F., Hennekens, C.H., Colditz, G.A., Johnson, M., Manson, J.E., Rosner, B. & Stampfer, M.J. (1999). Age at natural menopause and risk of cardiovascular disease. *Arch Intern Med, 159*, 1061-1066.

[45] Mondul, A.M., Rodriguez, C., Jacobs, E.J. & Calle, E.E. (2005). Age at natural menopause and cause-specific mortality. *Am J Epidemiol, 162*, 1089-1097.

[46] Colditz, G.A., Willett, W.C., Stampfer, M.J., Rosner, B., Speizer, F.E. & Hennekens, C.H. (1987). Menopause and the risk of coronary heart disease in women. *N Engl J Med, 316*, 1105-1110.

[47] Mack, W.J., Slater, C.C., Xiang, M., Shoupe, D., Lobo, R. & Hodis, H. (2004). Elevated subclinical atherosclerosis associated with oophorectomy is related to time since menopause rather than type of menopause. *Fertil Steril, 82*, 391-397.

[48] Howard, B.V., Kuller, L., Langer, R., Manson, J.E., Allen, C., Assaf, A., Cochrane, B.B., Larson, J.C., Lasser, N., Rainford, M., Van Horn, L., Stefanick, M.L. & Trevisan, M. (2005). Risk of cardiovascular disease by hysterectomy status, with and without oophorectomy: the Women's Health Initiative Observational Study. *Circulation, 111*, 1462-1470.

[49] Rexrode, K.M., Manson, J.E., Lee, I.M., Ridker, P.M., Sluss, P.M., Cook, N.R. & Buring J.E. (2003). Sex hormone levels and risk of cardiovascular events in postmenopausal women. *Circulation, 108*, 1688-1693.

[50] Rossouw, J.E., Anderson, G.L., Prentice, R.L., LaCroix, A.Z., Kooperberg, C., Stefanick, M.L., Jackson, R.D., Beresford, S.A., Howard, B.V., Johnson, K.C., Kotchen, J.M. & Ockene, J. (2002). Risks and benefits of estrogen plus progestin in healthy postmenopausal women: principal results From the Women's Health Initiative randomized controlled trial. *JAMA, 288*, 321-333.

[51] Hulley, S., Grady, D., Bush, T., Furberg, C., Herrington, D., Riggs, B. & Vittinghoff, E., for the Heart and Estrogen/progestin Replacement Study (HERS) Research Group. (1998). Randomized trial of estrogen plus progestin for secondary prevention of coronary heart disease in postmenopausal women. *JAMA, 280*, 605-613.

[52]   Grady, D., Herrington, D., Bittner, V., Blumenthal, R., Davidson, M., Hlatky, M., Hsia, J., Hulley, S., Herd, A., Khan, S., Newby, L.K., Waters, D., Vittinghoff, E. & Wenger, N., HERS Research Group. (2002). Cardiovascular disease outcomes during 6.8 years of hormone therapy: Heart and Estrogen/progestin Replacement Study follow-up (HERS II). *JAMA, 288*, 49-57.

[53]   Third report of the National Cholesterol Education Program (NCEP) Expert Panel on detection, evaluation, and treatment of high blood cholesterol in adults (Adult Treatment Panel III). (2002). *Circulation, 106*, 3143-3421.

[54]   Mosca, L., Grundy, S.M., Judelson, D., King, K., Limacher, M., Oparil, S., Pasternak, R., Pearson, T.A., Redberg, R.F., Smith, S.C. Jr, Winston, M. & Zinberg, S. (1999). Guide to preventive cardiology for women: AHA/ACC Scientific Statement Consensus Panel statement. *Circulation,* 99, 2480–2484. - Mosca, L., Banka, C.L., Benjamin, E.J., Berra, K., Bushnell, C., Dolor, R.J., Ganiats, T.G., Gomes, A.S., Gornik, H.L., Gracia, C., Gulati, M., Haan, C.K., MD; Judelson, D.R., Keenan, N., Kelepouris, E., Michos, E.D., Newby, K., Oparil, S., Ouyang, P., Oz, M.C., Petitti, D., Pinn, V.W., Redberg, R.F., Scott, R., Sherif, K., Smith, S.C. Jr, Sopko, G., Steinhorn, R.H., Stone, N.J., Taubert, K.A., Todd, B.A., Urbina, E. & Wenger, N.K., for the Expert Panel/Writing Group (2007). Evidence-Based Guidelines for Cardiovascular Disease Prevention in Women: 2007 Update: AHA Guideline. Circulation, *115*, 1481-1501.

[55]   Winkleby, M.A., Kraemer, H.C., Ahn, D.K., Varady, A.N. (1998). Ethnic and socioeconomic differences in cardiovascular risk factors: findings for women from the Third National Health and Nutritional Examination Survey, 1988-1994. *JAMA, 280*, 356-362.

[56]   Vittinghoff, E., Shlipak, M.G., Varosy, P.D., Furberg, C.D., Ireland, C.C., Khan, S.S., Blumenthal, R., Barrett-Connor, E., Hulley, S. & for the Heart and Estrogen/progestin Replacement Study. (2003). Risk factors and secondary prevention in women with heart disease: the Heart and Estrogen/progestin Replacement Study. *Ann Intern Med, 138*, 81-89.

[57]   Sullivan, A.K., Holdright, D.R., Wright, C.A., Sparrow, J.L., Cunningham, D. & Fox, K.M. (1994). Chest pain in women: clinical, investigative, and prognostic features. *BMJ, 308*, 883-886.

[58]   Rich-Edwards, J.W., Manson, J.E., Hennekens, C.H. & Buring, JE. (1995). The primary prevention of coronary heart disease in women [see comments]. *N Engl J Med, 332*, 1758-1766.

[59]   Miller, V.T. (1994). Lipids, lipoproteins, women and cardiovascular disease. *Atherosclerosis, 108*, S73-S82.

[60]   Orth-Gomer, K., Mittleman, M.A., Schenck-Gustafsson, K., Wamala, S.P., Eriksson, M., Belkic, K., Kirkeeide, R., Svane, B., Ryden, L. (1997). Lipoprotein(a) as a determinant of coronary heart disease in young women. *Circulation, 95*, 329-334.

[61]   Criqui, M.H., Heiss, G., Cohn, R., Cowan, L.D., Suchindran, C.M., Bangdiwala, S., Kritchevsky, S., Jacobs, D.R. Jr, O'Grady, H.K. & Davis, C.E. (1993). Plasma triglyceride level and mortality from coronary heart disease. *N Engl J Med, 328*, 1220-1225.

[62]   Ridker, P.M., Rifai, N., Cook, N.R., Bradwin G. & Buring J.E. (2005). Non-HDL
        cholesterol, apolipoproteins A-I and B100, standard lipid measures, lipid ratios, and
        CRP as risk factors for cardiovascular disease in women. *JAMA, 294*, 326-333.

[63]   Bengtsson, C., Bjorkelund, C., Lapidus, L., Lissner, L. (1993). Associations of serum
        lipid concentrations and obesity with mortality in women: 20 year follow up of
        participants in prospective population study in Gothenburg, Sweden. *BMJ, 307*, 1385-
        1388.

[64]   Kane, J.P., Malloy, M.J., Ports, T.A., Phillips, N.R., Diehl, J.C. & Havel, R.J. (1990).
        Regression of coronary atherosclerosis during treatment of familial
        hypercholesterolemia with combined drug regimens. *JAMA, 264*, 3007-3012.

[65]   Scandinavian Simvastatin Survival Study Group. (1994). Randomised trial of
        cholesterol lowering in 4444 patients with coronary heart disease: the Scandinavian
        Simvastatin Survival Study (4S). *Lancet, 344*, 1383-1389.

[66]   Miettinen, T.A., Pyorala, K., Olsson, A.G., Musliner, T.A., Cook, T.J., Faergeman,
        O., Berg, K., Pedersen, T. & Kjekshus, J., for the Scandinavian Simvastatin Study
        Group. (1997). Cholesterol-lowering therapy in women and elderly patients with
        myocardial infarction or angina pectoris: findings from the Scandinavian Simvastatin
        Survival Study (4S). *Circulation, 96*, 4211-4218.

[67]   Lewis, S.J., Sacks, F.M., Mitchell, J.S., East, C., Glasser, S., Kell, S., Letterer, R.,
        Limacher, M., Moye, L.A., Rouleau, J.L., Pfeffer, M.A. & Braunwald, E., for the
        CARE Investigators. (1998). Effect of pravastatin on cardiovascular events in women
        after myocardial infarction: the Cholesterol and Recurrent Events (CARE) trial. *J Am
        Coll Cardiol, 32*, 140-146.

[68]   Nissen, S.E., Tuzcu, E.M., Schoenhagen, P., Brown BG, Ganz P, Vogel RA, Crowe,
        T., Howard, G., Cooper, C.J., Brodie, B., Grines, C.L., DeMaria, A.N. &
        REVERSAL Investigators. (2004). Effect of intensive compared with moderate lipid-
        lowering therapy on progression of coronary atherosclerosis: a randomized controlled
        trial. Reversal of Atherosclerosis with Aggressive Lipid Lowering (REVERSAL).
        JAMA, 291, 1071-1080.

[69]   Zuanetti, G., Latini, R., Maggioni, A.P., Santoro, L. & Francosi, M.G., for the GISSI-
        2 Investigators. (1993). Influence of diabetes on mortality in acute myocardial
        infarction: data from the GISSI-2 study. *J Am Coll Cardiol, 22*, 1788-1794.

[70]   Kanaya, A.M., Herrington, D., Vittinghoff, E., Lin, F., Bittner, V., Cauley, J.A. &
        Hulley, S. (2005). Impaired fasting glucose and cardiovascular outcomes in
        postmenopausal women with coronary artery disease. *Ann Intern Med, 142*, 813-820.

[71]   Huxley, R., Barzi, F. & Woodward, M. (2006). Excess risk of fatal coronary heart
        disease associated with diabetes in men and women: meta-analysis of 37 prospective
        cohort studies. *BMJ, 332*, 73-78.

[72]   Hu, G., Jousilahti, P., Qiao, Q., Peltonen, M., Katoh, S. & Tuomilehto, J. (2005). The
        gender-specific impact of diabetes and myocardial infarction at baseline and during
        follow-up on mortality from all causes and coronary heart disease. *J Am Coll Cardiol,
        45*, 1413-1418.

[73] Haffner, S.M., Lehto, S., Ronnemaa, T., Pyorala K., Laakso M. (1998). Mortality from coronary heart disease in subjects with type 2 diabetes and in nondiabetic subjects with and without prior myocardial infarction. *N Engl J Med, 339*, 229-234.

[74] DeSanctis, R.W. Clinical manifestations of coronary artery disease: chest pain in women. In: Wenger, N.K, Speroff, L. & Packard, B., editors. *Cardiovascular health and disease in women.* Greenwich CT: Le Jacq Communications; 1993; 67-72

[75] Singer, D.E., Nathan, D.M., Anderson, K.M., Wilson, P.W.F. & Evans, J.C. (1992). Association of HbA1c with prevalent cardiovascular disease in the original cohort of the Framingham Heart Study. *Diabetes, 41*, 202-208.

[76] Blake, G.J., Pradhan, A.D., Manson, J.E., Williams, G.R., Buring, J.E., Ridker, P.M., Glynn, R.J. (2004). Hemoglobin A1c level and future cardiovascular events among women. *Arch Intern Med, 164*, 757-761.

[77] Fried, LP; Becker, DM. Smoking and cardiovascular disease. In: Douglas PS, editor. *Cardiovascular Health and Disease in Women.* Philadelphia: Saunders: 1993; 217-230.

[78] Willett, W.C., Green, A., Stampfer, M.J., Speizer, F.E., Colditz, G.A., Rosner, B., Monson, R.R., Stason, W. & Hennekens, C.H. (1987). Relative and absolute excess risks of coronary heart disease among women who smoke cigarettes. *N Engl J Med, 317*, 1303-1309.

[79] Burt, V.L., Whelton, P., Roccella, E.J., Brown, C., Cutler, J.A., Higgins, M., Horan, M.J. & Labarthe, D. (1995). Prevalence of hypertension in the US adult population. Results from the Third National Health and Nutrition Examination Survey, 1988-1991. *Hypertension, 25*, 305-313.

[80] Cornoni-Huntley, J., LaCroix, A.Z. & Havlik, R.J. (1989). Race and sex differentials in the impact of hypertension in the United States. The national health and nutrition examination survey I epidemiologic follow-up study. *Arch Intern Med, 149*, 780-788.

[81] Collins, L., Douglas, PS. Acute myocardial infarction in women. In: Gersh B, Rahimtoola S editors. *Acute Myocardial Infarction.* New York: Chapman and Hall; 1996.

[82] Mason, P.J., Manson, J.E., Sesso, H.D., Albert, C.M., Chown, M.J., Cook, N.R., Greenland, P., Ridker, P.M. & Glynn, R.J. (2004). Blood pressure and risk of secondary cardiovascular events in women: the Women's Antioxidant Cardiovascular Study (WACS). *Circulation, 109*, 1623-1629.

[83] ALLHAT Officers and Coordinators for the ALLHAT Collaborative Research Group. The Antihypertensive and Lipid-Lowering Treatment to Prevent Heart Attack Trial. (2002). Major outcomes in high-risk hypertensive patients randomized to angiotensin-converting enzyme inhibitor or calcium channel blocker vs diuretic: the Antihypertensive and Lipid-Lowering Treatment to Prevent Heart Attack Trial (ALLHAT). *JAMA, 288*, 2981-2997.

[84] Willett, W.C., Manson, J.E., Stampfer, M.J., Colditz, G.A., Rosner, B., Speizer, F.E. & Hennekens, C.H. (1995). Weight, weight change, and coronary heart disease in women. Risk within the 'normal' weight range. *JAMA, 273*, 461-465.

[85] Manson, J.E., Willet, W.C., Stampfer, M.J., Colditz, G.A., Hunter, D.J., Hankinson, S.E., Hennekens, C.H. & Speizer, F.E. (1995). Body weight and mortality among women. *N Engl J Med, 333*, 677-685.

[86] Lobo, R.A. Hormones, hormone replacement therapy, and heart disease. In: Douglas PS, editor. *Cardiovascular Health and Disease in Women*. Philadelphia: Saunders; 1993; 153-173.

[87] Li, T.Y., Rana, J.S, Manson, J.E., Willett, W.C., Stampfer, M.J., Colditz, G.A., Rexrode, K.M. & Hu, F.B. (2006). Obesity as compared with physical activity in predicting risk of coronary heart disease in women. *Circulation, 113*, 499-506.

[88] Jousilahti, P., Tuomilehto, J., Vartiainen, E., Pekkanen, J. & Puska, P. (1996). Body weight, cardiovascular risk factors, and coronary mortality: 15 year follow-up of middle-aged men and women in eastern Finland. *Circulation, 93*, 1372-1379.

[89] Yanovski, S.Z., Bain, R.P. & Williamson, D.F. (1999). Report of a National Institutes of Health-Centers for Disease Control and Prevention workshop on the feasibility of conducting a randomized clinical trial to estimate the long-term health effects of intentional weight loss in obese persons [see comments]. *Am J Clin Nutr, 69*, 366-372.

[90] Lissner, L., Odell, P.M., D'Agostino, R.B., Stokes, J., Kreger, B.E. & Belanger, A.J., (1991). Variability of body weight and health outcomes in the Framingham population. *N Engl J Med, 324*, 1839-1844.

[91] Folsom, A.R., French, S.A., Zheng, W., Baxter, J.E. & Jeffery, R.W. (1996). Weight variability and mortality: the Iowa Women's Health Study. *Int J Obes Relat Metab Disord, 20*, 704-709.

[92] Olson, M.B., Kelsey, S.F., Bittner, V., Reis, S.E., Reichek, N., Handberg, E.M. & Merz, C.N. (2000). Weight cycling and high-density lipoprotein cholesterol in women: evidence of an adverse effect: a report from the NHLBI-sponsored WISE study: Women's Ischemia Syndrome Evaluation Study Group. *J Am Coll Cardiol, 36*, 1565-1571.

[93] Barnard, N.D., Scialli, A.R., Bertron, P., Hurlock, D., Edmonds, K. & Talev, L. (2000). Effectiveness of a low-fat vegetarian diet in altering serum lipids in healthy premenopausal women. *Am J Cardiol, 85*, 969-972.

[94] Hu, F.B., Stampfer, M.J., Manson, J.E., Rimm, E., Colditz, G.A., Rosner, B.A., Hennekens, C.H. & Willett, W.C. (1997). Dietary fat intake and the risk of coronary heart disease in women. *N Engl J Med, 337*, 1491-1499.

[95] Fung, T.T., Willett, W.C., Stampfer, M.J., Manson, J.E., Hu, F.B. (2001). Dietary patterns and the risk of coronary heart disease in women. *Arch Intern Med, 161*, 1857-1862.

[96] Liu, S., Buring, J.E., Sesso, H.D., Rimm, E.B., Willet, W.C. & Manson, J.E. (2002). A prospective study of dietary fiber intake and risk of cardiovascular disease among women. J Am Coll Cardiol, 39, 49-56.

[97] Iso, H., Stampfer, M.J., Manson, J.E., Rexrode, K., Hu, F., Hennekens, C.H., Colditz, G.A., Speizer, F.E. & Willett, W.C. (2001). Prospective study of fat and protein intake and risk of intraparenchymal hemorrhage in women. *Circulation, 103*, 856-863.

[98]   Fuchs, C.S., Stampfer, M.J., Colditz, G.A., Giovannucci, E.L., Manson, J.E. &
       Kawachi, I. (1995). Alcohol consumption and mortality among women. *N Engl J
       Med, 332*, 1245-1250.

[99]   Rimm, E.B., Willett, W.C., Hu, F.B., Sampson, L., Colditz, G.A. & Manson J.E.
       (1998). Folate and vitamin B6 from diet and supplements in relation to risk of
       coronary heart disease among women. *JAMA, 279*, 359-364.

[100] Executive Summary of The Third Report of The National Cholesterol Education
       Program (NCEP) Expert Panel on Detection, Evaluation, And Treatment of High
       Blood Cholesterol In Adults (Adult Treatment Panel III). (2001). *JAMA, 285*, 2486-
       2497.

[101] Ninomiya, J.K., L'Italien, G., Criqui, M.H., Whyte, J.L., Gamst, A. & Chen, R.S.
       (2004). Association of the metabolic syndrome with history of myocardial infarction
       and stroke in the third national health and nutrition examination survey. *Circulation,
       109*, 42-46.

[102] Marroquin, O.C., Kip, K.E., Kelley, D.E., Jphnson B.D., Shaw L.J., Bairey Nerz
       C.N., Sharat B.L., Pepine C.J., Sopko G. & Reis S.E. (2004). Metabolic syndrome
       modifies the cardiovascular risk associated with angiographic coronary artery disease
       in women: a report from the Women's Ischemia Syndrome Evaluation. *Circulation,
       109*, 714-721.

[103] Kip, K.E., Marroquin, O.C., Kelley, D.E., Johnson, B.D. & Kelsey, S.F. (2004).
       Clinical importance of obesity versus the metabolic syndrome in cardiovascular risk
       in women: a report from the Women's Ischemia Syndrome Evaluation (WISE) study.
       Circulation, 109, 706-713.

[104] Petitti, D.B. (2003). Clinical practice: combination estrogen-progestin oral
       contraceptives. *N Engl J Med, 349*, 1443-1450.

[105] Chasan-Taber, L. & Stampfer, M.J. Epidemiology of oral contraceptives and
       cardiovascular disease. *Ann Intern Med, 128*, 467-477.

[106] Stadel, B.V. (1981). Oral contraceptives and cardiovascular disease (first of two
       parts). *N Engl J Med, 305*, 612-618.

[107] Royal College of General Practitioners' Oral Contraception Study. (1981). Further
       analyses of mortality in oral contraceptive users. *Lancet, 1*, 541-546.

[108] Croft, P. & Hannaford, P.C. (1989). Risk factors for acute myocardial infarction in
       women: evidence from the Royal College of General Practitioners' Oral
       Contraception Study. *BMJ, 298*, 165-168.

[109] Rosenberg, L., Palmer, J.R., Rao, R.S. & Shapiro, S. (2001). Low-dose oral
       contraceptive use and the risk of myocardial infarction. *Arch Intern Med, 161*, 1065-
       1070.

[110] WHO Collaborative Study of Cardiovascular Disease and Steroid Hormone
       Contraception. (1997). Acute myocardial infarction and combined oral
       contraceptives: results of an international multicentre case-control study. *Lancet, 349*,
       1202-1209.

[111] Mant, J., Painter, R. & Vessey, M. (1998). Risk of myocardial infarction, angina, and
       stroke in users of oral contraceptives: an updated analysis of a cohort study. *Br J
       Obstet Gynaecol, 105*, 890-896.

[112] Sidney, S., Siscovick, D.S., Petitti, D.B., Schwartz, S.M., Quesenberry, C.P. & Psaty, B.M. (1998). Myocardial infarction and use of low-dose oral contraceptives: a pooled analysis of 2 US studies. *Circulation, 98*, 1058-1063.

[113] Schwingl, P.J., Ory, H.W. & Visness, C.M. (1999). Estimates of the risk of cardiovascular death attributable to low-dose oral contraceptives in the United States. *Am J Obstet Gynecol, 180*, 241-249.

[114] Scarabin, P.Y., Vissac, A.M., Kirzin, J.M., Bourgeat, P., Amiral, J. & Agher, R. (1999). Elevated plasma fibrinogen and increased fibrin turnover among healthy women who both smoke and use low-dose oral contraceptives--a preliminary report. *Thromb Haemost, 82,* 1112-1116.

[115] Holschermann, H., Terhalle, H.M., Zakel, U., Maus, U., Parviz, B. & Tillmanns, H. (1999). Monocyte tissue factor expression is enhanced in women who smoke and use oral contraceptives. *Thromb Haemost, 82*, 1614-1620.

[116] Lewis, M.A., Spitzer, W.O., Heinemann, L.A.J. & Thorogood M. (1996). Third generation oral contraceptives and the risk of myocardial infarction: An international case-control study. BMJ, 312, 88-90.

[117] Dunn, N., Thorogood, M., Faragher, B., de Caestecker, L., MacDonald, T.M., McCollum, C., Thomas, S. & Mann, R. (1999). Oral contraceptives and myocardial infarction: results of the MICA case-control study. *BMJ, 318*, 1579-1583.

[118] Tanis, B.C., van den Bosch, A.A.J., Kemmeren, J.M., Cats, V.M., Helmerhorst, F.M., Algra, A., van der Graaf Y., & Rosendaal, F.R. (2001). Oral contraceptives and the risk of myocardial infarction. *N Engl J Med, 345*, 1787-1793.

[119] Baillargeon, J.P., McClish, D.K., Essah, P.A. & Nestler, J.E. (2005). Association between the current use of low-dose oral contraceptives and cardiovascular arterial disease: a meta-analysis. *J Clin Endocrinol Metab, 90*, 3863-3870.

[120] Schiff, I., Bell, W.R., Davis, V., Kessler, C.M., Meyers, C. & Nakajima, S. (1999). Oral contraceptives and smoking, current considerations: Recommendations of a consensus panel. *Am J Obstet Gynecol, 180*, S383-S384.

[121] Stampfer, M.J., Willett, W.C., Colditz, G.A., Speizer, F.E. & Hennekens, C.H. (1988). A prospective study of past use of oral contraceptive agents and risk of cardiovascular diseases. *N Engl J Med, 319*, 1313-1317.

[122] Merz, C.N., Johnson, B.D., Berga, S., Braunstein, G., Reis, S.E. & Bittner, V. (2006). Past oral contraceptive use and angiographic coronary artery disease in postmenopausal women: data from the National Heart, Lung, and Blood Institute-sponsored Women's Ischemia Syndrome Evaluation. *Fertil Steril, 85*, 1425-1431

[123] Haynes, SG; Czajkowski, SM. Psychosocial and environmental correlates of heart disease. In: Douglas PS, editor. *Cardiovascular Health and Disease in Women*. Philadelphia: Saunders; 1993; 269.

[124] Wamala, S.P., Mittleman, M.A., Schenck-Gustafsson, K. & Orth-Gomer, K. (1999). Potential explanations for the educational gradient in coronary heart disease: a population-based case-control study of Swedish women. *Am J Public Health, 89*, 315-321.

[125] Wilson P.W., D'Agostino R.B., Levy D., Belanger, A.M., Silbershatz, H. & Kannel, W.B. (1998). Prediction of coronary heart disease using risk factor categories. *Circulation, 97*, 1837-1847.

[126] D'Agostino, R.B., Grundy, S., Sullivan, L.M. & Wilson, P. (2001). Validation of the Framingham Coronary Heart Disease Prediction Scores: Results of a Multiple Ethnic Groups Investigation. *JAMA, 286*, 180-187.

[127] Orencia, A., Bailey, K., Yawn, B.P. & Kottke, T.E. (1993). Effect of gender on long-term outcome of angina pectoris and myocardial infarction/sudden unexpected death. *JAMA, 269*, 2392-.

[128] Kannel, W.B. & Vokonas, P.S. (1992). Demographics of the prevalence, incidence, and management of coronary heart disease in the elderly and in women. *Ann Epidemiol, 2*, 5-14.

[129] Lerner, D.J. & Kannel, W.B. (1986). Patterns of coronary heart disease morbidity and mortality in the sexes: 26-year follow-up of the Framingham population. *Am Heart J, 111*, 383-390.

[130] Diamond, G.A. & Forrester, J.S. Analysis of probability as an aid in the clinical diagnosis of coronary- artery disease. *N Engl J Med, 300*, 1350-1358.

[131] Weiner, D.A., Ryan, T.J., McCabe, C.H., et al. (1979). Exercise stress testing. Correlations among history of angina, ST- segment response and prevalence of coronary-artery disease in the Coronary Artery Surgery Study (CASS). *N Engl J Med, 301*, 230-235.

[132] Alexander, K.P., Shaw, L.J., Delong, E.R., Mark, D.B. & Peterson, E.D. (1998). Value of exercise treadmill testing in women. *J Am Coll Cardiol, 32*, 1657-1664.

[133] D'Antono, B., Dupuis, G., Fortin, C., Arsenault, A., & Burelle, D (2006). Angina symptoms in men and women with stable coronary artery disease and evidence of exercise-induced myocardial perfusion defects. *Am Heart J*, 151, 813-819.

[134] Pepine, C.J., Abrams, J., Marks, R.G., Morris, J.J., Scheidt, S.S. & Handberg, E. (1994). Characteristics of a contemporary population with angina pectoris. *Am J Cardiol, 74*, 226-231.

[135] Arnold, A.L., Milner, K.A. & Vaccarino, V. (2001). Sex and race differences in electrocardiogram use (The National Hospital Ambulatory Medical Care survey). *Am J Cardiol, 88*, 1037-1040.

[136] Orencia, A., Bailey, K., Yawn, B.P. & Kottke, T.E. (1993). Effect of gender on long-term outcome of angina pectoris and myocardial infarction/sudden unexpected death. *JAMA, 269*, 2392-2397.

[137] White, H.D., Barbash, G.I., Modan, M., Simes, J., Diaz, R., Hampton, J.R., et al. (1993). After correcting for worse baseline characteristics, women treated with thrombolytic therapy for acute myocardial infarction have the same mortality and morbidity as men except for a higher incidence of hemorrhagic stroke. The Investigators of the International Tissue Plasminogen Activator/Streptokinase Mortality Study. *Circulation, 88*, 2097-2103.

[138] Gibbons, R.J., Balady, G.J., Bricker, J.T., et al. (2002). ACC/AHA 2002 guideline update for exercise testing: summary article: a report of the American College of Cardiology/American Heart Association Task Force on Practice Guidelines

(Committee to Update the 1997 Exercise Testing Guidelines). *Circulation, 106*, 1883-1892.

[139] Gibbons, R.J., Abrams, J., Chatterjee, K., et al. (2003). ACC/AHA 2002 guideline update for the management of patients with chronic stable angina. ACC/AHA 2002 Guideline Update for the Management of Patients With Chronic Stable Angina—Summary Article: a report of the American College of Cardiology/American Heart Association Task Force on Practice Guidelines (Committee on the Management of Patients With Chronic Stable Angina). *Circulation, 107*, 149-158.

[140] Shaw, L.J., Miller, D.D., Gillespie, K.N., Younis, L.T., Chaitman, B.R. & Romeis, J.C. (1995). A gender-specific hazard-based clinical and noninvasive coronary risk scoring system for patients with suspected coronary artery disease. *Clin Perform Qual Health Care, 3*, 209-217.

[141] Sketch, M., Mohiuddin, S., Lynch, J., Zencka, A. & Runco, V. (1975). Significant sex differences in the correlation of electrocardiographic exercise testing and coronary angiography. *Am J Cardiol, 36*, 169-173.

[142] Mora, S., Redberg, R.F., Cui, Y., Whiteman, M.K., Flaws, J.A., Sharrett, A.R. & Blumenthal, R.S. (2003). Ability of exercise testing to predict cardiovascular and all-cause death in asymptomatic women: a 20-year follow-up of the Lipid Research Clinics prevalence study. *JAMA, 290*, 1600-1607.

[143] Marwick, T., Anderson, T., Williams, M.J., Haluska, B., Melin, J.A., Pashkow, F. & Thomas, J.D. (1995). Exercise echocardiography is an accurate and cost-efficient technique for detection of coronary artery disease in women. *J Am Coll Cardiol, 26*, 335-341.

[144] Bateman, T.M., O'Keefe, J.H., Dorg, V.M. & Bamhart, C. (1994). Prognostic significance of nonischemic SPECT stress myocardial perfusion scintigraphy in women. *J Nucl Med, 35*, 60P.

[145] Giri, S., Shaw, L.J., Murthy, D.R., Travin, M.I., Miller, D.D. & Hachamovitch, R. (2002). Impact of diabetes on the risk stratification using stress single-photon emission computed tomography myocardial perfusion imaging in patients with symptoms suggestive of coronary artery disease. *Circulation, 105*, 32-40.

[146] Chae, S.C., Heo, J., Iskandrian, A.S., Wasserleben, V. & Cave, V. (1993). Identification of extensive coronary artery disease in women by exercise single-photon emission computer tomographic (SPECT) thallium imaging. *J Am Coll Cardiol, 21*, 1305-1311.

[147] Johnson, L.L. (1995). Sex specific issues relating to nuclear cardiology. *J Nucl Cardiol, 2*, 339-348.

[148] Osbakken, M.D., Okada, R., Boucher, C.A. et al. (1984). Comparison of exercise perfusion and ventricular function imaging: An analysis of factors affecting the diagnostic accuracy of each technique. *J Am Coll Cardiol, 3*, 272-283.

[149] Shaw, L.J., Miller, D.D., Romeis, J.C., Kargl, D. & Younis, L.T. (1994). Gender differences in the noninvasive evaluation of patients with suspected coronary artery disease. *Ann Intern Med, 120*, 559-566.

[150]   Goodgold, H.M., Rehder, J.G., Samuels, L.D. & Chaitman, B.R. (1987). Improved interpretation of exercise thallium-201 scintigraphy in women: Characterization of breast attenuation artifacts. *Radiology, 165*, 361-366.

[151]   Stratmann, H.G., Williams, G.A., Wittry, M.D., Chaitman, B.R. & Miller, D.D. (1994). Exercise technetium-99m sestamibi tomography for cardiac risk stratification of patients with stable chest pain. *Circulation, 89*, 615-622.

[152]   Williams, M.J., Marwick, T.H., O'Gorman, D. & Foale, R.A. (1994). Comparison of exercise echocardiography with an exercise score to diagnose coronary artery disease in women. *Am J Cardiol, 74*, 435-438.

[153]   Cheitlin, M.D., Armstrong, W.F., Aurigemma, G.P., Beller, G., Bierman, F.Z., Davis, J.L., Douglas, P.S., Faxon, D.P., Gillam, L.D., Kimball, T.R., Kussmaul, W.G., Pearlman, A.S., Philbrick, J.T., Rakowski, H. & Thys, D.M. (2003). ACC/AHA/ASE 2003 Guideline Update for the Clinical Application of Echocardiography: Summary Article: a report of the American College of Cardiology/American Heart Association Task Force on Practice Guidelines (ACC/AHA/ASE Committee to Update the 1997 Guidelines for the Clinical Application of Echocardiography). *Circulation, 108,* 1146-1162.

[154]   Marwick, T., D'Hondt, A.M., Baudhuin, T., Willemat, A., Wijns, W. & Detry, J. (1993). Optimal use of dobutamine stress for the detection and evaluation of coronary artery disease. Combination with echocardiography or scintigraphy or both? *J Am Coll Cardiol, 22*, 159-167.

[155]   Secknus, M.A. & Marwick, T.H. (1997). Influence of gender on physiologic response and accuracy of dobutamine echocardiography. *Am J Cardiol, 80*, 721-724.

[156]   Lewis, J.F., Lin, L., McGorray, S. & Pepine, C.J. (1999). Dobutamine stress echocardiography in women with chest pain. Pilot phase data from the National Heart, Lung and Blood Institute Women's Ischemia Syndrome Evaluation (WISE). *J Am Coll Cardiol, 33*, 1462-1468.

[157]   Arruda-Olson, A.M., Juracan, E.M., Mahoney, D.W., McCully, R.B., Roger, V.L. & Pellikka, P.A. (2002). Prognostic value of exercise echocardiography in 5,798 patients: is there a gender difference?. *J Am Coll Cardiol, 39*, 625-631.

[158]   Melin, J.A., Wijns, W., Vanbutsele, R.J., Robert, A., De Coster, P., Brasseur, L.A., Beckers, C. & Detry, J.M. (1985). Alternative diagnostic strategies for coronary artery disease in women: Demonstration of the usefulness and efficiency of probability analysis. *Circulation, 71*, 535-542.

[159]   Mieres, J.H., Shaw, L.J., Arai, A., Matthew J. Budoff, M.J., Scott D. Flamm, S.D., Gregory Hundley, G., Thomas H. Marwick, T.H., Mosca, L., Patel, A.R., Quinones, M.A., Redberg, R.F., Taubert, K.A., Taylor, A.J., Thomas, G.S., & Wenger, N.K., (2005). Role of noninvasive testing in the clinical evaluation of women with suspected coronary artery disease: consensus statement from the Cardiac Imaging Committee, Council on Clinical Cardiology, and the Cardiovascular Imaging and Intervention Committee, Council on Cardiovascular Radiology and Intervention, American Heart Association. *Circulation, 111*, 682-696.

[160]   Buchthal, S.D., den Hollander, J.A., Bairey Merz, C.N., Rogers, W.J., Pepine, C.J., Reichek, N., Sharaf, B.L., Reis, S., Kelsey, S.F. & Pohost, G.M. (2000). Abnormal

myocardial phosphorus-31 nuclear magnetic resonance spectroscopy in women with chest pain but normal coronary angiograms. *N Engl J Med, 342*, 829-835.

[161] Glaser, R., Herrmann, H.C., Murphy, S.A., Demopoulos, L.A., DiBattiste, P.M., Cannon, C.P. & Braunwald, E. (2002). Benefit of an early invasive management strategy in women with acute coronary syndromes. *JAMA, 288*, 3124-3129.

[162] Braunwald, E., Antman, E.M., Beasley, J.W., et al. (2002). ACC/AHA. Committee on the Management of Patients With Unstable Angina. ACC/AHA 2002 guideline update for the management of patients with unstable angina and non-ST-segment elevation myocardial infarction – summary article: a report of the American College of Cardiology/American Heart Association task force on practice guidelines (Committee on the Management of Patients With Unstable Angina). J *Am Coll Cardiol, 40*, 1366-1374.

[163] Mosca, L., Appel, L.J., Benjamin, E.J., Berra, K., Chandra-Strobos, N., Fabunmi, R.P., Grady, D., Haan, C.K. & Hayes SN, (2004). Evidence-based guidelines for cardiovascular disease prevention in women. *Circulation, 109*, 672-692.

[164] Daly, C., Clemens, F., Lopez Sendon, J.L, Tavazzi, L., Boersma, E., Danchin, N. & Delahaye, F. (2006). Gender differences in the management and clinical outcome of stable angina. *Circulation, 113*, 490-498.

[165] Antiplatelet Trialists' Collaboration. (1994). Collaborative overview of randomised trials of antiplatelet therapy— I: Prevention of death, myocardial infarction, and stroke by prolonged antiplatelet therapy in various categories of patients. [published erratum appears in BMJ 1994; 308:1540]. *BMJ, 308*, 81-106.

[166] de Gaetano, G. (2001). Low-dose aspirin and vitamin E in people at cardiovascular risk: a randomised trial in general practice. Collaborative Group of the Primary Prevention Project. *Lancet, 357*, 89-95.

[167] Ridker, P.M., Cook, N.R., Lee, I.M., Gordon D., Gaziano J.M. & Manson J.E. (2005). A randomized trial of low-dose aspirin in the primary prevention of cardiovascular disease in women. *N Engl J Med, 352*, 1293-1304.

[168] Becker, D.M., Segal, J., Vaidya, D., Yanek, L.R., Herrera-Galeano, J.E., Bray, P.F. & Moy, T.F. (2006). Sex differences in platelet reactivity and response to low-dose aspirin therapy. *JAMA, 295*, 1420-1427.

[169] Clarke, K.W., Gray, D., Keating, N.A. & Hampton, J.R. (1994). Do women with acute myocardial infarction receive the same treatment as men? *BMJ, 309*, 563-566.

[170] Pfeffer, M.A., Braunwald, E., Moyé, L.A, Basta, L., Brown, E.J. Jr, Cuddy, T.E. & Davis, B.R. (1992). Effect of captopril on mortality and morbidity in patients with left ventricular dysfunction after myocardial infarction: Results of the survival and ventricular enlargement trial. *N Engl J Med, 327*, 669-677.

[171] Pedersen, T.R., Kjekshus, J., Berg, K., Olsson, A.G., Wilhelmsen, L. & Wedel, H. (1996). Cholesterol lowering and the use of healthcare resources: Results of the Scandinavian Simvastatin Survival Study. *Circulation, 93*, 1796-1802.

[172] Herrington, D.M., Vittinghoff, E., Lin, F., et al. (2002). Statin therapy, cardiovascular events, and total mortality in the Heart and Estrogen/Progestin Replacement Study (HERS). *Circulation, 105*, 2962-2967.

[173] Lewis, S.J., Sacks, F.M., Mitchell, J.S., et al, for the CARE Investigators. (1998). Effect of pravastatin on cardiovascular events in women after myocardial infarction: The Cholesterol and Recurrent Events (CARE) trial. *J Am Coll Cardiol, 32*, 140-146.

[174] MRC/BHF Heart Protection Study of cholesterol lowering with simvastatin in 20536 high-risk individuals: a randomised placebo-controlled trial. (2002). *Lancet, 360*, 7-22.

[175] Cannon, C.P., Braunwald, E., McCabe, C.H., Rader, D.J., Rouleau, J.L., Belder, R., et al. (2004). Intensive versus moderate lipid lowering with statins after acute coronary syndromes. *N Engl J Med, 350*, 1495-1504.

[176] Blomkalns, A.L., Chen, A.Y., Hochman, J.S., Peterson, E.D., Trynosky, K., Diercks, D.B., et al. (2005). Gender disparities in the diagnosis and treatment of non-ST-segment elevation acute coronary syndromes: large-scale observations from the CRUSADE (Can Rapid Risk Stratification of Unstable Angina Patients Suppress Adverse Outcomes With Early Implementation of the American College of Cardiology/American Heart Association Guidelines) National Quality Improvement Initiative. *J Am Coll Cardiol, 45*, 832-837.

[177] Maynard, C., Litwin, P.E., Martin, J.S. & Weaver, W.D. (1992). Gender differences in the treatment and outcome of acute myocardial infarction: Results from the myocardial infarction triage and intervention registry. *Arch Intern Med, 152*, 972-976.

[178] Karnash, S, Granger, CB, White, HD, Woodlief, L.H., Topol, E.J., Califf, R.M., for the GUSTO-I Investigators. (1995). Treating menstruating women with thrombolytic therapy: Insights from the Global Utilization of Streptokinase and Tissue Plasminogen Activator for occluded coronary arteries (GUSTO-I) trial. *J Am Coll Cardiol, 26,* 1651-1656.

[179] Rossouw, JE, Anderson, GL, Prentice, RL, LaCroix, A.Z., Kooperberg, C., Stefanick, M.L., Jackson, R.D., Beresford, S.A., Howard, B.V., Johnson, K.C., Kotchen, J.M., Ockene, J. (2002). Risks and benefits of estrogen plus progestin in healthy postmenopausal women: principal results From the Women's Health Initiative randomized controlled trial. *JAMA, 288*, 321-333.

[180] Hulley, S, Furberg, C, Barrett-Connor, E, Cauley, J., Grady, D., Haskell, W., Knopp, R., Lowery, M., Satterfield, S., Schrott, H. & Vittinghoff, E., (2002). Noncardiovascular disease outcomes during 6.8 years of hormone therapy. Heart and Estrogen/progestin Replacement Study follow-up (HERS II). *JAMA, 288*, 58-64.

[181] Anderson, G.L., Limacher, M., Assaf, A.R., et al., (2004). Effects of conjugated equine estrogen in postmenopausal women with hysterectomy: the Women's Health Initiative randomized controlled trial. *JAMA, 291*, 1701-1712.

[182] Prentice, R.L., Langer, R.D., Stefanick, M.L., et al. (2006). Combined analysis of women's health initiative observational and clinical trial data on postmenopausal hormone treatment and cardiovascular disease. *Am J Epidemiol, 163*, 589-599.

[183] Cauley, J.A., Seeley, D.G., Browner, W.S., Ensrud, K., Kuller, L.H., Lipschutz, R.C., et al. (1997). Estrogen replacement therapy and mortality among older women. The Study of Osteoporotic Fractures. *Arch Intern Med., 157*, 2181-2187.

[184] Clarke, S.C., Kelleher, J., Lloyd-Jones, H., Slack, M. & Schofiel PM. (2002). A study of hormone replacement therapy in postmenopausal women with ischaemic heart disease: the Papworth HRT atherosclerosis study. *BJOG, 109*, 1056-1062.

[185] Manson, J.E. & Martin, K.A. (2001). Clinical practice. Postmenopausal hormone-replacement therapy. *N Engl J Med.*, 345, 34-40.

[186] Mosca L., Collins P., Herrington D.M., Mendelsohn M.E., Pasternak R.C., Robertson R.M., Schenck-Gustafsson K., Smith S.C., Taubert K.A. & Wenger N.K. (2001). Hormone replacement therapy and cardiovascular disease: a statement for healthcare professionals from the American Heart Association. *Circulation, 104*, 499-503.

[187] Daly, C., Clemens, F., Lopez Sendon, J.L., Tavazzi, L., Boersma, E., Danchin, N., et al. (2006). Gender differences in the management and clinical outcome of stable angina. *Circulation, 113*, 490-498.

[188] Lehmann, J.B., Wehner, P.S., Lehmann, C.U. & Savory, L.M. (1996). Gender bias in the evaluation of chest pain in the emergency department. *Am J Cardiol, 77*, 641-644.

[189] Anand, S.S, Xie, C.C., Mehta, S., Franzosi, M.G., Joyner, C., et al. (2005). Differences in the management and prognosis of women and men who suffer from acute coronary syndromes. *J Am Coll Cardiol, 46*, 1845-1851.

[190] King, K.M., Ghali, W.A., Faris, P.D., et al. (2004). Sex differences in outcomes after cardiac catheterization: effect modification by treatment strategy and time. *JAMA, 291*, 1220-1225.

[191] Watanabe, C.T., Maynard, C. & Ritchie, J.L. (2001). Comparison of short-term outcomes following coronary artery stenting in men versus women. *Am J Cardiol, 88*, 848-852.

[192] Jacobs, A.K. (2003). Coronary revascularization in women in 2003: sex revisited. *Circulation, 107*, 375-377.

[193] Schunkert, H., Harrell, L. & Palacios, I.F. (1999). Implications of small reference vessel diameter in patients undergoing percutaneous coronary revascularization. *J Am Coll Cardiol, 34*, 40-48.

[194] Jaffe, R. & Strauss, B.H. (2007). Late and very late thrombosis of drug-eluting stents. Evolving Concepts and Perspectives. *J Am Coll Cardiol, 50*, 119-127.

[195] Lansky, A.J., Hochman, J.S., Ward, P.A, Mintz, G.S., Fabunmi, R., & Berger, P.B. (2005). Percutaneous coronary intervention and adjunctive pharmacotherapy in women: a statement for healthcare professionals from the American Heart Association. *Circulation, 111*, 940-953.

[196] O'Connor, G.T., Morton, J.R., Diehl, M.J., Olmstead, E.M., Coffin, L.H., Levy, D.G., Maloney, C.T., Plume, S.K., Nugent, W., Malenka, D.J., et al. (1993). Differences between men and women in hospital mortality associated with coronary artery bypass graft surgery. *Circulation, 88*, 2104-2110.

[197] Hogue, C.W. Jr, Barzilai, B., Pieper, K.S., et al. (2001). Sex differences in neurological outcomes and mortality after cardiac surgery: A Society of Thoracic Surgery National Database Report. *Circulation, 103*, 2133-2137.

[198] Jacobs, A.K., Kelsey, S.F., Brooks, M.M., Faxon, D.P., Chaitman, B.R., Bittner, V. & Mock, M.B. (1998). Better outcome for women compared with men undergoing coronary revascularization: a report from the bypass angioplasty revascularization investigation (BARI). *Circulation, 98,* 1279-1285.

[199] Ness, R.B., Harris, T., Cobb, J., Flegal, K.M., Kelsey, J., Balanger, A. & Stunkard, A.J. (1993). Number of pregnancies and the subsequent risk of cardiovascular disease. *N Engl J Med, 328,* 1528-1533.

[200] Lawlor, D.A., Emberson, J.R., Ebrahim, S., Lawlor, D.A., Emberson, J.R., Ebrahim, S., Whincup, P.H., Wannamethee, S.G., Walker, M. & Smith, G.D. (2003). Is the association between parity and coronary heart disease due to biological effects of pregnancy or adverse lifestyle risk factors associated with child-rearing? Findings from the British Women's Heart and Health Study and the British Regional Heart Study. *Circulation, 107,* 1260-1264.

[201] Karamermer, Y. & Roos-Hesselink, J.W. Coronary heart disease and pregnancy. *Future Cardiology, 2007, 3,* 559-567.

In: Heart Disease in Women
Editor: B. V. Larner and H. R. Pennelton

ISBN 978-1-60692-066-4
© 2009 Nova Science Publishers, Inc.

Chapter IX

Prognosis of Women with Acute Coronary Syndromes: An Overview

Andreja Sinkovic[*]

Department of Medical Intensive Care, General Hospital Maribor, Slovenia

Abstract

Background. Participation of women in studies of acute coronary syndromes, including acute ST-elevation myocardial infarction (MI) as well as unstable angina and/or non-ST-elevation MI is about 30-40% and is remaing constant during last 20 years. It is well known that in ST-elevation MI women, who are older than men and are mostly less agressively treated, experience worse outcome than men. The results of studies of unstable angina and/or non-ST-elevation MI also demonstrated that women are significantly older and with significantly more comorbidities. However, the results of the studies are controvesial, regarding the short- and long term prognosis. Some studies demonstarted significantly increased risk of 30-day and six-month adverse outcomes in women, when compared to men in spite of their similar treatments, but others similar outcomes with similar treatments in spite of older age.

Conclusions. In this review article the results of studies, regarding the outcomes of women compared to men in acute coronary syndromes are discussed, especially the use of treatments, including coronary interventions, misuse or errors in medical treatments, as well as future perspectives in women with coronary artery disease in the new millenium.

Introduction

Cardiovascular disease is the leading cause of death in the population of the western countries in general in spite of increased preventive, diagnostic and therapeutic measures

---

[*] Correspondence:Ljubljanska 5, 2000 Maribor, Slovenia, Phone: +386-2-3212471, fax: +386-2-3312393, e-mail: andreja.sinkovic@guest.arnes.si.

provided during the last decades [1-3]. The mortality rate from cardiovascular disease in men is declining steadily during the last twenty years, but this has remained unchanged in women. In addition, higher proportion of women in the aging population is among the causes for increasing cardiovascular mortality in women each year in comparison to men. Increasing prevalence of obesity and diabetes in women means increasing prevalence and clustering of risk factors for atherosclerosis in women and therefore for coronary heart disease. In future higher prevalence of diabetes and obesity in women will likely contribute significantly to the occurence of atherosclerosis and coronary heart disease in women at an younger age [4-7].

Comparing women and men with coronary artery disease there are some clear gender differences, but also biases. Clear gender differences were identified in epidemiology and clinical presentation, risk factors, the use of diagnostic and therapeutic interventions, medications used and in outcome [4,5,8]. In addition, women were evaluated less intensively, less agressively, less frequently or even misdiagnosed at grater frequency as men for the same disease as demonstrated by some studies and registries [9-11]. Most differences and bias can be attributed to differences in baseline characteristics, but frequently encountered worse outcome in cardiovascular disease in women may not be explained entirely by comorbidities and older age [4-6,8].

Definition and Clasification of Acute Coronary Syndromes (ACS)

ACS are most important acute clinical manifestations of coronary artery disease. They are presenting with chest pain and changes on ECG, either with or without persistent ST-segment elevation, reflecting ether subendocardial or transmural myocardial ischemia (Figure 1). They are usually caused by total occlusion or subtotal stenosis of a coronary artery, caused by the formation of occlusive thrombus on ruptured, eroded or inflamed atherosclerotic plaque that results in myocardial ischemia. If myocardial ischemia, being the consequence of occlusive coronary atherothrombosis, lasts sufficiently long (> 20 minutes) the ischemic myocardial area becomes necrotic in the next few hours. Clinically, besides persistent or recurrent chest pain, not responding to sublingual nitroglicerin the ECG signs of ishemia evolve within hours to ECG signs of myocardial necrosis or myocardial infarction (MI) with the formation of Q-wave and/or negative T-wave in addition to the increase of serum troponin T or I levels. Serum troponins are most senssitive and specific markers of myocardial necrosis or infarction, but also predictors of outcome in patients with ACS [12-14].

In majority of patients with ACS and persistent ST- elevation on ECG there is usually evolution of Q-wave MI, but in minority of non-Q MI. In ACS patients without persistent ST-elevation there is either evolution to non-Q MI or thre is unstable angina. In non-Q MI there is additionally an increase of biomarkers of ischemic necrosis, but not in unstable angina [12].

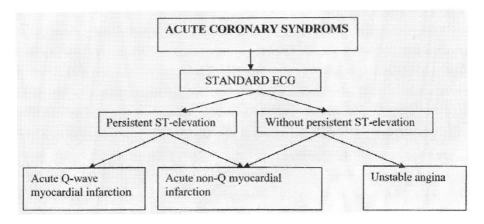

Figure 1. Shematic classification and consequences of ACS.

Epidemiology of ACS

According to annual statistical report provided by American Heart Association for the year 2003 there were approximately 870.000 individuals discharges from hospitals in USA diagnosed as ACS, among them about 497.000 men and 382.000 women. When including secondary discharge diagnosis the corresponding number of hospital discharge for ACS was even 1.555.000 hospitalizations annualy, icluding 846.000 for MI and 650.000 for unstable angina. The estimates for ST-elevation ACS range from 30-45%. According to annual report of American Heart Association 42 % of patients suffer ACS with ST-segment elevation on ECG and 51 % ACS without ST-elevation on ECG, whereas in 6.5 % of patients ACS ECG changes are nonspecific [4].

According to European GRACE registry admission and discharge diagnosis differ. On admission 44% of patients are diagnosed as unstable angina, 36% as evolving acute MI, 9% are admitted to rule out an acute MI, and 7% as chest pain. However, at discharge 30% of patients are diagnosed as ST-elevation MI, 25% as non-ST-elevation MI, 38% as unstable angina, 4% as other cardiac causes and 3% as noncardiac cause for chest pain [2]. When comparing north American and European registries there are obviously no significant differences in epidemiology of ACS in general [2,4,5].

And what are the consequences of ACS? According to Euroheart Survey ACS in European countries in about 64 % of patients with ST-elevation ACS develope Q-MI, 22.2 % non-Q MI and unstable angina 13 %. In ACS patients without persistent ST-segment elevation in 7,9 % Q-MI is the consequence, in 26.9 % non-Q MI and in 65.1 % unstable angina [3]

Only 50 % of patients with evolving MI have typical chest pain and ST-segment elevation on ECG in at least two contiguous leads, but in the rest of patients nonspecific ECG changes are registered. Normal ECG does not exclude an ACS as even in 6 % of them myocardial necrosis is demonstated by some other methods [1-3].

In Europe, where the percentage of population over 40 years is exceeding 45%, the incidence of an acute MI is about 1 - 2.0 per 1000 population and of unstable angina up to 2.5 per 1000 population [7]. The age-adjusted risk of coronary artery disease in women is approximately 1/3 that for men [4,5,8]. European women < 65 years of age suffer ST-elevation ACS in 39% in comparison to 51% of men in the same age group. This difference is significant. However, older women (> 65 years of age) get ACS with ST-elevation in 36% in comparison to 38% of elderly men (> 65 years of age) [8].

In USA, where the total prevalence of coronary heart disease in 2003 was 6.9% (13.200.000), there was a significant difference in prevalence of coronary artery disease between men and women, in men being 8.4% (7.200.000) and in women 5.6% (6.000.000), respectively. In the same time the total prevalence of MI was 3.5% (7.200.000) and again there were striking differences between men and women, as the prevalence of MI in men was 5% (4.200.000) and 2.3% in women [4].

In USA estimated annual incidence of new coronary events is 700.000 and of recurrent events about 500.000, of first acute MI approximatelly 565.000 and of recurrent MI 300.000. Coronary heart disease is responsible for more than half of all cardiovascular events in men and women under the age of 75 years. The average age of first acute MI is 65.8 years for men and 70.4 years for women. The life time risk to develope coronary heart disease after the age of 40 is 49% for men and 32% for women. Women are 10 years behind men for MI and sudden cardiac death. In this way the annual average age-adjusted coronary artery disease incidence rates per 1000 population are up to 12.5% in men and up to 5.1% in women. The annual incidence rate for the first MI in men is about 19/1000 population for the age group 65-74 years, 28/1000 population for the age group 75-84 years and 50.6 for the age over 85 years. In women in the same age groups the annual incidence rates for MI are 6.8%, 14.2% and 33.2%, respectively. The annual statistics demonstrate significant differences in the annual incidence rate for the first MI between the genders in all age groups, as well as increasing incidence rate of first MI with age in both genders [4,5].

Data from randomised trials demonstrated that women represented only about 1/3 of the ACS population, in trials with thrombolytic agents even less – 18% in TIMI II trial, 24% in GUSTO 1 trial [10,11]. As in registries, in randomized trials women were significantly older than men [11].

The Outcome and Prognosis of ACS in Women and Comparison to Men

Coronary heart disease represents the single most important cause of death worldwide. However, death rate due to coronary heart disease in the developed countries declined during the last 15 years for about 33%. Coronary heart disease causes 1 of 5 deaths annually. According to the US statistics the overall death rate for coronary heart disease in 2003 was 162/100.000 population, whereas in 2004 150.5/100.000 population. In 2003 the overall death rate for coronary heart disease for women was up to 160/100.000 and up to 240/100.000 for men. In 2004 overall death rate for coronary heart disease for women was up to 148.6 and about 222.2 for men per 100.000 population. According to this data there is trend to lower death rate for coronary artery disease im and in women. According to the statistics over 80% of population, who die due to coronary artery disease, is over 65 years of age [4,5].

In-hospital mortality for acute MI declined from 1990 till 1999 from 12.2% to 9.4% in the US [4]. However, still 25% of men and 38% of women die within 1 year after initial acute MI. As women are older, when suffering their first MI, they are more likely to die within the next few weeks. At the same time women < 50 years of age die twice as likely after an acute MI than men of the same age. About 50% of men and women < 65 years of age, who have an acute MI, will die within the next 8 years. 64% of women in comparison to 50% of men dying suddenly of coronary heart diseasedo not have any preceeding warning symptoms and signs [4].

In the thrombolytic era ISIS-3 trial in 1992, comparing the efficacy of three randomized fibrinolytic agents - streptokinase, tissue plasminogen activator, or anisoylated plasminogen-streptokinase activator complex, demonstrated that 30-day mortality of women was significantly increased in comparison to men [9].

In GUSTO 1 trial in 1993 also demonstated significantly increased relative risk of 30-day mortality as well as of heart failure, shock and reinfarction within 30 days in women in comparison to men [10].

According to Fibrinolytic Therapy Trialists Collaborative Group (FTT) meta-analysis in 1994 women had 60% greater 35-day mortality rate than men irrespective of the use of thrombolytic agents [11].

In the large randomized trial GUSTO-IIb some years later again significantly fewer women than men constituted the ACS population, but 30-day mortality of women with ACS in general was still significantly higher than in men. However, GUSTO-IIb demonstrated only a nonsignificant trend toward an increased risk of death and reinfarction among women as compared with men in ST-elevation ACS and similar 30-day reinfarction rate women and in men [10,15]. According to GUSTO-IIb mortality and reinfarction rate in women and men were equal in non-ST-elevation MI, but in unstable angina the outcome was even significantly better in women than in men. [15].

A report from TIMI IIIB, evaluating the outcome in unstable angina and non-Q-wave MI, demonstated similar outcomes in women and men, that was related to the less severe coronary artery disease in women rather than to gender itself in spite of older age in women [16].

According to European data in the last 10 years the in-hospital outcome or discharge diagnosis of patients admitted to the hospitals as ACS with or without ST-elevation were either acute Q-MI, non-Q MI or unstable angina [8]. In women the discharge diagnosis Q-MI was significantly less common in comparison to younger men, being 28% in women and 40% in younger men. The discharge diagnosis non-Q MI was equally present in women (25%) and men (23%), but unstable angina was significantly more common in women (47%) than in men (37%). However, any type of an infarct was significantly less common in women (53%) than in men (63%) [8].

According to recent data short-term outcome of women diagnosed as ACS in general is significantly worse in comparison to men, mostly due to increased combined mortality and reinfarction rate within 30-days of ST-elevation MI. However, the outcome in non-ST-elevation MI is equal in women and men and in unstable angina the outcome is even in favour of women compared to men [17].

Long-term outcome of ACS patients did not demostrate any difference in 5-year mortality between women and men with unstable angina [18-20]. However, 5-year mortality was significantly increased after acute MI in women (38.8%), when compared to men (26.8%) [21].

What Are the Reasons for Differences in Outcome between the Genders?

Registries and majority of randomized trials demostrated many significant and non-significant differences between the genders regarding pre-treatment data and treatment modalities. Significant differences were mostly in age, comorbidities, medication received and invasive procedures performed [4,5,8,17]. As mentioned before, in the recent years it was demonstrated that women are 10 years behind men regarding ACS, especially in acute MI, where median age of women is about 71 years of age and of men 61 years. On the other hand median age of women with unstable angina is 67 years and of men 62 years (p < 0.01) [17]

In all types of ACS there are some significant differences between the genders regarding comorbidities. The differences are striking in diabetes, arterial hypertension and obesity, all three being more common in women than in men. Among risk factors for atherosclerosis, smoking is still more likely in younger men than in women. [16-18,22-24]. Majority of comorbidities, registered more frequently in women, are well-established risk factors for atherosclerosis and for cororonary artety disease. Dyslipidemias are another well-established and important risk factors of atherosclerosis, that are also registered more frequently in women than in men [16-18,22]. Women are subjects to the same atherogenic risk factors as men, though their significance in women are different. Gender-related differences in the lipid status before the menopause are well known, especially the differences in the levels of total and LDL-cholesterol, which are low before menopause and increase later to reach maximul levels in women between ages 55 to 65 years. HDL-cholesterol levels are higher in women than in men irrespective of age and low HDL-cholesterol levels are well-known significant independent atherogenic risk factor [22,25]. Triglicerides are more significant atherogenic risk factor for women than for men and elevated trigliceris in women posess greater atherogenic risk than in men. In addition it represents a component of metabolic syndrome, a novel and important risk factor for atherosclerosis [4,5,22,25].

Atypical chest pain in addition to ECG changes is an other important difference between men and women with ACS. Women eyperience other atypical symptoms such as fatigue, indigestion, nausea, etc. more frequently than men. These differences in clinical presentation of ACS may contribute to misdiagnosis or even delays in diagnostic and therapeutic interventions in women with ACS [26-29].

There are evidences that cardiac biomarkers, especially in non-ST-elevation ACS, are differentially expressed in men and women. CRP and natriuretic peptide are more frequently increased in women and troponins in men [30].

Comparing the differences between the genders in the use of medical therapy before hospital admission due to ACS, it was demonstrated that in women beta-blockers, calcium antagonists and diuretics were significantly more likely prescribed than in men [8,20,31].

In addition to diabetes, hypertension and obesity, other comorbidities such as congestive heart failure, chronic obstructive pulmonary disease, etc are more frequently encountered in women than in men [21].

Recent trials adressing the differences in outcome between the genders demonstrated, that after adjustment for baseline characteristics there were any sex-specific differences in 1-year mortality among survivors of acute MI, unstable angina, stable angina or nonspecific chest pain on admission. Female gender was even associated with decreased 1-year mortality, especially in unstable angina [17,19]. A possible explanation for this observation is the higher prevalence of normal coronary arteries in women with ACS as demonstated by several other studies before [8,15-18, 24].

In the past and also in recent years there are reports that women are undertreated, or treated less agressively or even that treatment is withheld in comparison to men. [19,31,27].

According to European data published in GRACE registry in 2002 in ST-elevation ACS any kind of reperfusion therapy was equally received in women (62%) and in men (65%), either as fibrinolytic therapy (40% in women and 39% in men) or primary percutaneous coronary intervention (21% in women and 25% in men) [8]. However, in older age groups, women received reperfusion therapy significantly less likely than men (53% vs 43%) [8]

Recently, Kaul P et al in his large observational study included more than 50.000 patients with suspected ACS and demonstrated that indeed women less likely than men underwent coronary revascularization procedure during the year following their first visit to the emergency unit as. However, seemingly less agressive approach to treatment among women had no impact on their 1-year mortality [17].

In non-ST-elevation ACS there are even evidences that women have an improved long-term outcome after very early agressive revascularization with coronary stenting of the culprit lesion as the primary revascularization strategy as compared with men. [18,24]. Other studies did not demonstrate any significant reduction of the risk for the future events among women in comparison to men by the use of invasive strategy in non-ST-elevation ACS in spite of less severe disease in comparison to men [20].

In European survey of ACS in 2002 interactions between age and sex with respect to clinical presentation were observed, with younger females having more unstable angina and less ST-elevation ACS [8]

According to coronary angiography data in GRACE registry in 2002 coronary angiography is performed less likely in women than in men irrespective of age. Coronary angiography studies also demonstrated that younger women have significantly better angiograms in comparison to younger men, though the frequency of 3-vessel disease increases with age in both genders irrespective of age [8]. The results of studies regarding the use of percutaneous coronary interventions are controversial. Some studies demonstrated unequal use of percutaneous coronary interventions, while others - especially European ones their equal use in both genders, though CABG was performed less likely in women than in men [15,8,17].

Several prospective studies of invasive therapy in ACS patients also demonstrated that coronary artery disease is less severe in women than in men as there are significantly less severe stenotic coronary lesions and less extensive atherosclerosis changes of the coronary arteries in women than in men. This was found in ST-elevation, non-ST-elevation ACS and in unstable angina [15,20,33].

The later onset and slower progression of atherosclerosis in women was suspected to be influenced by the loss of estrogen hormones after menopause. In the past, hormone replacement therapy (HRT) was suggested as the primary prevention of cardiovascular disease in women. In early observational and cohort studies cardioprotective role of HRT in general seemed to be promising. However, later HERS and ERA trials showed no benefit from HRT in the reduction of death or coronary events over 4 years [34,35].

Large randomized trials, including the Women's Health Initiative (WHI), assessing the long-term effect of various HRT regimens on coronary and non-coronary outcomes among women, demonstrated an increased risk of nonfatal MI, of death from coronary disease, excess risk of stroke and of venous thromboembolism, resulting in an over-all increased relative risk of an adverse outcome from cardiovascular disease of 22%. At present the use of HRT is not recommended in postmenopausal women. The evidences to recommend for or against the use of unopposed estrogen for chronic disease prevention in women after hysterectomy are inconclusive [36,37]. Combined continuous HRT treatment is advised for distressing menopausal symptoms, but not routinely for all postmenopausal women. The slightly increased risk of cardiovascular disease and breast cancer outweigh the benefits in asymptomatic women. HRT should not be used in postmenopausal women to prevent future cardiovascular events. For distressing postmenopausal symptoms women should take HRT as short as possible and to use the lowest effective dose [37].

Conclusions

Biologically women are less likely to develop ACS at younger ages than men. When they have an ACS at a younger age then it is more likely unstable angina than ST-elevation or non-ST-elevation MI. The onset of MI is about 10 years later than in men in spite of more comorbitities such as diabetes, arterial hypertension, obesity and dyslipidemias. Women are less agressively treated than men, though coronary angiography demonstrates usually less extensive and less severe coronary artery disease in all ACS forms in women. Female gender is associated with increased risk for 30-day mortality in ST-elevation MI and similar 30-day mortality in non-ST-elevation MI and even decreased risk in unstable angina in comparison to men. In women, surviving MI, the risk for long-term mortality is increased in comparison to men. In spite of being treated less agressively by invasive procedures prognosis of women with ACS in general is promising as there is even decreased 1-year mortality in comparison to men possibly due to the higher prevalence of normal coronary arteries in women with ACS as demonstated by several studies.

Regarding epidemiology the prevalence and incidence of coronary artery disease, including ACS and MI in women is still high. Fortunatelly, women are 10 years behind men in the clinical manifestation of coronary artery disease and have better prognosis than men, especially when contemporary diagnostic and therapeutic interventions are used.

References

[1]   Fox KAA, Cokkinos DV, Deckers J, Keil U, Steg PG on behalf of the ENACT. The ENACT study: A pan-european survey of acute coronary syndromes. *Eur. Heart J.* 2000; 21:1440-9.

[2]   Fox KAA, Goodman SG, Klein W, Brieger D, Steg PG, Dabbous O, Avezum A for the GRACE Investigators. Management of acute coronary syndromes. Vaiations in practice and outcome. Findings from the Global Registry of Acute Coronary Events (GRACE). *Eur. Heart J.* 2002; 23:1177-89.

[3]   Hasdai D, Behar S, Wallentin L, Dauchin N, Gitt AK, Boersma E, Fioretti PM, Simoons ML, Battler AA. Prospective survey of the characteristics, treatments and outcomes of patients with acute coronary syndromes in Europe and the Mediterranean basin. The Euro Heart Survey of Acute Coronary Syndromes (Euro Heart Survey ACS). *Eur. Heart J.* 2002; 23:1190-201.

[4]   Thom T, Haase N, Rosamond W, Howard VJ, Runsfeld J, Manolio T, Zheng Z-J, Flegal K, O'Donnell C, Kittnet S, Lloyd-Jones D, Goff DC, Hong Y, Members of the statistics committee and stroke statistics subcommittee, Adams R, Friday G, Furie K, Gorelick P, Kissela B, Marler J, Meigs J, Roger V, Sidney S, Sorlie P, Steinberger J, Wasserthiel-Smoller S, Wilson M and Wolf P. Heart Disease and stroke statistics – 2006 update: a report from the American Heart Association statistics committee and stroke statistics subcommittee. *Circulation* 2006; 113:85-151.

[5]   Rosamond W, Flegal K, Friday G, Ho M, Howard V, Kissela B, Kittner S, Lloyd-Jones D, McDermott M, Meigs J, Moy C, Nichol G, O'Donnell CJ, Roger V, Rumsfeld J, Sorlie P, Steinberger J, Thom T, Wasserthiel-Smoller S, Hong Y, for the American Heart Association statistics committee and stroke statistics subcommittee. Heart disease and stroke statistics -2007 update. A report from the American Heart Association statistics committee and stroke subcommittee. *Circulation* 2006; 115:69-171.

[6]   Wenger NK, Shaw LJ, Vaccario V. Coronary heart disease in women: Update 2008. *Clin. Pharmacol. Ther.* 2007 Nov 28 [Epub ahead of print].

[7]   Taylor MJ, Scuffham PA, McCollam P, Newby DE. Acute coronary syndromes in Europe: 1-year costs and outcomes. *Curr. Med. Res. Opin.* 2007; 23:495-503.

[8]   Rosengren A, Wallentin L, Gitt AK, Behar S, Battler A, Hasdai D. Sex, age, and clinical presentation of acute coronary syndromes. *Eur. Heart J.* 2004; 25:663-70.

[9]   Third International Study of Infarct Survival (ISIS-3) Collaborative Group. A randomized trial of streptokinase vs tissue plasminogen activator vs anistreplase and of aspirin plus heparin vs aspirin alone among 41,299 cases of suspected acute myocardial infarction. *Lancet* 1992; 339:753-70.

[10]   The GUSTO Investigators. An international randomized trial comparing four thrombolytic strategies for acute myocardial infarction. *N Engl. J. Med.* 1993; 329:673-82.

[11]   Fibrinolytic Therapy Trialists Collaborative Group. Indications for fibrinolytic therapy in suspected acute myocardial infarction: collaborative overview of early mortality and major morbidity result from all randomized trials of more than 1000 patients. *Lancet* 1994; 343:311–22.

[12] Erhardt L, Herlitz J, Bossaert L, Halinen M, Keltai M., Koster R., Marcassa C, Quinn T and van Weert H.. Chest Pain (Management of). *Eur. Heart J.* 2002; 23:1153-76.

[13] Van de Werf F, Ardissino D, Betriu A, Cokkinos DV, Falk E, Fox KAA, Julian D, Lengyel M, Neumann FJ, Ruzyllo W, Thygesen C, Underwood RS, Vahanian A, Verheugt FWA, Wijns W. Management of acute myocardial infarction in patients presenting with ST-segment elevation. *Eur. Heart J.* 2003; 24:28-66.

[14] Bassand JP, Hamm CW, Ardissino D, Boersma E, Budaj A, Fernandez-Aviles F, Fox KAA, Hasdai D, Ohman EM, Wallentin L, Wijns W. Non-ST-segment Elevation Acute Coronary Syndromes (Guidelines for the Diagnosis and Treatment of. *Eur. Heart J.* 2008; 28:1598-660.

[15] Hochman JS, Tammis JE, Thompson TD, et al for the global use of strategies to open occluded coronary arteries in acute coronary syndromes IIb investigators. Sex, clinical presentation, and outcome in patients with acute coronary syndromes. *N Engl. J. Med.* 1999; 341:226-32.

[16] Hochman JS, McCabe CH, Stone PS, et al. for the TIMI investigators. Outcome and profile of women and men presenting with acute coronary syndromes: a report from TIMI IIIB. *J. Am. Coll Cardiol* 1997; 30:141-8

[17] Kaul P, Chang WC, Westrhout C, Graham MM, Armstrong PW. Differences in admission rates and outcomes between men and women presenting to emergency departments with coronary syndromes. *CMAJ* 2007; 177:1193-9.

[18] Mueller C, Neumann F-J, Roskamm H, et al. Women do have an improved long-term outcome after non-ST-elevation acute coronary syndromes treated very early and predominantly with percutaneous coronary intervention. *J. Am. Coll Cardiol.* 2002; 40:245-50

[19] Roger VL, Farkouh ME, Weston SA, et al. Sex differences in evaluation and outcome of unstable angina. *JAMA* 2000; 283:646-52.

[20] Lagerquist B, Safstrom K, Stahle E, Wallentin L, Swahn E and the FRISC II Study Group Investigators. Is early invasive treatment of unstable coronary artery disease equally effective for both women and men? *J. Am. Coll Cardiol.* 2001; 38:41-8.

[21] Chang W-C, Kaul P, Westerhout CM, Graham MM, Fu Y, Chowdbury T, Armstrong PW. Impact of sex on long-term mortality from acute myocardial infarction vs unstable angina. *Arch Intern. Med.* 2003; 163:2476-84.

[22] Sinkovic A, Marinsek M, Svensek F. Women and men with unstable angina and/or non-ST-elevation myocardial infarction. *Wien Klin Wochenschr* 2006; 118(Suppl): 52-57.

[23] Bowker TJ, Turner RM, Wood DA, et al. A national survey of acute myocardial infarction and ischemia (SAMII) in the U.K.: characteristics, management and in-hospital outcome in women compared to men in patients under 70 years. *Eur. Heart J.* 2000; 21:1458-63.

[24] Glaser R, Herrmann HC, Murphy SA, et al. Benefit of an early invasive management strategy in women with acute coronary syndromes. *JAMA* 2002; 288:3124-29.

[25] Stangl V, Baumann G and Stangl K. Coronary atherogenic risk factors in women. *Eur. Heart J.* 2002; 23:1738-52.

[26] Patel H, Rosengren A, Ekman I. Symproms in acute coronary syndromes: Does sex make a difference? *Am. Heart J.* 2004; 148:27-33.

[27] Fodor JG, Tzerovska R, Dorner T and Rieder A. Do we diagnose and treat coronary heart disease differently in men and women. *Wien Med. Wochenschr* 2004; 154:423-5.

[28] Andreotti F, Conti E, Sanna T, Crea F, Zecchi P,Maseri A. Acute coronary syndromes in women: pathophysiology and therapeutic options. *Cardiologia* 1999; 44(suppl 19):511-4.

[29] De Von HA, Johnson Zerwic J. Symptoms of acute coronary syndrome: are there gender differences? A review of the literature. *Heart Lung* 2002; 31:235-45.

[30] Wiviott SD, Cannon CP, Morrow DA, Murphy SA, Gibson CM, McCabe CH, Sabatine MS, Rifai N, Giugliano RP, DiBattiste PM, Demopoulos LA, Antmann EM, Braunwald E. Diffential expression of cardiac biomarkers by gender in patients with unstable angina/non-ST-elevation myocardial infarction. A TACTICS-TIMI 18 (treat angina with aggrastat and determine cost of therapy with an invasive or conservative strategy – thrombolysis in myocardial infarction 18) substudy. *Circulation* 2004; 109:580-6.

[31] Klein W. Gender differences in clinical trials in coronary heart disease: response to drug therapy. *Eur. Hear J.* 1996; 17:1786-90.

[32] Feldman T, Silver R. Gender differences and the outcome of interventions for acute coronary syndromes. *Cardiol Review* 2000; 8:240-7.

[33] Scheifer SE, Arora UK, Gersh BJ, Weissman NJ: Sex differences in morphology of coronary artery plaque assessed by intravascular ultrasound. Coron Artery Dis 2001;12:17-20.

[34] Hulley S, Grady D, Bush TL, Furberg CD, Herrington DM, Riggs B, et al. Randomized trial of estrogen plus progestin for secondary prevention of coronary heart disease in postmenopausal women. *JAMA* 1998; 280:605-13.

[35] Herrington DM, Reboussin DM, Brosnihan KB, Sharp PC, Shumaker SA, Snyder TE, et al. Effects of estrogen replacement on the progression of coronary-artery atherosclerosis. *N Engl. J. Med.* 2000; 343:522-9.

[36] US Preventive Services Task Force. Postmenopausal hormone replacement therapy for the primary prevention of chronic conditions: recommendations and rationale. Rockville (MD): The Task Force; 2002. Available: www.ahrq.gov/clinic/3rduspstf/hrt/hrtrr.htm

[37] Abramson BL, Derzko C, Lalonde A, Reid R, Turek M, Wielgosz A. Hormone replacement therapy and cardiovascular disease: a joint statement. *Can. J. Cardiol.* 2002; 18:723-4.

In: Heart Disease in Women
Editor: B. V. Larner and H. R. Pennelton

ISBN 978-1-60692-066-4
© 2009 Nova Science Publishers, Inc.

Chapter X

The Effects of Aging on the Electrophysiological Properties of the Atrial Myocardium in Women with and without Paroxysmal Atrial Fibrillation

Osmar Antonio Centurión, Akihiko Shimizu and Shojiro Isomoto*

Division of Electrophysiology and Arrhythmias, Cardiovascular Institute,
Sanatorio Migone-Battilana, Asunción, Paraguay

Abstract

Introduction: The presence of electrophysiological abnormalities of the atrial myocardium with increasing age could explain the differences in the genesis of atrial fibrillation in women with paroxysmal atrial fibrillation (PAF). Aging could influence not only the atrial response to premature atrial depolarizations but also the morphology of atrial electrograms.

Material and Methods: Programmed atrial stimulation with single extrastimulus was performed in 102 female patients, 48 of them had normal sinus node function and did not have PAF (Group I), and 54 of them had PAF, idiopathic or associated to other arrhythmias (Group II). Programmed atrial stimulation was performed from the right atrial appendage at double diastolic threshold with stimulus duration of 2 ms with a computarized cardiac stimulator.

Results: The incidence of induction of repetitive atrial firing (68% vs 36%; $p<0.02$), fragmented atrial activity (85% vs 47%; $p<0.005$), and sustained PAF (43% vs 5%; $p<0.001$) was significantly higher in Group II than in Group I. The zone of induction of repetitive atrial firing (34 ± 33 vs 10 ± 19 ms; $p<0.005$), fragmented atrial activity (49 ± 40 vs 12 ± 15 ms; $p<0.001$), and interatrial conduction delay (51 ± 32 vs 26 ± 28 ms; $p<0.02$) was significantly wider in Group II than in Group I. The induction rate and the respective

---

* Address for correspondence: Osmar Antonio Centurión, Eligio Ayala 1293. Asunción, Paraguay,FAX: 595-21-205630,E-mail: osmar@rieder.net.py.

zones of these electrophysiologic parameters had a significantly positive correlation with age in Group II.

Conclusions: Our results shed light on the mechanisms responsible for developing atrial fibrillation in aging women. The electrophysiological indicators of augmented atrial vulnerability are significantly altered with increasing age in women with paroxysmal atrial fibrillation. There is a significantly greater predisposition to atrial fibrillation in aging women because they develop a significantly greater augmented atrial vulnerability with increasing age.

Key words: Paroxysmal atrial fibrillation, repetitive atrial firing, fragmented atrial activity, interatrial conduction delay, atrial vulnerability in women

Introduction

The everchanging technology and novel approaches to diagnosis and treatment of diseases has led to a growing number of elderly people. It is estimated that about 25% of the population worldwide will be over 65 years old by year 2035 [1-5]. It is very difficult to attribute a certain condition to the aging process because it is often impossible to separate physiological aging from the development of pathological changes due to a comorbid disease. The atrial myocardial cells in the elderly appear to be more susceptible to arrhythmias when calcium homeostasis is disturbed and especially under certain conditions that enhance calcium loading. Experimental studies clearly suggest that overload in ionized calcium in the senescent human atrial myocardial cells may play an important role in arrhythmogenesis [6, 7].

Strong evidence of abnormalities of the conduction system in an apparently healthy elderly population has been demonstrated. Prolongation of the PR interval, high prevalence of atrioventricular nodal and His-Purkinje disease, and unexplained sinus node abnormalities were consistently found in older apparently healthy individuals [8-11]. It is well known that atrial fibrillation is not an electrophysiologically homogeneous process. There are several predisposing factors which may provide the background for this tachyarrhythmia to occur. Elderly subjects are particularly prone to develop atrial fibrillation, and changes of the atrial muscle with advancing age may be a factor accounting for this phenomenon. It was reported that atrial fibrillation in some aged patients was associated with loss of muscle fibers in the sinoatrial node and its approaches without any clear pathological cause [12]. Muscle loss with advancing age was found to be accompanied by an increase in fibrous tissue in both the sinoatrial node and the internodal tracts [12-16]. It was strongly suggested that muscle loss and increase of fibrosis in the atria is a slow but continuous process starting around 60 years of age [14]. Since aging has a profound effect on structural changes of the atrial muscle, it seems reasonable to assume that there may be detectable age induced changes in atrial electrophysiological properties in women. Therefore, we performed programmed atrial stimulation with single extrastimulus and analyzed the atrial vulnerability and atrial responses, namely, repetitive atrial firing, fragmented atrial activity, interatrial conduction delay and their respective zones of induction in women with and without PAF. To our best knowledge, this is the first study designed to clarify the influence of advancing age on the electrophysiological properties of the atrial myocardium in women with and without paroxysmal atrial fibrillation.

Material and Methods

Study Patients

One hundred and two nonconsecutive patients referred to the Nagasaki University Hospital and Sanatorio Migone Battilana for electrophysiological evaluation of their arrhythmias underwent detailed programmed atrial stimulation that was performed from the right atrial appendage at double diastolic threshold with stimulus duration of 2 ms with a computarized cardiac stimulator during the course of their studies. No patient with organic heart disease, or congestive heart failure was admitted in this study protocol. No patient showing atrial enlargment on echocardiography was included in this investigation.

The study patients comprised 102 female patients, 48 of them had normal sinus node function and did not have atrial fibrillation (Group I). The age in group I ranged from 18 to 83 years and the mean age was 55.8±16.5. In this Group I, there were 27 patients with atrioventricular nodal reentrant tachycardia, 16 had the Wolff-Parkinson-White syndrome, and the remaining 5 had ventricular tachycardia. On the other hand, 54 female patients had paroxysmal atrial fibrillation, idiopathic or associated to other arrhythmias (Group II). The age in group II ranged from 19 to 80 years and the mean age was 57.0±14.1. In this Group II, there were 28 patients with idiopathic PAF, 16 patients with sick sinus syndrome, and the remaining 10 had the Wolff-Parkinson-White syndrome. The PAF of all the patients in Group II was well documented by means of conventional electrocardiography (ECG), bedside ECG monitoring, or at least two ambulatory 24 hs Holter recordings. The sinus node recovery time was measured in all patients after an atrial overdrive pacing at rates of 70 to 210/min, for a period of one minute at each level [17, 18].

Electrophysiologic Study

All patients were studied in the postabsortive, nonsedated state after they had given informed consent. The present investigation complies with the declaration of Helsinki. Electrophysiologic evaluation was performed after approval of the study plan by the regional Ethics Committee. All drugs were discontinued at least 72 hours before the procedure. No patient received amiodarone.

The Programmed atrial stimulation protocol was performed with cuadripolar catheter electrodes (N° 6F USCI, Div. C.R. Bard, Billerrica, MA, USA) that were inserted percutaneously into the femoral and subclavian veins and were advanced into the heart under fluoroscopic guidance. The distance between the electrodes was 10 mm and the width of the electrode ring was 2 mm. All the right atrial endocardial electrograms were recorded during sinus rhythm at a fixed gain setting accompanied by a 0.2 mV=3 mm calibration signal, and were filtered at 50 to 1000 Hz. The baseline of recordings was stable for each patient. The atrial endocardial electrogram and three surface ECGs (I, aVF, V1) were displayed on a multichannel oscilloscope (polygraph MIC-8800T, Fukuda-Denshi Inc., Tokyo, Japan) and simultaneously recorded at a paper speed of 100 mm/s on a twelve-channel, ink-jet recorder (Siemens-Elema 804, Siemens-Elema, Solna, Sweden). Particular attention was paid to assure that all instruments were properly isolated and grounded.

Definitions

S1 and A1 refer to the driving stimulus and the atrial electrogram, respectively, of the basic drive beat. S2 and A2 refer to the stimulus artifact and the atrial electrogram, respectively, of the induced premature beat (Figure 1). The coupling interval between S1 and S2 was decreased in 10 msec steps until S2 was no longer captured. The ERP of the right atrial appendage was defined as the longest S1-S2 interval that did not elicit an atrial depolarization. The conduction time from the stimulus artifact to the distal electrode pair placed at the coronary sinus was measured as the interatrial conduction time during a single premature stimulation performed from the right atrial appendage. The atrial response zone was defined as the range of S1-S2 intervals that resulted in the respective atrial response. When the atrial response was not induced, the respective atrial response zone was expressed as zero.

Repetitive atrial firing (RAF): According to Wyndham et al [19], repetitive atrial firing is defined as the occurrence of two or more successive atrial complexes with a return cycle of <250 msec and a subsequent cycle length of <300 msec (Figure 1).

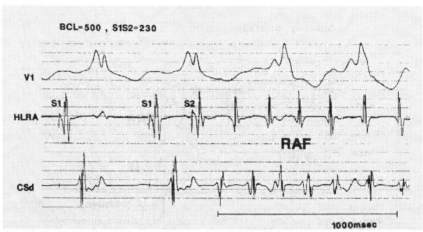

An example of the induction of repetitive atrial firing (RAF) as defined in the text. Surface electrocardiographic lead V1 is shown together with intracardiac electrograms from the high lateral right atrium (HLRA), and distal coronary sinus (CSd). S1 and S2 are, respectively, the driving and premature stimulus artifacts. The basic drive cycle length (BCL) was 500 ms and the coupling interval (S1 S2 interval) was 230 ms. Reprinted with permission from Konoe A, Fukatani M, Tanigawa M, et al. Electrophysiological abnormalities of the atrial muscle in patients with manifest Wolff-Parkinson-White syndrome associated with paroxysmal atrial fibrillation. PACE 1992;15:1040-1052.

Figure 1. Induction of repetitive atrial firing (RAF).

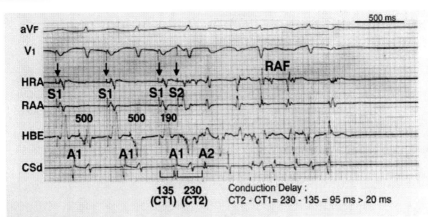

An example of the induction of fragmented atrial activity (FAA) as defined in the text. Surface electrocardiographic lead V1 is shown together with intracardiac electrograms from the high lateral right atrium (HLRA), and distal coronary sinus (CSd). S1 and S2 are, respectively, the driving and premature stimulus artifacts. The basic drive cycle length (BCL) was 500 ms and the coupling interval (S1 S2 interval) was 230 ms. There is a prolongation of the duration of atrial activity from 110 to 200 ms in the HLRA. CD indicates interatrial conduction delay. Reprinted with permission from Konoe A, Fukatani M, Tanigawa M, et al. Electrophysiological abnormalities of the atrial muscle in patients with manifest Wolff-Parkinson-White syndrome associated with paroxysmal atrial fibrillation. PACE 1992;15:1040-1052.

Figure 2. Induction of fragmented atrial activity (FAA).

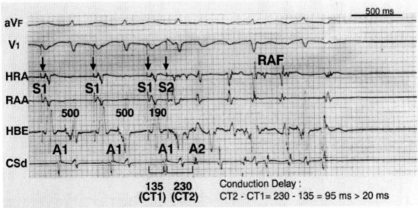

Atrial extrastimulus testing in a patient with paroxysmal AF showing atrial conduction delay (CD). S1 and A1 refer to the driving stimulus and the atrial electrogram, respectively, of the basic drive beat. S2 and A2 refer to the stimulus artifact and the atrial electrogram, respectively, of the induced premature beat. The atrial extrastimulus was programmed at a coupling interval of 190 ms with a driving cycle length of 500 ms. The S1-A1 interval in the distal coronary sinus was 135 ms. At the premature beat, S2-A2 interval prolonged to 230 msec. The maximum CD in this patient was 95 msec. This atrial CD led to repetitive atrial firing (RAF). HRA indicates high right lateral atrium; RAA, right atrial appendage; HBE, His bundle area; and CSd, distal coronary sinus. Reprinted with permission from Isomoto S, Centurión OA, Shibata R, et al. The effects of aging on the refractoriness and conduction of the atrium in patients with lone paroxysmal atrial fibrillation revealed with programmed atrial stimulation. Rev Soc Parag Cardiol 2005;3:25-30.

Figure 3. Induction of interatrial conduction delay (CD).

Fragmented atrial activity (FAA): Ohe et al. [20] defined fragmented atrial activity elicited by atrial extrastimuli as the occurrence of disorganized atrial activity >150% of the duration of the local atrial electrogram of the basic beat recorded in the RA (Figure 2).

Interatrial conduction delay (IACD): According to the definition of Shimizu et al.[21] an intra-atrial conduction delay was defined as an increase in the S2 through A2 interval of the extrastimulus ≥20 msec compared with the S_1 through A_1 of the basic drive (Figure 3).

The zones of induction of these electrophysiological parameters (RAF, FAA, IACD) were defined as the range of S1-S2 intervals that resulted in one of these parameters. Once a premature extrastimulus delivered at a critical coupling interval resulted in RAF, FAA, or IACD, earlier premature stimuli evoked them until the ERP was reached thus the zones of these electrophysiological parameters were calculated as the difference between the longest coupling interval eliciting them and the ERP. When one of these parameters was not induced, the zone was expressed as zero. The correlation between age and each of these electrophysiological parameters was investigated dividing each of the two groups by age, those less than 60 years old, and those over 60 years of age.

Data Analysis

The results are expressed as the mean values±standard deviation. Statistical significance was determined by using the student's t test for unmatched pairs. Prevalence was compared using the chi-square test. Correlation coefficients were determined by linear regression analysis.

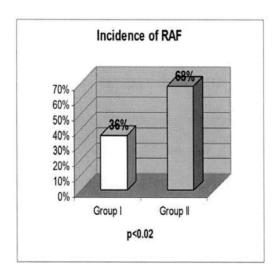 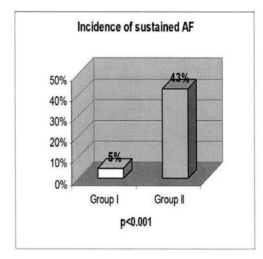

Figura 4. Incidence of induction of repetitive atrial firing (RAF), and the incidence of induction of sustained atrial fibrillation in women with paroxysmal atrial fibrillation (Group II) and women without it (Group I).

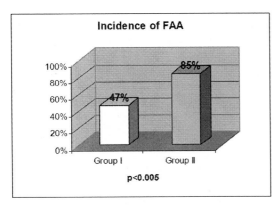 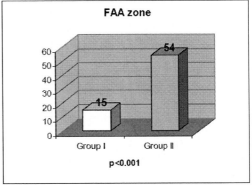

Figura 5. Incidence of induction of fragmented atrial activity (FAA), and the zone of induction of FAA in women with paroxysmal atrial fibrillation (Group II) and women without it (Group I). See text for details.

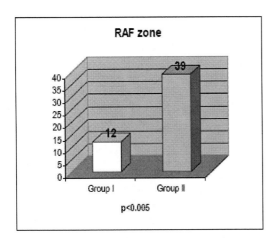 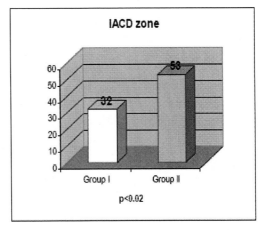

Figure 6. The zone of induction of repetitive atrial firing (RAF), and the zone of induction of interatrial conduction delay (IACD) in women with paroxysmal atrial fibrillation (Group II) and women without it (Group I). See text for details.

Results

Once a premature extrastimulus delivered at a critical coupling interval resulted in RAF, FAA, or IACD, earlier premature stimuli evoked them until the ERP was reached thus the zones of these electrophysiological parameters were calculated as the difference between the longest coupling interval eliciting them and the ERP. The incidence of induction of repetitive atrial firing (68% vs 36%; p<0.02) (Figure 4), fragmented atrial activity (85% vs 47%; p<0.005) (Figure 5), and sustained atrial fibrillation (43% vs 5%; p<0.001) was significantly higher in Group II than in Group I. The zone of induction of repetitive atrial firing (34±33 vs 10±19 ms; p<0.005), fragmented atrial activity (49±40 vs 12±15 ms; p<0.001), and interatrial conduction delay (51±32 vs 26±28 ms; p<0.02) (Figure 6) was significantly wider in Group II than in Group I.

The Influence of Age in Group I

The induction rate of repetitive atrial firing, fragmented atrial activity, and interatrial conduction delay and their respective zones of induction did not show a significant correlation with age in women from Group I. However, the longest coupling interval of the extrastimulus that induced these electrophysiologic parameters showed a slightly significant positive correlation with age in women from Group I. The longest coupling interval that induced RAF had a correlation coefficient (r) of r=0.417 <0.01. The longest coupling interval that induced FAA had a correlation coefficient (r) of r=0.567 <0.01. The longest coupling interval that induced IACD had a correlation coefficient (r) of r=0.453 <0.01 in women from Group I.

The Influence of Age in Group II

The induction rate of repetitive atrial firing, fragmented atrial activity, and interatrial conduction delay and their respective zones of induction showed a significant correlation with age in women with PAF. The longest coupling interval of the extrastimulus that induced these electrophysiologic parameters showed a significant positive correlation with age in women with PAF. The longest coupling interval that induced RAF had a correlation coefficient (r) of r=0.624 <0.001. The longest coupling interval that induced FAA had a correlation coefficient (r) of r=0.683 <0.001. The longest coupling interval that induced IACD had a correlation coefficient (r) of r=0.537 <0.005 in women with PAF.

Discussion

More successful recognition and treatment of cardiovascular risk factors and diseases continues to decrease mortality and increase the proportion of elderly population. Ecocardiographic measurements performed in elderly patients confirm the histologic evidence of increasing prevalence of left ventricular wall hypertrophy in aging population. The resulting left ventricular diastolic dysfunction with aging may increase the size of the left atrium predisposing elderly patients to develop atrial fibrillation. However, none of our study patients had atrial enlargement on echocardiography. Some investigators have observed that normal histological changes in the atrial muscle occur with advancing age. These include a reduction in the number of myocardial cells within the sinus node, a generalized loss of atrial myocardial fibers in the vicinity of the internodal tracts, as well as an increase in the quantity of connective tissue which leads to an apparent loss of myocardial fiber continuity [12-14]. The process of aging and its effect on the histologic appearance of the conduction system of the heart have been scantly described. It is very difficult to attribute a certain condition to the aging process because it is often impossible to separate physiological aging from the development of pathological changes due to a comorbid disease. Atrial fibrillation is a common arrhythmia, and its incidence rise sharply with age. The increase in prevalence of AF in older persons has been reported to be associated with degeneration of the atrial muscle. [22-24]. Spach and Dolber [24] found evidence in the human atrial muscle of age-related electrical uncoupling of the side-to-side connections between bundles, related to the proliferation of extensive collagenous tissue septa in intracellular spaces. We have previously demonstrated that aging affects the electrophysiological properties of the atrial muscle induced by programmed atrial stimulation in the patients without documented episodes of AF [22], which may agree with the findings obtained from pathological studies. On the other hand, the effect of aging on the atrial electrophysiological properties in women with paroxysmal AF is unclear.

Abnormal responses of the atrium can be elicited by programmed stimulation, such as repetitive atrial firing, fragmented atrial activity, and intraatrial conduction delay, and have been observed more frequently in patients with PAF than in those without it [25-28]. Shorter atrial effective refractory period has been also shown to be of electrophysiological significance in the genesis of AF [28]. An understanding of these electrophysiological abnormalities is important when choosing effective antiarrhythmic agents against AF. Davies and Pomerance reported that atrial fibrillation in some aged patients was associated with loss of muscle fibers in the sinoatrial node and its approaches without any clear pathological cause [12]. Erickson and Lev have shown degenerative changes in the conduction system with age [29].

It was demonstrated a clinical evidence of abnormalities of the conduction system in an apparently healthy elderly population. Prolongation of the PR interval, high prevalence of atrioventricular nodal and His-Purkinje disease, and unexplained sinus node abnormalities were consistently found in older apparently healthy individuals [8-11]. With this histological and clinical background in mind, changes in the electrophysiologic properties of the atrial muscle with advancing age can be anticipated to be observed in elderly women. As a matter of fact, dispersion and lengthening of atrial refractoriness with aging have been reported [29-31]. The demonstration of electrophysiologic changes in the atrial muscle with age [32-34] is consistent with the concept that electrophysiologic functional changes are related to histologic changes of the conduction system of the heart with advancing age. It was suggested that aging modifies atrial refractoriness in a nonuniform manner, inducing a progressing increment of dispersion of atrial refractoriness [30-37]. It was reported that aging induces a lengthening of atrial refractoriness only at the high right atrium, but not at the mid and low right atrium. It was also demonstrated a nonuniform anisotropic atrium with advancing age [23, 24]. However, the influence of age on the electrophysiological properties of the atrial myocardium in women with and without paroxysmal atrial fibrillation has not been described so far. Our results indicate that aging also influences the characteristics of several parameters of atrial vulnerability in women with and without paroxysmal atrial fibrillation.

In the present study, we have found a significantly higher incidence of induction of repetitive atrial firing, fragmented atrial activity, and sustained atrial fibrillation in women with paroxysmal atrial fibrillation than in women without it. The zone of induction of repetitive atrial firing, fragmented atrial activity, and interatrial conduction delay was also significantly wider in women with PAF than in women without it. Our previous studies have demonstrated that these electrophysiological parameters of atrial vulnerability are good indices of a tendency to develop AF [38-44]. We have also found that the induction rate of repetitive atrial firing, fragmented atrial activity, and interatrial conduction delay and their respective zones of induction showed a significant correlation with age in women with PAF. The longest coupling interval of the extrastimulus that induced these electrophysiologic parameters also showed a significant positive correlation with age in women with PAF.

There are certain limitations that should be considered. First, only the right atrial ERP was measured, and therefore the atrial responses of other areas of the atrium to programmed pacing are unknown. Second, the control subjects in the present study were not really "normal" since they all suffered from some form of arrhythmia and about one third of them had WPW syndrome. Patients with an anomalous atrioventricular connection are known to have predisposition to develop PAF [45-52]. However, there was no clinical evidence of PAF in any of these WPW patients of the Group I. Although we performed at least two ambulatory 24 hs ECG Holter recordings, several conventional ECG and bedside ECG monitoring, PAF was not detected in these patients. Third, it is well established that asymptomatic episodes are common in patients with AF [53, 54], and clinical evaluation based on the presence or absence of documented AF may be of limited value. However, these are common limitations in many studies. Besides these mentioned limitations, the present study demonstrated a significantly higher atrial vulnerability in women with PAF than in women without it. Although there is a better understanding in the genesis of AF in these days, the precise pathophysiological bases for AF initiation and maintenance have not been resolved yet. As newer and more sophisticated technology become available, controversies about AF genesis have reemerged. New advances may be relevant to the ultimate understanding of the mechanisms of AF initiation by the interaction of the propagating wavefronts with anatomic or functional obstacles in their paths.

Conclusions

Our results shed light on the mechanisms responsible for developing atrial fibrillation in aging women. The electrophysiological indicators of augmented atrial vulnerability are significantly altered with increasing age in women with paroxysmal atrial fibrillation. There is a significantly greater predisposition to atrial fibrillation in aging women because they develop a significantly greater augmented atrial vulnerability with increasing age.

References

[1]   Selzer A. Atrial fibrillation revisited. *N Engl. J. Med.* 1982;306:1044-1045.
[2]   Albers GW, Atwood JE, Hirsh J, et al. Stroke prevention in nonvalvular atrial fibrillation. *Ann. Intern. Med.* 1991;115:726-727.

[3]   Kannek WB, Abbot RD, Savage DD, et al. Epidemiologic features of chronic atrial fibrillation: The Framingham study. *N Engl. J. Med.* 1982;306:1018-1022.

[4]   Feinberg WM, Blackshear JL, Laupacis A, et al. Prevalence, age distribution, and gender of patients with atrial fibrillation: Analysis and implications. *Arch Intern. Med.* 1995;155:469-473.

[5]   Laupacis A, Albers G, Dalen J, et al. Antithrombotic therapy in atrial fibrillation. *CHEST* 1998;114:579S-589S.

[6]   Escande D, Coulombe A, Faibre JF, et al. Two types of transient outward currents in adult human atrial cells. *Am. J. Physiol.* 1987;252:142H-148H.

[7]   Van wagoner DR, Pond AL, McCarthy PM, et al. Outward K+ current densities and Kv 1.5 expression are reduced in chronic human atrial fibrillation. *Circ. Res.* 1997;80:772-781.

[8]   Fleg JL, Dhirenda ND, Lakatta EG. Right bundle branch block: Long term prognosis in apparently healthy men. *J. Am. Coll Cardiol.* 1983;1:887-892.

[9]   Fleg JL, Kennedy HL. Cardiac arrhythmias in a healthy elderly population. *CHEST* 1982;81:302-307.

[10]   Tresh DD, Fleg JL. Unexplained sinus bradycardia: Clinical significance and long-term prognosis in apparently healthy persons older than 40 years. *Am. J. Cardiol.* 1986;58:1009-1013.

[11]   Maurer MS, Shefrin EA, Fleg JL. Prevalence and prognostic significance of exercise induced supraventricular tachycardia in apparently healthy volunteers. *Am. J. Cardiol.* 1995;75:788-792.

[12]   Davies M.J., Pomerance A. Pathology of atrial fibrillation in man. *Br. Heart J.* 1972; 34:520-25.

[13]   Lev M. Aging changes in the human sinoatrial node. *J. Geront* 1954; 9:1.

[14]   Davies M.J., Pomerance A. Quantitative study of aging changes in the human sinoatrial node and aintenodal tracts. *Br. Heart J.* 1972; 34:150-152.

[15]   Hudson REB. The human pacemarker and its pathology. *Br. Heart J.* 1960; 22: 153.

[16]   Centurion O.A., Fukatani M., Konoe A., Tanigawa M., Shimizu A., Isomoto S., Kaibara M., Hashiba K. Different distribution of abnormal endocardial electrograms within the right atrium in patients with sick sinus syndrome. *Br. Heart J.* 1992; 68: 596-600.

[17]   Mandel W., Hayakawa H., Danzig R., Marcus H. S. Evaluation of sino-atrial node function in man by overdrive suppression. *Circulation* 1971; 44: 59-65.

[18]   Narula O. S., Samet P., Javier R. P. Significance of the sinus node recovery time. *Circulation* 1972; 45: 140-158.

[19]   Wyndham C, Amat-y-Leon F, Wu D, Denes P, Dhingra R, Simpson R, Rosen KM. Effects of cycle length on atrial vulnerability. *Circulation* 1977;55:260-267.

[20]   Ohe T, Matsuhisa M, Kamakura S, Yamada J, Sato I, Nakajima K. Relation between the widening of the fragmented atrial activity zone and atrial fibrillation. *Am. J. Cardiol.* 1953;53:1219-22.

[21]   Shimizu A, Fukatani M, Tanigawa M, Mon M, Hashiba K. Intra-atrial conduction delay and fragmented atrial activity in patients with paroxysmal atrial fibrillation. *Jpn. Circ. J.* 1959;53:1023-30.

[22] Isomoto S., Fukatani M., Shimizu A., Konoe A., Tanigawa M., Centurion O.A., Seto S. et al. The influence of advancing age on the electrophysiological changes of the atrial muscle induced by programmed atrial stimulation. *Jpn. Circ. J.* 1.992; 56: 776-82.

[23] Spach M. S., Dolber P. C. anderson P. A. W. Multiple regional differences in cellular properties that regulate repolarization and contraction in the right atrium of adult and newborn dogs. *Circ. Res.* 1.989; 65: 1.594-1.611.

[24] Spach M. S., Dolber P. C. Relating extracellular potentials and their derivatives to anisotropic propagation at microscopic level in human cardiac muscle. Evidence for electrical uncoupling of side-to-side fiber connections with increasing age. *Circ. Res.* 1.986; 58: 356-371.

[25] Kumagai K, Akimitsu S, Kamahira K, Kawahira K, Kawanami F, Yamanouchi Y, Hiroki T, Arakawa K. Electrophysiological properties in chronic lone atrial fibrillation. *Circulation* 1991;84:1662-8.

[26] Centurion GA, Isomoto S, Fukatani M, Shimizu A, Konoe A, Tanigawa M, Kaibara M, Sakamoto R, Hano O, Hirata T, Yano K. Relationship between atrial conduction defects and fractionated atrial endocardial electrograms in patients with sick sinus syndrome. *PACE* 1993:16:2022-33.

[27] Centurion OA, Shimizu A, Isomoto S, Konoe A, Hirata T, Hano O, Kaibara M, Yano K. Repetitive atrial firing and fragmented atrial activity elicited by extrastimuli in the sick sinus syndrome with and without abnormal atrial electrograms. *Am. J. Med. Sci.* 1994;307:247-54.

[28] Cosio FG, Palacios J, Vidal JM, Cocina EG, Gomez-Sanchez MA, Tamargo L. Electrophysiologic studies in atrial fibrillation. Slow conduction of premature impulses: a possible manifestation of the background for reentry. *Am. J. Cardiol.* 1953;51:122-30.

[29] Erickson E.E., Lev M. Aging changes in the human AV node, bundle and bundle branches. *J. Gerontol* 1.952; 7: 1.

[30] Michelucci A., Padeletti L., Fradella G.A., Lova R. M., Monizzi D., Giomo A., Fantini F. Ageing and atrial electrophysiologic properties in man. Int. *J. Cardiol* 1.984; 5: 75-81.

[31] Dubrow I. W. Fisher E. A., Denes P., Hastreiter A. R. The influence of age on cardiac refractory periods in man. *Pediatr. Res.* 1.976; 10: 135-139.

[32] Roberts N. G., Gillette P. C. Electrophysiologic study of the conduction system in normal children. *Pediatrics* 1.977; 60: 858-63.

[33] Escande D., Loisance D., Planche C., Coraboeuf E. Age-related changes of action potential plateau shape in isolated human atrial fibers. *An J. Physiol.* 1.985; 249: H843-H850.

[34] Centurión OA, Shimizu A, Isomoto S, Konoe A, Kaibara M, Hayano M, et al. Influence of advancing age on fractionated right atrial endocardial electrograms. *Am. J. Cardiol.* 2005;96:239-242.

[35] Spach M, Miller WT, Geselowitz DB, Barr RC, Kootsey JM, Johnson EA. The discontinuous nature of propagation in normal canine cardiac muscle: evidence for recurrent discontinuities of intracellular resistance that affect the membrane currents. *Circ. Res.* 1951;45:39-54.

[36] Spach MS, Miller WT, Dolber PC, Kootsey JM, Sommer JR, Mosher CE Jr.: The functional role of structural complexities in the propagation of depolarization in the atrium of the dog: cardiac conduction disturbances due to discontinuities of effective axial resistivity. *Circ. Res.* 1952;50:175-91.

[37] Spach MS, Barr RC, Serwer GA, Kootsey JM, Johnson EA. Extracellular potential related to intracellular action potentials in the dog Purkinje system. *Circ. Res.* 1972;30:505-11.

[38] Shimizu A, Konoe A, Tanigawa M, Isomoto S, Fukatani M, Centurion OA, Yano K, Hashiba K. Electrophysiologic characteristics of repetitive atrial firing: atrial extrastimulus at four sites. *Jpn. J. Cardiac. Pacing Electrophysiol.* 1993;9:126-31.

[39] Hashiba K, Centurión OA, Shimizu A. Electrophysiologic of human atrial muscle in paroxysmal atrial fibrillation. *Am. Heart J.* 1996;131:778-789.

[40] Shimizu A, Centurión OA. Electrophysiological properties of the human atrium in atrial fibrillation. *Cardiovasc. Res.* 2002;54:302-314.

[41] Shimizu A, Fukatani M, Tanigawa M, Kaibara M, Konoe A, Isomoto S, Centurion GA, Yano K, Hashiba K. Mechanism of the suppression of repetitive atrial firing by isoproterenol: comparison with disopyramide. *Int. J. Cardiol.* 1994;43:175-83.

[42] Isomoto S, Shimizu A, Konoe A, Tanigawa M, Kaibara M, Centurion OA, et al. Effects of intravenous verapamil on atrial vulnerability. *Jpn. Circ. J.* 1994;58:1-8.

[43] Shimizu A, Fukatani M, Konoe A, Isomoto S, Centurion OA, Yano K. Electrophysiologic effects of new class III antiarrhythmic agent (E4031) on the conduction and refractoriness of the in-vivo human atrium. *Cardiovasc. Res.* 1993;27:1333-8.

[44] Centurion OA, Isomoto S, Shimizu A, Konoe A, Kaibara M, Hirata T, et al. The effects of aging on atrial endocardial electrograms in patients with paroxysmal atrial fibrillation. *Clin. Cardiol.* 2003;26:435-438.

[45] Konoe A, Fukatani M, Tanigawa M, Isomoto S, Kadena M, Sakamoto T, et al. Electrophysiological abnormalities of the atrial muscle in patients with manifest Wolff-Parkinson-White syndrome associated with paroxysmal atrial fibrillation. *Pacing Clin. Electrophysiol.* 1992;15:1040-1052.

[46] Sarubbi B. The Wolff-Parkinson-White electrocardiogram pattern in athletes: how and when to evaluate the risk for dangerous arrhythmias: The opinion of the paediatric cardiologist. *J. Cardiovasc. Med.* 2006;7(4):271-278.

[47] Aytemir K, Amasyali B, Kose S, Kilic A, Abali G, Oto A, et al. Maximum P-wave duration and P-wave dispersion predict recurrence of paroxysmal atrial fibrillation in patients with Wolff-Parkinson-White syndrome after successful radiofrequency catheter ablation. *J. Interv. Card Electrophysiol.* 2004;11:21-7.

[48] Hamada T, Hiraki T, Ikeda H, Kubara I, Yoshida T, Ohga M, et al. Mechanism for atrial fibrillation in patients with Wolff-Parkinson-White syndrome. *J. Cardiovasc. Electrophysiol.* 2002;13:223-229.

[49] Zhang Y, Wang L. Atrial vulnerability is a major mechanism of paroxysmal atrial fibrillation in patients with Wolff-Parkinson-White syndrome. *Med. Hypotheses.* 2006;67:1345-1347.

[50] Hsieh MH, Tai CT, Chiang CE, Tsai CF, Chen YJ, Chan P, et al. Double atrial potentials recorded in the coronary sinus in patients with Wolff-Parkinson-White syndrome: a possible mechanism of induced atrial fibrillation. *J. Interv. Card Electrophysiol.* 2004;11:97-103.

[51] Kalarus Z, Kowalski O, Lenarczyk R, Prokopczuc J, Pasyk S. Electrophysiological features of orthodromic atrioventricular reentry tachycardia in patients with Wolff-Parkinson-White syndrome and atrial fibrillation. *PACE* 2003;26:1479-1488.

[52] Soylu M, Demir AD, Ozdemir O, Soylu O, Topaloglu S, Korkmaz S, et al. Increased P wave dispersion after the radiofrequency catheter ablation in overt preexcitation patients: The role of atrial vulnerability. *Int. J. Cardiol.* 2004;95:167-170.

[53] Yamashita T, Murakawa Y, Hayami N, Sezaki K, Inoue M, Fukui E, Omata M. Relation between aging and circadian variation of paroxysmal atrial fibrillation. *Am. J. Cardiol.* 1998;82;1364-1367.

[54] Page RL, Wilkinson WE, Clair WK, McCarthy EA, Pritchett EL. Asymptomatic arrhythmias in patients with symptomatic paroxysmal atrial fibrillation and paroxysmal supraventricular tachycardia. *Circulation* 1994;89:224-227.

In: Heart Disease in Women   ISBN 978-1-60692-066-4
Editor: B. V. Larner and H. R. Pennelton   © 2009 Nova Science Publishers, Inc.

Chapter XI

Women and Angina Pectoris: Emergency Department and Diagnostic Difficulties in an Undeveloped Community

Esed Omerkic[1] and Fahir Barakovic[2]

[1] Emergency, Health center Zivinice, Bosnia and Herzegovina
[2] Tuzla, Bosnia and Herzegovina

Abstract

Background: Angina pectoris is the result of myocardial ischemia caused by an imbalance between myocardial blood supply and oxygen demand. In women, more often than men, coronary heart disease may manifest with atypical presentations. Beside conventional, psychosocial factors are especially expressed in our country as risk factors which lead to disease of coronary arteries, separately in women. Diagnosing this condition in the emergency department (ED) under circumstances where an electrocardiogram (ECG) is the only one exact method that may show myocardial ischemia is very difficult. Methods and Results: In the undeveloped municipality of Zivinice the population is about 70,000 people. About 20% of them are refuges from East Bosnia, mainly women and younger people. We analyzed data in 2007 from the Emergency Department (ED) of the Health center Zivinice. ED in this year had accepted 32.570 or about 46.5% population of this community, respectively 89 patients per day. We investigated a number of patients who had a diagnosis of angina pectoris, their symptoms, risk factors and co morbidity, and which portion were female. During the time of investigation, the number of patients with conditions and risk factors to develop CHS (coronary heart disease), and symptoms which may be seen in angina pectoris, were 6.937 or 21.3%. Almost two-thirds of these patients were female with average age 61.5 (±11.2) years. During the period of research in the ED 910 women were registered with a diagnosis of stable angina pectoris. Even in 275 of these women, an electrocardiogram was performed for the first time in their life on the occasion of an examination. In eleven of them, without significant ECG changes, biomarkers of cardiac damage (troponin and creatin kynaze) were elevated and they were hospitalized under diagnoses of acute coronary syndrome. On average, refugee women develop angina pectoris for 5.4 years before domicile women. The three most frequent risk factors were menopause, hypertension and psychosocial factors; smoking was a relatively rare risk factor. Leading symptoms in these women were weakness and breathlessmess, more frequently than palpitations, and in only one woman angina pectoris was presented with chest pain. In more than two-thirds of female patients with established diagnosis of angina pectoris, the leading symptoms were atypical, compared with men where less than one-third had atypical symptoms. Conclusions: Besides presence of conventional risk factors, big role in the development of angina pectoris psychosocial factors play a big role in the development of angina pectoris especially in women refugees from Eastern Bosnia. The possibility of missed diagnoses of angina pectoris and inappropriate medical decisions is high, and their percentage in such circumstances is approximately 15%. We need to adequately reorganize emergency medical services to improve quality and quantity, together with strong support from the local community and state.

Introduction

Angina pectoris is the result of myocardial ischemia caused by an imbalance between myocardial blood supply and oxygen demand. Most patients with angina pectoris report retrosternal chest discomfort rather than chest pain.[1] Women have a slightly higher rate of mortality from coronary heart disease (CHD) compared with men, in part because of an older age at presentation and a frequent lack of classic anginal symptoms.[2] Vasospastic and microvascular angina pectoris are more frequent in women than men, as well as in syndrome X where symptoms are cleared in cases when coronary arteries are normal. The frequency of atypical presentations is also more common among women compared with men. In women, more often than men, coronary heart disease may manifest with atypical presentations, such as silent ischemia, weakness, breathlessness, palpitations, or acute coronary syndrome and sudden cardiac death.[3,4,5] Sudden cardiac death frequently is the first symptom of coronary heart disease in women.[6] The prevalence of angina pectoris increases with age that is a strong independent risk factor for mortality and is greater in women than in men. Women were 10 years older than men at the time of initial coronary heart disease and were more likely to have comorbid conditions such as diabetes and hypertension.[1,7] Low incidence of coronary heart disease in young women (≤ 40 years) may be attributed to a cardioprotective role of their hormonal status, especially estrogen. Cessation of hormonal activity of the ovaries leads to drastic increase of coronary heart disease in women. However, a consensus on the use of adjuvant hormonal therapy during menopause has not been established. Substitute hormonal therapy may be recommended during adaptation time in cases when hypertension, obesity, climacteric symptoms, osteoporosis and psychophysical activity come to reduce quality of life. In the menopausal period are registered significant disorders of serum level of lipids, blood pressures, intolerance of glucose and vascular reactions. These changes significantly increased the risk of developing coronary heart disease. Women's obesity is expressive in middle and older age, like diabetes, that significantly increases risk from a fatal event in CHD. Syndrome X is more frequent in women and understood as clear symptomatology of angina pectoris with entirely normal coronary arteries on coronarography.[1,8,9] Use of acetylsalicylic acid decreased number of cerebrovascular events in women, but not the number of myocardial infarctions.[10] CHD has been the leading cause of death in the last 30 years worldwide, causing about 12 million deaths per year. According to data from 2000[h], 983.,229 women and 967.,258 men died from CHD in Europe. In Bosnia and Herzegovina from cardiovascular disease is about 56% per year; it is the leading cause of death in general mortality.[11,12,13].Psychosocial factors are especially expressed in our country as risk factors which lead to the disease of coronary arteries, separately in women. These factors are posttraumatic stress disorders (PTSD) as consequences of war from 1992 to 1995, unemployment, being a refugee, lack of most fellow-creatures, depression, phobic anxiety and general lacking of society and social perspective.[14,15]

Methods and Results

In the undeveloped of municipality of Zivinice, there live about 70,000 people. About 20% of them are refugees from East Bosnia, mainly women and younger people. We analyzed data in 2007[t] from the Emergency Department (ED) of the Health center in Zivinice. The Emergency Department in this year accepted 32,570 or about 46.5% of the population of this community, respectively 89 patients per day, because their acute health disorders and illness, psychophysical trauma and/or exacerbation of chronic diseases. The ages of the patients were as follows: 7.882 (24.20%) were 1 to 18 years; 13.826 (42.45%) were from 19 to 65 years; and 10.862 (33.35%) of patients were over 65 years. We investigated the number of patients who had a diagnosis of angina pectoris, symptoms, risk factors and co morbidity, and determined how many were female. Physicians established a diagnosis of angina pectoris and other forms of coronary heart disease – acute coronary syndrome and sudden cardiac death - on the basis of history, symptomatology, physical examination and electrocardiogram (ECG), without the possibility of any other routine diagnostics procedures or laboratory findings of markers of myocardial ischemia or necrosis. Diagnosing these conditions under such circumstances where electrocardiogram is the only one exact method that may show myocardial ischemia is very difficult. Even in a developed country like the US, the percentage of missed diagnoses of acute coronary syndrome in EDs is 2 to 8%. ECG is useful for evaluating persons with angina pectoris, but findings are variable among them. In such circumstances where the ECG is the only one exact method for diagnosis of myocardial ischemia, the number of missed diagnoses of angina pectoris probably is very high. Indications for performing an ECG was the presence of any pain from ear to umbilicus, retrosternal chest discomfort, weakness, breathlessness, palpitations, nausea and other atypical symptoms. An ECG was performed in all patients with previous established diagnosis of diabetes, hypertension, hyperlipidemia, angina pectoris and previous myocardial infarction. In women with symptoms of anxiety, depression or panic disorders we also performed an ECG.

During the time of investigation, the number of patients with conditions and risk factors to develop CHD, and symptoms which may be seen in angina pectoris, were 6.937 or 21.3%. Almost two-thirds of these patients (4.356 or 62.8%) was female with average age 61.5

($\pm$11.2) years. In 2.905 or 66.7% women, the ECG was normal, but 1.451 or 33.3% women had changed ECG (Table 1).

Table 1. ECG changes

Sudden Cardiac Death (SCD)	6
- pulseness ventricular tachycardia (VT)	1
- ventricular fibrillation (VF)	1
- pulseness electrical activity (PEA)	1
- asystole	3
Acute Coronary Syndrome (ACS)	83
- Acute Myocardial Infarction (AMI) with ST Elevation (STEMI)	23
- Left Bundle Branch Block (LBBB) of recent origin	4
- Unstable Angina Pectoris (Horizontal ST Depression)	56
Signs of Chronic Myocardial Infarction	25
ECG signs of Stable Angina Pectoris	811
- T-wave inversion	645
- T-wave alternation	327
- Non specific changes of ST segment	255
- Changes of QRS complex	175
Others ECG changes (with and/or without ECG signs of CHD)	1.115
- Sinus tachycardia	250
- Sinus bradycardia	70
- Supraventricular extrasystole	128
- Ventricular extrasystole	70
- AV block	55
- Branch block	180
- Intraventricular disturbances of conduction	160
- Atrial flutter/fibrillation	115
- ECG signs of left ventricular hypertrophy	245
- Others (rare)	95

During 2007 were transported to the ED six female patients without vital signs of life, and there was established a diagnosis of sudden cardiac death. Witnesses and escort are not offering any form of life support to these women. Average time from the moment of out-of-hospital cardiac arrest (OHCA) to arrival in ED has been too long – 21 ($\pm$15) minutes. In four of these women ECG registered asystole and in these cases medical staff are not called to do cardiopulmonary resuscitation (CPR) because of the absence of breathing longer than five minutes – 30 ($\pm$17). In woman with pulseless electrical activity (PEA), CPR has been unsuccessful. Post mortem, in this case, the pathologist establishes as cause of death a rupture of the aneurism of the abdominal aorta. After advanced cardiac life support and defibrillation in one woman with VF has been established sinus rhythm with signs of massive acute myocardial infarction. Unfortunately, she died during transportation to the Intensive Care Unit (ICU) at the University Clinical Center Tuzla.

According to data about causes of death in 2007 from the Epidemiology Department of the Health center in Zivinice in this year 92 persons died due to sudden cardiac death, in relationship 50:50% according to sex. Average ages of these persons were 69,1 (±12) years. On average, men suffer sudden cardiac death 7 years earlier than women (65.6 vs. 72.6). Compared with males, the curve of SCD in females regularly followed advanced age (Figure 1), and more than two-thirds of them died after their seventieth year of life (72 vs. 43%). Thirteen women died before their seventieth year; in ten of them (77%) sudden cardiac death was the first symptom of coronary heart disease according to the history taken from family members and/or witnesses of SCD.

In 83 female patients, a physician established a diagnosis of acute coronary syndrome. After therapy with MONA Protocol and their stabilization, all these women had been transported to the ICU. Average age of these women was 66.5 (±12) years. In this same period we registered 74 men with a diagnosis of ACS, their average age was 58 (±15) years. On average, men develop acute coronary syndrome 8.5 years before women.

Signs of chronic myocardial infarction (wide and deep Q cog) on ECG in this period were found in 25 women. Only five of them had knowledge of this, but 20 women with the average age of 64 (±8.5) were unaware of the event and time of an AMI. Among these 20 chronic myocardial infarctions, 16 of them had inferior localization. Retrospectively, on the basis of history, we concluded that these women in a space of time between three months and five years had atypical symptoms which frequently may be seen in stomach diseases, colds, overwork and/or other similar conditions. In the same period we registered 5 men (vs. 20 women) with unknown chronic myocardial infarction with average age 54 (±12) years.

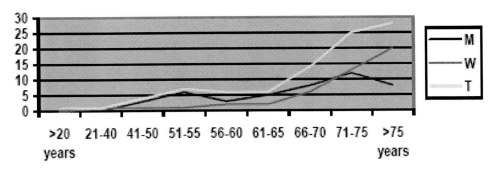

M – Men; W – Women; T – Total

Figure 1. Sudden cardiac death - relationship between men's and women's age.

During the period of research in the ED were registered 910 women with a diagnosis of stable angina pectoris. Before examination in the ED, 580 of them already had verified diagnosis of ischemic heart disease. In 330 cases diagnosis (or suspicion) of angina pectoris was established for the first time in the ED on the basis of medical history, symptomatology, physical examination and ECG changes, without other laboratory data. However, even in 275 of these women electrocardiogram was performed for the first time in their lives on the occasion of an examination. Average age of all these women was 58.4 (±14.2) years and every one of them had three or more risk factors responsible for the development of coronary heart disease (Table 2). The most frequent three risk factors were menopause, hypertension and psychosocial factors; smoking was a relatively rare risk factor. In the same period we registered only 217 men with a diagnosis of stable angina pectoris. On an average, men become angina pectoris 6.6 years before women and their average age was 51.8 (±12.6) years. Three frequent risk factors in men were hypertension, smoking and inadequate physical activity.

Table 2. Medical history of risk factors presence

RISK FACTOR	NUMBER	%
Hypertension	565	62,1
Diabetes	257	28,2
Smoking	91	10,0
Hyperlipidaemia	135	14,8
Obesity	320	35,1
Family history of CHD	348	38,2
Inadequate physical activity	335	36,8
Menopause	687	75,5
Psychosocial factors	390	42,

More than one-third or 315 (34.6%) of these women were refugees that kept away from East Bosnia because of war from 1992 to 1995, and who lived in a territory of municipal Zivinice last for the 12 to 15 years. Average age of these women was 56.7 (±11.5) years younger, on average, by 5.4 years than domicile women with angina pectoris which required medical help in ED during 2007. Their average age was 61.1 (±12.8) years. 35% of these refugee women (vs. 20% domicile) had previously established any of several psychiatric diagnoses, frequently depression and posttraumatic stress disorder after a disaster event, or symptoms were ascribed as consequences of climacteric condition by general physicians. Even in 40% of these women, mainly younger than 50 years, they had never previously had any cardiologic examination and procedures, including ECG.

After observation and therapy in 855 (93.9%) women with established diagnosis of stable angina pectoris were sent back home because of a lack of symptoms, with advice about the necessity of being examined by a cardiologist. Despite therapy, 55 (6,1%) women were directed to the Clinic of Internal Medicine in Tuzla because of the continuing existence of symptoms or their worsening. In eleven of them (20.0%), without significant ECG changes, biomarkers of cardiac damage (troponin and creatin kynaze) were elevated and they were hospitalized under diagnoses of acute coronary syndrome. All these women had diabetes and hypertension, and three of them were younger than 50 years. Leading symptoms in these women were weakness and breathlessness more frequently than palpitations, and in only one woman angina pectoris was presented with chest pain.

However, in more than two-thirds of female patients with an established diagnosis of angina pectoris found in leading symptoms were atypical, which is different men where atypical symptoms had been found in less than one-third of them, and their symptoms were mainly classical- chest pain and retrosternal discomfort.

Discussion

Bosnia and Herzegovina belonged, unfortunately, in a group of several other undeveloped countries in Europe, with a high degree of unemployment, misery and illiteracy, mainly as consequences of aggression and war from 1992 to 1995. The level of health protection of inhabitants is low because of insufficient human and technical resources. Other problems include inadequate medical education of people, non-existing programs of disease prevention, especially cardiovascular, and non-existing widespread recognition of a healthy lifestyle. These problems are particularly marked in primary health protection and in EDs, which are a part of that.[2]

Besides the reasons listed above, underlying factors responsible for high mortality due to cardiovascular diseases are ignorance of risk factors for their origin, bad quality of nutriment, inadequate therapy and management of hypertension and diabetes. By the way, Bosnia and Herzegovina belonged in a small group countries where state television advertised cigarette smoking. In addition to the presence of conventional risk factors, a big role in CVD is played by psychosocial factors like prolonged posttraumatic stress disorders, loneliness, depression, phobic anxiety, lacking of societal and social perspective, unemployment, and a general bad economic and political situation in the country.[1,14,15,16]

Psychosocial factors as an evidenct risk factor for CVD origin, CHD and especially sudden cardiac death, are particularly expressed in women who were refugees from Eastern Bosnian areas during war and genocide in which ten of thousands of people perished and executed about, mainly males from 14 to 70 years of age, their sons, fathers, husbands… The biggest number of them found recourse in a territory of municipal Zivinice where they are at this moment permanent residents, a majority of them are middle aged.

A significant percentage of these women have previously established some type of psychiatric diagnosis, so physicians often ascribed their symptoms to these conditions. In view of the age of origin of cardiovascular diseases in women moving to earlier years of life and a more frequent presence of atypical clinical features of angina pectoris, the possibility of missed diagnoses is high even in the more developed emergency departments, and let alone in an ED where ECG is presented as the only one exact parameter for diagnosis CHD, respectively of angina pectoris.[2,17]

Exactly that situation exists in the department of emergency medical service (EMS) of municipal Zivinice where all day, only one medical team (physician and two medical technicians/nurses), worked without the presence of EMS on call, with an average number of patients of 89 per day. It's understood that the physician had about 16 minutes for examination and establishing diagnosis for one patient. In view of poor resources like that, the possibility of establishing missed diagnoses and medical decisions on incomplete information is high. According to researches in developed countries about the percentage of missed diagnoses of coronary heart diseases in EDs, in our circumstances that percentage is, more or less, about 15% in our opinion. A mitigating circumstance, for patients and physicians, is evidence of a lower number of possible fatal events and consequences of missed diagnoses in patients with atypical symptoms of angina pectoris or acute coronary syndrome and without significant ECG changes, especially in women [4,16,17,18].

To reduce medical errors and their consequences, we need a fast adequate approach to the reorganization of emergency medical services in the sense of quality and quantity. First of all, work must be done on prevention of the disease, through mass information which educates the population about risk factors and symptoms. The leading role in this task must be taken by physicians of general and family medicine together with strong support from the local community and the state.[2]

In our concrete case, in view of the population number and patients, the ED must have at least three medical teams at every moment, including EMS on call. Without this persons with an event of SCD had practically no chance of survival [19,20]. For diagnosis of angina pectoris and acute coronary syndrome, besides ECG, fast access to a laboratory is necessary with the possibility of determining basic findings like complete blood count, cardiac enzymes, serum electrolyte levels, glucose level, lipids and chest x-ray. Until these fundamental medical needs are not accessible, we are aware of the danger of the existence of high possibilities to make large errors in medical diagnostics and decisions in such circumstances [2,3,5,18].

Conclusion

Angina pectoris plays an important role in female pathology. The incidence, history, clinical features, evaluation and therapy of coronary heart disease have important differences when comparing women and men. Besides the presence of conventional risk factors, big role in the origin of CHD is played by psychosocial factors, which are especially expressed in women refugees from Eastern Bosnia. The possibility of establishing missed diagnoses of angina pectoris and inappropriate medical decisions is high, and their percentage in such circumstances is approximately 15%. We need to adequately perceive the problem of angina pectoris in women, and educate women and medical staff with the aim of decreasing risk factors and improving lifestyle. Also, we need an adequate approach to reorganization of emergency medical services in the sense of quality and quantity, together with strong support from the local community and state.

References

[1]   Gibbons RJ, Abrams J, Chatterjee K, et al. ACC/AHA 2002 guideline update for the management of patients with chronic stable angina-summary article: a report of the American College of Cardiology/American Heart Association Task Force on practice guidelines (Committee on the Management of Patients. *J. Am. Coll Cardiol.* 2003;41 (1):159-68.

[2]   Omerkic E, Barakovic F, Masic I. The examination space of time from the beginning symptoms of the acute coronary syndrome to the time of the urgent treatment. *Med. Arh* 2006; 60(6): 356-359.

[3]   Barclay L. Acute Coronary Syndromes May Be Misdiagnosed in Women. *Arch Intern. Med.* 2007;167:2396, 2405-2413.

[4] Lee TH, Goldman L. Evaluation of the Patient with Acute Chest Pain. *N Engl. J. Med.* 2000; 342: 1187-95.

[5] Erhardt L, Herlitz J, Bossaert L et al. Task force on the management of chest pain. Task Force Report. *Eur. Heart J.* 2002; 21: 1153-76.

[6] Kannel WB, Wilson PWF, D'Agostino RB, Cobb J. Sudden coronary death in women. *Am. Heart J.* 1998; 136: 205-212.

[7] Vaccarino V, Krumholz HM, Berkman LF, Horowitz RI. Sex differences in mortality after myocardial infarction. *Circulation* 1995; 91: 1861.

[8] Anonymous. European guidelines on cardiovascular disease prevention in clinical practice: executive summary. *Eur. Heart J.* 2007; 28: 2375.

[9] Cannon RO. Chest pain with normal coronary angiograms. *N Engl. J. Med.* 1993; 328(23): 1706.

[10] Ridker P, Cook NR, Lee IM. A randomized trial of low-dose aspirin in the primary prevention of cardiovascular disease in women. *N Engl. J. Med.* 2005; 352: 1293.

[11] Sutcliffe SJ, Fox KF, Wood DA, et al. Incidence of coronary heart disease in health authority in London: review of a community register. *BMJ* 2003; 326: 20.

[12] Levi F, Lucchini F, Negri E, La Vecchia C. Trend in mortality from coronary heart and cerebrovascular diseases in Europe and other areas of the world. *Heart* 2002; 88: 119-124.

[13] Raljevic E, Rudic A, Dilic M, Masic I, Smajkic. Trends of cardiovascular diseases in Bosnia and Herzegovina and some European countries. *Med. Arh* 2004; 58(2): 35-37.

[14] Everson-Rose SA, Lewis TT. Psychosocial Factors and Cardiovascular Diseases. *Annu. Rew. Publ. Health* 2005; 26: 469-500

[15] Albert CM, Chae CU, Rexrode KM, Manson JE, Kawachi I. Phobic Anxiety and Risk of Coronary Heart Disease and Sudden Cardiac Death Among Women. *Circulation* 2005; 111: 480-487.

[16] Ryden L, Standl E, Bartnik M, den Berghe GV, Betteridge J, de Boer MJ, Cosentino F, Jonsson B, Laakso M, Malmberg K, Priori S, Ostergren J, Tuomilehto J, Thrainsdottir I. Guidelines on diabetes, pre-diabetes, and cardiovascular diseases: executive summary. The Task Force on Diabetes and Cardiovascular Diseases of the European Society of Cardiology (ESC) and of the European Association for the Study of Diabetes (EASD). *Eur. Heart J.* 2007; 28: 88-136.

[17] Salerno SM, Alguire PC, Waxman HS. Competency in Interpretation of 12-Lead Electrocardiograms: A Summary and Appraisal of Published Evidence. *Ann. Inter. Med.* 2003; 138: 751-760.

[18] Pope JH, Aufderheide TP, Ruthazer R et al. Missed Diagnoses of Acute Cardiac Ischemia in the Emergency Department. *N Engl. J. Med.* 2000; 342: 1163-70.

[19] Anonymous. European Resuscitation Council Guidelines for Resuscitation 2005. *Resuscitation* 2005; 67S1: S1-S2

[20] Ibrahim WH. Recent advances and controversies in adult cardiopulmonary resuscitation. *Postgrad. Med.* J. 2007; 83: 649-654.

Index

B

D

F

I

N

O

P

Q

T

U

V

X

Y

W